Child Development Centre
March 1995.

2095
R45–
BPA

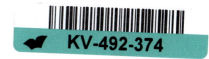

Neurological Problems in Childhood

To my teachers and colleagues during 50 years of medical practice

Neurological Problems in Childhood

Neil Gordon MD, FRCP(Lond and Ed), HonFCST

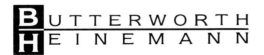
BUTTERWORTH
HEINEMANN

Butterworth-Heinemann Ltd
Linacre House, Jordan Hill, Oxford OX2 8DP

ℛ A member of the Reed Elsevier Group

OXFORD   LONDON   BOSTON
MUNICH   NEW DELHI   SINGAPORE   SYDNEY
TOKYO   TORONTO   WELLINGTON

First published 1993

British Library Cataloguing in Publication Data
Gordon, Neil
    Neurological Problems in Childhood
    I. Title
    618.928

ISBN 0 7506 0898 6

Printed and bound in Great Britain by The University Press, Cambridge

Contents

Foreword

Dr Neil Gordon is the wise grand old man of UK paediatric neurology. Originally starting from general neurology—with an early interest in, and deep empathy for, developmentally deviating and disabled children—he created a leading international child neurology centre in Manchester throughout the 50s, 60s and 70s. This centre had a particularly family and society-centred concept. Neil Gordon's approach is to give equal emphasis to the three pillars of the field: developmental paediatrics, the diagnosis and treatment of neurological diseases, and the care of the handicapped child. This credo has been underlined by the large number of articles, annotations and research contributions he has had published over the years.

In the early 70s, Neil Gordon took on the important task of surveying the main and most essential clinical areas in the field, with practical guidelines, the paediatric neurology for the general clinician. This resulted in the *Clinics in Developmental Medicine* Nos 59/60 in the Spastics International Medical Publications Series, published in 1976. This bible for the general paediatrician and public health physician has been most useful and appreciated over the years. But 'paediatric neurology is a rapidly expanding subject, and one in which there is much to learn', as Neil Gordon himself emphasized at the end of his original introduction to the book. This has proved to be true, especially over the last 15 years. It is now an extreme advantage to have an updated, new version concerned with 'Neurological Problems in Childhood'. The strength of this book lies in the well-balanced and explicit analyses and compilations of symptoms and signs, and how to deal with them in the examination room. In addition, new knowledge and biological data have been compiled in an understandable and practical way. This has only been possible through an admirable melting together of essentials for the general clinician in his daily work; one of the hardest tasks for a textbook writer today. Neil Gordon is to be warmly congratulated on a sucessful result, so useful for so many!

Bengt Hagberg
Professor of Paediatrics
Consultant Child Neurologist
at East Hospital
Gothenburg, Sweden

Preface

Involvement of the nervous system is a very frequent association of almost any illness in childhood. For example, common infections such as those of the upper respiratory tract may lead to otitis media and hence to possible damage to hearing, and such damage involves a nervous system which is growing and developing. The input of the auditory system plays its part in the functional maturation of the nervous system and hence in the development of the child into the adult. It has been estimated that about one third of all paediatric consultations involve hazards to the nervous system.

Yet paediatric neurology is a young specialty, and the numbers of paediatric neurologists in most countries is small. Most of paediatric neurology will therefore be practised by general paediatricians, and this may be no bad thing. Unlike most other specialties, paediatrics pays attention not to a particular system of the body but to a group of people. The paediatrician looks at the whole child and all the organ systems, but he or she needs a very thorough knowledge of neurology to be fully effective. This book is written for the doctor training in paediatrics, both in hospital and community practice, or in neurology, who is not necessarily going to practise paediatric neurology at a later date, as well as for those in other disciplines.

Paediatric neurology is based on three main pillars: developmental paediatrics; the diagnosis and treatment of neurological diseases; and the care of the handicapped child. Abnormalities in the growing child cannot be assessed without a sound knowledge of normal growth and development. Early diagnosis is often essential if a progressive disability is to be avoided by prompt treatment, and in no other aspect of medicine is prevention more important: a delay in diagnosis often makes cure impossible and results in a lifetime of handicap. In diagnosis and treatment, the paediatric neurologist will often need all the resources of a well-equipped hospital. Neurological disorders account for many of the chronic disabilities of childhood, and, once the diagnosis has been confirmed, even if the cause is unknown or untreatable medically or surgically, efforts must be made to help these children reach their maximum potential. This frequently entails co-operation between a number of specialists, and the paediatric neurologist can only work efficiently as a member of a team. Within the medical field, advice may be needed from the audiologist, ophthalmologist, orthopaedic specialist, psychiatrist and others. Psychologists, teachers, speech therapists, physiotherapists, occupational therapists and social workers will all take part in this team approach which is so rightly stressed in the care of the handicapped child. Also, among all these experts, the role of the parents must not be forgotten.

It is not intended to cover every aspect of paediatric neurology in this book, but emphasis has been laid on those conditions which occur frequently among children attending paediatric neurology clinics, and on some of those diseases which raise particular problems. A number of topics have been omitted, for example neonatal neurology, which is now a specialty in its own right. Others, such as clinical genetics, which has expanded greatly in the past few years, receive limited mention. There are a number of good books devoted entirely to these subjects. A number of topics in acute neurology, such as bacterial meningitis, are not included, partly because they are the concern of every paediatrician, and partly because the paediatric neurologist is usually only involved in their complications. Eyebrows may be raised over some of the subjects discussed. The author's excuse is that the material has been gathered over many years, rather than written at any particular point of time, and certain conditions have a special importance to him. References have been chosen which illustrate special points, and which have proved useful in practice.

The work of a paediatric neurology department has to be based on the hospital, and on a centre for assessment and care. The latter should not just be a diagnostic unit but should combine investigation with treatment, assessment with education. An individual child may react to his or her disabilities in many different ways, and his or her response to the teaching situation can provide vital clues in the search for the best type of education. The different ways in which disabled children make use of their potential may relate in particular to emotional factors, and it must be borne in mind that handicapped children are more, not less, liable to emotional disorders. Some of the difficulties can be related to unrealistic educational programmes which concentrate on goals that are too academic and not practical enough.

Paediatric neurology must reach out into the community if it is to be really effective, with joint clinics held in district general hospitals, and in special schools, with other specialists. In the UK this is recognized in training programmes for consultant paediatricians working in the community, although how such teaching is to be accomplished is still to be decided. Paediatric neurology is not a specialty of rarities, but mainly of common conditions affecting many children. Also, to a greater degree than in most specialties, it does overlap many other disciplines, both within medicine and in the fields of sociology and education.

Paediatric neurology is a rapidly expanding subject, and one in which there is much to learn; perhaps this is one of its greatest attractions.

Acknowledgements

The help of a number of colleagues is greatly appreciated, especially their generous help in providing knowledge which I lacked.

Dr Werner Schutt has made a major contribution to the discussions on the care and welfare of the handicapped child, and I wish particularly to express my indebtedness for all the help he gave in the chapters on developmental abnormalities of the brain and spinal cord, disorders and diseases of the motor system, and cerebral palsy. I am also most grateful to Dr Richard George for reviewing the chapter on infections of the nervous system.

A number of illustrations have been used from the previous text *Paediatric Neurology for the Clinician* which have been acknowledged; and for the many additions my thanks are due to Dr Stuart Green, Dr S. Chapman, Dr F. Raafat and Dr J.E. Wraith for all their work.

In updating, revising and re-organizing the text, and extracting that which was irrelevant to the intentions of the present book, the help that Dr Stuart Green has given has been invaluable. He is not to blame for any inadequacies in this book, but for any merits there may be he certainly deserves great credit. Without his help the book would never have been attempted, and I am deeply grateful to him for taking on such a difficult and onerous task. I would also like to thank Mr Jack Waring for all the help he has given in preparing the text with the use of a word processor.

1 The neurological examination

Any neurological examination must take account of the patient's age and be modified accordingly. This is particularly relevant to the neonate and the infant. A working knowledge of developmental sequences is therefore essential. The following examination schemes stress the developmental differences at varying ages, but the chronological divisions are partly a matter of convenience, as there is no sharp division between one stage and another.

There are a number of books devoted to the details of the neurological examination, such as those by Paine and Oppé (1966) and Prechtl (1977), which can be referred to for additional information.

The history

A good history is often more important than the examination, and this is especially true in the field of paediatric neurology. The information will often be obtained from parents, teachers and others concerned with the care of the child, but it must not be forgotten that even the very young child is often capable of giving a description of symptoms. A particularly good example is the diagnosis of epilepsy. A clear description of attacks can often establish their nature, whether they are epileptic or due to other causes such as reflex anoxia and, if epileptic, the type of seizure, which is so important to prognosis and treatment. Dunea (1990) quotes Sir William Osler when discussing the importance of the history. His aphorism was 'listen to the patient, he is telling you the diagnosis.'

Questions should be limited if they are not to overwhelm the patient or the witness, and the skill of the experienced history-taker is in asking the right questions which will elicit the vital information. This skill can only be developed with practice. Sir Thomas Lewis expected his junior colleagues to know how to examine a patient but not necessarily to know how to obtain a satisfactory history. This is very much the 'art of medicine'; and, although difficult to measure, it is one of the criteria which establish a 'good doctor'.

Examination of the nervous system in the neonate

State of arousal

Assessment at this age is made by measuring the behavioural reactions to a variety of stimuli, and in the newborn these reactions are relatively crude. Much depends on the gestational age and the state of arousal at the time of the examination. The responses will vary according to whether the baby is placid or irritable, fully awake or asleep. Prechtl and Beintema (1964) define six states of arousal:

1. Eyes closed, regular respiration and no movements
2. Eyes closed, irregular respiration and no gross movements
3. Eyes open and no gross movements
4. Eyes open, gross movements and no crying
5. Eyes open or closed and crying
6. Other states to be described.

The most reliable information is obtained when the baby lies quietly with his or her eyes open, and admittedly it is important to define these states, but it is important also to bear in mind that the baby's environment changes as soon as the examination begins.

It must be strongly emphasized that careful observation of the baby's posture, movement patterns and behavioural reactions is often more rewarding than the conventional neurological examinations practised on older children. With older children, the examination depends on the children's responses to commands and activities in which co-operation between the examiner and the patient is crucial.

Spontaneous motor activity

When lying supine, the baby will usually show a range of movements of the head and extremities which will vary with the state of arousal. Limb movements have been described as 'mass movements' by some and as 'athetoid' by others. These limb movements are usually symmetrical, though even at an early age a normal infant may show more activity on one side than another. The immature infant frequently makes rapid jerky movements involving the whole limb. These movements are usually bilateral, with writhing of the trunk. The infant born at term produces a smoother movement pattern, and movements of single limbs are seen much more frequently than in pre-term babies. Lack of movement may be due to depression or dysfunction of the nervous system, a muscular abnormality, or even a skeletal defect. All muscle groups can be affected, and lack of movement occurs in CNS depression (by hypoxia or drugs) or in conditions such as infantile spinal muscular atrophy and myasthenia gravis. It can be isolated to one limb, as in hemiplegia or spinal cord and nerve root lesions.

Hemisyndromes in the newborn period are seen fairly often, particularly after birth injury and hypoxia, and they may follow convulsions. The longer they persist the worse the prognosis is likely to be. The muscles of the affected side may be abnormally floppy or abnormally resistant to passive movement. The persistence of the tendon reflexes favours an upper motor neurone lesion, but in the presence of a severe hypotonia it is difficult to know if there is a true paralysis or not. Some recover fully, but a typical hemiplegia can develop as the baby grows older. Only repeated examination will establish the prognosis.

Excessive motor activity which is not relieved by a feed is a sign of cerebral irritation, and often occurs 24–48 hours after an anoxic or traumatic delivery. When associated with deep jaundice, 'windmilling' of arms and legs is a sign of kernicterus.

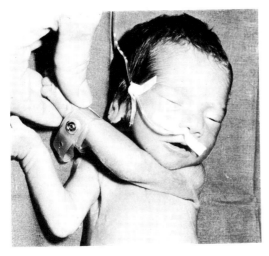

Figure 1.1   Scarf sign.

Resistance to passive movements—tone

The ease with which a limb is put through a range of passive movements is influenced by many factors, e.g. the baby's state of arousal, the gestational age and the integrity of the CNS. Infants delivered prematurely at 28 weeks have little or no resistance to passive movement and will lie in full extension at rest. The limbs are usually outstretched, and there is complete head lag when the body is pulled up from the supine position by the arms. The hypotonia is so marked that the arms can be wound around the neck (the scarf sign, Fig. 1.1), but as maturity increases it becomes more difficult to tuck the upper arm under the chin. As the infant grows these features diminish and resistance to passive movement increases. After the 36th week of gestation the extremities usually adopt a position of flexion at the elbows, hips and knees. Release after passive extension by the examiner will result in recoil to the original flexed position. The immature baby has poor head control, and, before 34 weeks' gestation, he or she has to be actively supported to prevent the neck from bending forward or backward excessively. At full term the alert infant will attempt to keep his or her head up and in the mid-line, though he or she succeeds only for short periods and the head oscillates widely. These oscillations are characteristic of the first 3 months of life, but become less as the child grows older.

The resistance to passive movement is generally greater in the extremities than in the trunk and neck. It is also more pronounced in the first 3 postnatal days than subsequently. Babies who have suffered from lack of oxygen are more likely to be hypotonic on the first day of life. Hypertonus does occur, and affected infants often pass from one state to another after 24–36 hours. The changing patterns in muscle tone are well illustrated by comparing the newborn infant with a child at 3 months, when both are held erect and are shaken gently. The neonate will show much head movement and the arms remain still. If the same manoeuvre is performed 3 months later, the head is held firmly and the arms are loose.

Increase of extensor tone in early infancy is likely to indicate a severe disorder, especially if the arms are markedly involved. The causes are many, and include raised intracranial pressure, infections of the nervous system, brain damage from anoxia and, occasionally, metabolic disorders. They cause the decerebrate rigidity by releasing the brain stem from the control of the mid-brain in the region of the red nucleus.

Neonatal reflexes

Neonatal reflexes are of interest because under normal circumstances they can be elicited only for a limited period during early life. They are important in that their absence soon after birth implies immaturity or depression of the nervous system, whilst persistence after the fourth month indicates maturational delay requiring further investigation (Paine, 1960). Milani-Comparetti and Gidoni (1967) also emphasize that normal development is dependent on the disappearance of various primitive reflexes and the appearance of a number of postural reflexes, although other evidence suggests that these relationships may be weak, if present at all (Touwen, 1976). Neural mechanisms are unlikely to entirely disappear but are dominated or covered by other mechanisms or possibly expanded or combined with others. This can explain their reappearance in the event of brain damage in later life. However, the persistence of primitive reflexes is a variable finding and must be interpreted in the context of the overall behaviour of the child. These reflexes are more fully described by Prechtl (1977), but a few are mentioned here.

Feeding reflexes

The sucking reflex   This is produced by inserting a teat (or finger) into the baby's mouth. Vigorous sucking results.

Rooting response and cardinal points reflexes   Stimulation of the baby's cheek by the mother's breast (or hand) will result in the head turning towards the stimulus. Stimulation of the centre of the upper lip will result in lifting the lip and baring the gum. Touching the angle of the mouth will cause the lips to pout to that side and stroking the lower lip will result in lowering of the lip and jaw.

Crawling and stepping movements

A number of characteristic movement patterns can be observed in the newborn child. While lying in the prone position he or she can be induced to crawl by touching the soles of the feet. This reaction is weak on the first day of life and is much more prominent after the third day, lasting until about the fourth or fifth week of life. When held erect and with the feet touching a horizontal surface the child will make high stepping movements. These can be best induced by tilting the body forward and by rocking the baby slightly from side to side.

Placing reaction

Stimulation of the dorsum of a foot will result in initial leg flexion followed by extension. This is most easily done at the edge of a table and causes the foot to be firmly placed on its surface. The response is progressively easier to evoke after the first day, but as the child grows older, it will be voluntarily resisted. It is called *réflexe d'enjambement* by the French and *Stehbereitschaft* by the Germans.

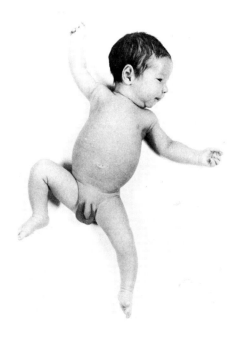

Figure 1.2   Asymmetrical tonic neck reflex.

Tonic neck reflexes

Two responses occur and are known as the symmetrical and the asymmetrical tonic neck reflexes.

The *symmetrical tonic neck reflex* is elicited by flexion and extension of the neck. Flexing the neck results in arm flexion and leg extension, whilst extending the neck results in arm extension and leg flexion. The reflex is thought to aid normal children to get on to hands and knees with the head up before they crawl and use their limbs independently. It is most easily elicited between the ages of 6 and 8 months, and its absence at this time, or exaggeration and persistence to an older age, are signs of a disorder of development. In the latter case it will interfere with crawling.

The *asymmetrical tonic neck reflex* is more easily observed and determines the characteristic fencing posture adopted by normal babies between 1 and 3 months of age when the head is turned to one side. This results in an increase in extensor tone of the arm on the side of the face and greater flexor tone of the arm nearest the occiput (Fig. 1.2). The legs often assume a similar postural pattern, though it is usually less obvious. The reflex is often difficult to elicit, especially in the first 2 weeks after delivery, and cannot be reliably reproduced during testing. Also, the baby should always be able to overcome the position by struggling, and if it is obligatory it is abnormal. Characteristically it persists in children with severe developmental delay and in those with cerebral palsy.

Labyrinthine reflexes

These are dependent on the functions of the semicircular canals and help to orientate the head in the erect position. The *tonic labyrinthine reflex* is of some importance, particularly in children with cerebral palsy, as it influences tone depending on body posture in relation to gravity. Flexor tone is increased by these reflexes when the child is prone, and extensor tone is increased when the child is supine. In some children with cerebral palsy, raising the head while they lie in the prone position will produce arm flexion, and the labyrinthine reflex is then seen to override the symmetrical tonic neck reflex which has the opposite effect, and the protective arm extension is lost.

Grasp reflex

Introducing a finger or pencil into the palm of the infant's hand from the ulnar side produces strong finger flexion and a tight grip strong enough to lift a small baby from the examining surface. When the head is in the mid-line the grip is equal in both hands, becoming stronger in the hand on the side of the occiput when the head is turned. It has been elicited in fetuses of 16 weeks' gestation, but Amiel-Tison (1968) comments that even at 28 weeks it is weak, consists of finger-flexion only, and is difficult to elicit repeatedly. Persistence after 3 months denotes delay in normal maturation or cerebral palsy. Stroking the dorsum of the fingers results in the opposite reaction with opening of the hand. The grasp reflex can also be elicited in the foot by stroking the sole behind the toes. The plantar grasp reflex persists for longer than the palmar reflex.

Crossed extensor reflex (allongement croise)

With one leg fixed and extended at the knee, the sole of that foot is stimulated with a pin. The contralateral limb will first flex and then extend with slight adduction.

Withdrawal reflex

Stimulation of an unfixed limb will result in simultaneous flexion of both limbs, even in the most immature babies.

Both the crossed extensor and the withdrawal reflexes will be absent or difficult to elicit in children with spinal cord lesions.

Moro response

Any sudden change in posture or a sudden loud noise will initiate a series of movements consisting of brief adduction followed by extension of the arms with the hands opening. There follows adduction of the arms with a return to the original flexed position. The response is best obtained by holding the baby on the forearms with the head in the observer's palms and the feet on his or her chest. The supported head is then allowed to drop backwards for 3–4 cm. Alternatively, the whole baby can be suddenly lowered while cradled in the arms.

The reflex can be evoked after the 29th week of gestation, but then the phase of adduction may be incomplete and the arms will fall back on to the cot. At full term it can be increased in babies who have cerebral irritation. This can also result in a decreased Moro response, particularly when the baby is hypertonic. For this reason it is often difficult to elicit the reaction a second time, particularly when the child is crying.

Babies who are hypotonic will also show a poor response. An asymmetrical response is most often due to head rotation to one side. A fractured clavicle or humerus may have the same effect, as will a peripheral nerve injury, such as an Erb's palsy. An asymmetrical Moro reflex may also be seen in an infant with a spastic hemiplegia. It gradually disappears at around 5 or 6 months of age.

A sudden noise or tapping the baby's body, will elicit a startle response which differs from the Moro reflexes. The elbows remain flexed and the hands do not open.

Galant reflex (trunk incurvation)

Stimulation of the skin on either side of the spine when the infant is held in ventral suspension with the examiner's hand supporting the abdomen results in bottom waggling and bending of the trunk to the stimulated side. This response can be obtained in very immature babies. It is absent in spinal cord injury.

Bauer's response

Crawling can be observed to occur spontaneously and can be reinforced by pressing the thumb gently on the soles of the feet. Crawling is absent or weak in infants whose general condition is depressed or who are suffering from muscle weakness.

Traction response

When the baby is lying supine and the trunk is pulled upward by traction on the wrists, the head will be pulled into the neutral position soon after the shoulders leave the couch (Fig. 1.3). The more immature the baby, the longer this response is delayed, and in babies born before the 33rd week of gestation the manoeuvre may result in an alarming degree of head extension.

Neck-righting reflex

Rotation of the head results in lateral rotation of the whole body. The reflex is first seen after about 34 weeks' gestation and is very easily detected in the first 3 months of life, after which time it gradually disappears, perhaps over a period of several years.

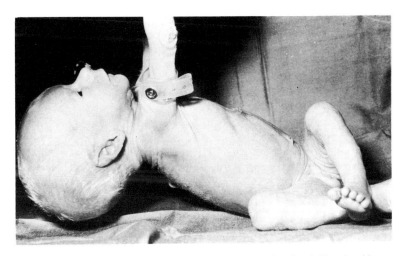

Figure 1.3 Start of the traction response (35 weeks' gestational age). Note head lag.

Tendon reflexes

The ease with which tendon reflexes are obtained will depend on whether there is increased or decreased muscle tone and whether there is CNS irritation or depression. The area from which the jerks can be obtained is greatly increased in diseases of the pyramidal tracts, and the biceps jerk can at times be elicited by tapping the forearm from the wrist upwards. Correspondingly, the knee jerk can be obtained by tapping the tibia from the ankle upwards. The earlier the tendon reflex can be elicited by this procedure, the greater the likelihood of a pyramidal tract lesion. Asymmetry of the tendon reflexes may be the only manifestation of a hemisyndrome.

Ankle clonus in the neonate does not have the same significance as clonus in children of 2 months of age and over. It can be found in children who subsequently develop normally, but when detected should always indicate a follow-up examination.

Habituation

Sokolov (1963) has described the orientating reflex as the organism's first brief response to any stimulus. Whether the neonate continues to respond to such a stimulus is related to the importance of the stimulus for successful functioning of the neonate. Thus the rooting response to a nipple touching the area round the mouth is likely to elicit a prolonged or repeated response. Other stimuli, such as a repeatedly flashing light or a repeated noise such as a rattle, may not be so meaningful, and may even impair reception of other potentially meaningful stimuli, and thus demand rapid cessation of response. Habituation to the orientating reflex is one indication of the ability to inhibit a response. This ability is a vital and yet easily disrupted human function, without which the neonate would continue responding to every stimulus indiscriminately.

Habituation can be tested in the neonate by repeatedly shining a flashlight into the baby's eyes while he or she is in light sleep (Prechtl, state 2), and watching for the decrement in response. The normal response is either a startle, other body movements or facial grimacing. Responses to a rattle or a bell can be tested in the same way. The method is outlined in detail by Brazelton (1973).

Habituation can also be tested for by repeating the glabellar tap or the Moro reflex several times, when it will be rapidly inhibited in the normal baby, but may persist in the presence of brain damage. However, this is thought by many to be unnecessarily discomforting for the infant, who, it must be remembered, is entirely at the paediatrician's mercy.

Examination of the eyes

Examining the eyes of neonates has its own problems, and it is at times difficult to induce them to open the eyelids. This can be done by raising the child into the vertical position or getting the child to suck a bottle. It can also be achieved by swinging the child around, as described by Paine (1960). This manoeuvre consists of cradling the baby on the examiner's forearms with the head supported by the hands. The examiner then rotates around his or her own axis two or three times. Not only do the eyes open, but the eyes will move in the direction of the rotation. On stopping, coarse nystagmus in the opposite direction will occur, which is a normal reaction unless prolonged. In the absence of some fixation there may be no nystagmus and the eyes may only deviate in the opposite direction. This *rotation test* will be absent when vestibular function is

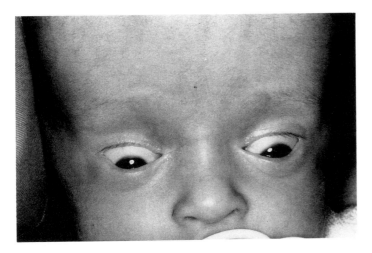

Figure 1.4   Setting-sun sign.

disturbed and there will be an abnormal response in ocular palsies. Strabismus is usually only noticed when marked, but conjugate deviation of the eyes and slow, roving eye movements are seen in children after a complicated delivery, and in those who show other signs of nervous system disturbance.

Congenital abnormalities of the eyes will also be identified, and fundoscopy may reveal retinal defects, pigmentation and haemorrhages.

Setting-sun sign

This sign can occur in normal babies in the first few weeks of life, especially on change of posture or removal of light. It is also found when kernicterus is present. It has two components: downward rotation of the eyeballs and retraction of the upper eyelids (Fig. 1.4). If it is marked and occurs among older infants it is strongly suggestive of raised intracranial pressure, particularly if combined with intermittent strabismus or undulating eye movements.

Eye reflexes

Routine examination of the eye reflexes is not often undertaken and, as with most reflex activities in the newborn, eye reflexes are critically influenced by the state of arousal of the child. In an alert but placid newborn they can give the first indication that the visual pathways are intact and that the range of eye movements is full.

Blink reflexes   Bright light, loud noise, tapping over the supra-orbital region or bridge of the nose will all elicit blinking of the eyelids, as will a light touch on the cornea. Blinking to light will occur even in sleep.

Pupil reflexes   A soft light will cause the pupil to react, though the reaction may be sluggish in the premature infant. A bright light causes the eyelids to shut. Pupil reactions to light are first seen in infants born at 29 weeks' gestation and become brisk after the 31st week. The myotonic pupil (Holmes-Adie syndrome) is sometimes a cause of diagnostic confusion. One or both pupils can be affected. The pupil is moderately dilated and the reaction to light, direct and consensual, is absent or very sluggish. On accommodation, if the child looks at a near object, the pupil will very slowly contract. On gazing into the distance, the pupil will equally slowly dilate. The tendon reflexes may or may not be absent. The vision of the affected eye can be blurred, and other symptoms of a disturbance of autonomic function, such as numbness of the hands, can occur.

The tonic pupil usually constricts to eye drops of 2.5 per cent methacholine, while the normal or Argyll-Robertson pupil (the pupil reacting to accommodation but not to light) is unaffected. This is due to supersensitivity to drugs of the acetylcholine group as a result of parasympathetic paralysis.

Doll's eye phenomenon (eye-righting reflex response)   Rotation of the head when the baby is awake results in the eyes remaining fixed in their original axis for a while without rotating with the head. In the first few weeks of life there may be a considerable time-lag before the eyes follow the head, but then they begin to move with the head as the eye-righting reflex ensures a rapid adjustment of the eye position with turning. If this does not occur it is an indication of brain damage. Although this reflex relies on stimuli from tendons, muscles and joints, the labyrinths also have a part to play.

In a child who is comatose, for example after a head injury, testing for the presence of *doll's eye movements* can be a useful measure of brain-stem function. The head is passively moved from side to side while the eyelids are held open. A positive reaction is turning of the eyes in the opposite direction to that of the head, and if there are no such doll's eye movements serious injury of the brain-stem must be suspected. Similarly, irrigating the ear with cold water should cause deviation to the side of the stimulated ear, with nystagmus to the opposite side, unless there is a gross impairment of function. The mnemonic COWS may be useful: cold opposite warm same, indicating cold water causes nystagmus to the opposite side and warm to the same side.

These are obviously two different phenomena. One is a reflex which is developing in the conscious baby, and may be better termed the eye-righting reflex; the other is a brain-stem response in the unconscious child which can be referred to as doll's eye movements. This may avoid confusion, as sometimes they are both called the doll's eye reflex.

Visual fixation

Newborn infants will fixate objects, especially moving objects, and this may be accompanied by momentary suppression of other motor activity. The human face appears to be the optimum stimulus. At the same time, the palpebral fissure may widen, the facial features relax and respirations become regular.

Cranial nerves

Nerve 2   As stated, vision in the newborn can be assessed crudely in a number of ways. The child will turn the head towards a diffuse light coming from one source (the Window test). The eyes of newborn babies will often follow a light or human face and they will also follow the dark and white stripes on a moving drum.

Nerves 3, 4 and 6   Examination of eye movements, as described above, can give a fair estimate of whether or not these nerves are intact. The observation of spontaneous movements is particularly important.

Nerve 5   Stimulation of the side of the face for the rooting response indicates that facial sensation is intact.

Nerve 7   Facial nerve palsies are quite common following forceps delivery and are usually transient. The feeding reflexes will again give additional information about whether or not the facial muscles are functioning normally.

Nerve 8   Babies will often startle and blink their eyes when exposed to loud noises. They will also quieten when hearing a soft, low-pitched, continuous vocalization from the mother or examiner, and may turn their gaze in the direction of the sound.

Nerves 9 and 10   Palatal movement is observed by noting the gag response.

Nerve 11   The sternomastoids are easily felt and examined when the head is allowed to fall back and when testing the traction response.

Nerve 12   Tongue movements are best noted on sucking and during examination of the mouth.

Estimation of maturity

Accurate assessment of dysmaturity is of particular importance in view of the risks these babies run of developing complications, and in order to establish a reliable prognosis.

Developmental changes are so consistent in newborn infants that many observers use them to determine gestational maturity where this is in doubt in babies born

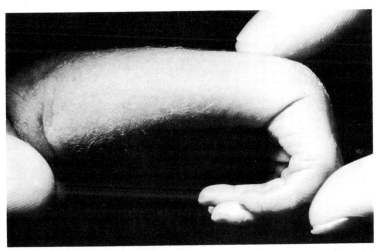

Figure 1.5   Square-window sign (the more mature the baby the narrower the angle). One of the 10 neurological criteria on the Dubowitz scale for the assessment of gestational age.

before term, or in those who are 'small for dates' (Farr, 1968). Muscle tone, posture, reflex activity and behavioural reactions change with advancing gestation, and an infant born at 36 weeks shows different patterns from those seen at 32 or 40 weeks' gestation. In skilled hands gestational age can be determined in this way with an accuracy of 2-week stages, which approximates those estimations based on birthweight and physical or radiological examination. Dubowitz and his colleagues have developed a scheme for the neurological assessment of pre-term and full-term newborn infants, whereby the inexperienced observer can objectively record criteria of neurological function in a standardized way. The Dubowitz scale is based on 10 neurological criteria (Fig. 1.5) and 11 external criteria, the combined score of the two giving the most reliable estimation of gestational age (Dubowitz, Dubowitz and Goldberg, 1970; Dubowitz and Dubowitz, 1981).

Estimations are likely to be most accurate if information from all sources is used, including the mother's menstrual history and sonar scan, but all are subject to variation. Neurological evaluation will be particularly helpful where the menstrual history is uncertain and the birthweight influenced by placental insufficiency. In turn, neurological signs will be affected by conditions that either depress or irritate the CNS.

It is particularly rewarding to study movement patterns, postural reactions, reflex behaviour and muscle tone. All show changing characteristics with increasing maturity.

Posture and muscle tone

The characteristic posture of flexion of the full-term newborn infant has already been described. As the child matures, flexor tone increases and joints adopt the appropriate posture in a definite sequence (Brett, 1965). At 28 weeks flexion begins first at the hips, so that by 32 weeks the legs often come to lie almost parallel to the trunk. At 34 weeks the knees flex as well, and at 36 weeks the elbows are bent.

In ventral suspension, with the examiner's hand under the abdomen, the immature baby will show marked back and neck flexion with a drooping head. The limbs hang loosely in extension. With progressive maturation the back straightens, the head is pulled up and the limbs become more flexed. As already mentioned, there is also a steady improvement in head control on pulling the baby into the sitting position.

Movement patterns

In contrast to the non-purposive 'athetoid' movements seen in the baby born at 40 weeks' gestation, the immature infant frequently makes rapid jerky movements involving the whole limb. They are often bilateral, and are associated with writhing of the trunk. The movement of the mature infant is smoother and more often isolated to one limb. The increased resistance to passive extension of the limbs and an increased tendency for the limb to recoil to the original flexed position as the child matures must be mentioned again at this point.

Reflex activity and assessment of maturity

Details of the neonatal reflexes have been given previously, but many of them do not help in determining gestational age.

Robinson (1966) found that the following reflexes appeared at predictable times:

1. Pupil reaction to light, 29–31 weeks' gestation
2. Glabellar tap reflex, 32–34 weeks' gestation
3. Traction response, 33–36 weeks' gestation
4. Neck-righting reflex, 34–37 weeks' gestation
5. Head turning to diffuse light, 32–36 weeks' gestation.

The feeding reflexes (sucking and rooting) are of particular importance to infants and are difficult to elicit before the 34th week of gestation. Satisfactory feeding patterns will become established only when they have appeared.

Studies have shown that the motor nerve conduction velocity of the ulnar and tibial nerves can be correlated with gestational age, and encephalographic evoked responses to photic stimuli have shown a latency that was inversely related to gestational age (Engel and Benson, 1968).

Examination of the nervous system of the infant

Developmental assessment

There have been a number of other notable contributors to the detailed study of the nervous system in early life and the methods by which its function can be put to the test; for instance, André-Thomas, Chesni and Saint-Anne Dargassies in France (1960) and Peiper in Germany (1964).

Neurological examination of infants after the neonatal period must take account of expected levels of function and skill at a given age, and the examiner must be familiar with the norms laid down by Gesell and Amatruda (1947); Sheridan (1975); Illingworth (1962, 1972) and others. Such developmental screening can usually be carried out under the following headings: general history; developmental history; general inspection; posture and gross motor performance; vision and fine manipulation; hearing and language; and everyday skills and social responses. The most important aspects of development are: the child's gradual acquisition of the erect posture and subsequent ambulation; the increasing awareness of objects, individuals and activities in the surroundings; the development of hand function; and the acquisition of speech. Developmental screening is not a substitute for the neurological examination but an indication that a more detailed investigation may be needed. Also, no exact correlation exists between the results of developmental assessment scales and intelligence tests carried out at a later age. Great care must be taken not to jump to conclusions, and a number of children with low development quotients in early life turn out to be of average intelligence. Discrepancies between different aspects of development must be borne in mind; for example, a significant number of mentally retarded children show normal motor development, and some children with cerebral palsy have normal intelligence.

Like individuals at any age, young infants respond to a friendly approach and it is as important to talk to the child during the examination as it is to talk to the parents. Much information is obtained from the parents' account, and if this is obtained first it gives the child time to adapt to the situation. The examination should confirm the history and is best done in a play situation. The parent's lap is a secure and comfortable place, but it can also be restricting and much will be gained if the examiner and his or her patient can descend to the carpet. A more reliable record of the child's abilities is likely to be obtained within a familiar home setting in the company of siblings than by a strange person working in a hospital environment. Accurate information is often best elicited by two examiners, one of whom will attract the child's attention while the other performs the test. This applies particularly to tests of hearing and vision, visual fields, and during fundoscopy. A rough estimate of the visual fields can be obtained by bringing a dangling object from behind the baby's head and noting when the eyes deviate towards it. Fundoscopy is greatly helped by allowing the baby to suck on a bottle.

Observation is often more rewarding than manual palpation, and it is often more accurate to assess increase in tone by observing poverty of movement than by the conventional method of assessment by passive movement. This applies particularly to children under the age of 12 months. It is also worth remembering that when testing for responses to visual or auditory stimuli, the examination should be set up in such a way that the reaction to the first presentation of the stimuli can be accurately observed, as familiarity with the test object or sound will cause it to be ignored on subsequent presentation, and the results of the examination will remain in doubt.

The following observations have been adapted from the monograph on children's developmental progress by Sheridan (1975); and in the light of her experience the developmental examination has recently been presented by Egan (1990).

One month

Posture and movement   Movements are still jerky and the arms are more active than the legs; the hands are often fisted; the fingers fan out during extensor limb movement. Asymmetric tonic neck reflex often induces the fencing position at rest; there is some head lag on lifting, but momentary head support when the baby is held vertically; the back still shows a single curve when the baby is held in a sitting position.

Vision   The baby stares at diffuse light and blinks at bright light; and will follow a light or a small ball for short distances.

Hearing   The baby may momentarily stop spontaneous movements when spoken to or when a bell is rung.

Speech   He or she cries lustily when hungry or uncomfortable; makes guttural noises when content; and coos in response to the mother's voice from about 6 weeks of age.

Social behaviour   Stops crying when picked up or spoken to; gradual increase in alertness and awareness; sleeps most of the time when not handled or fed.

Three months

Posture and movement   The limbs are more pliable and movements smoother and more continuous; the arms are waved symmetrically; the hands are open and approximated in the mid-line after about 16 weeks to grasp a toy put into one hand by the mother; the baby kicks the legs together or alternately; very little head lag occurs when the baby is pulled to a sitting position; the head is held erect for short periods (Fig.1 6); the back is straighter, but still has a primary spinal curve; when lying in the prone position the head is raised well up, and at 4 months the baby will support the trunk with the arms; the hand is open and he or she may playfully claw the surface of

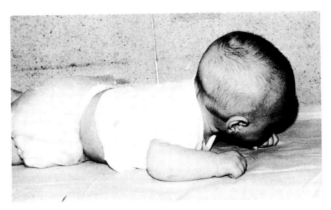

Figure 1.6   Head control at 4 months.

the table; he or she may hold a rattle placed in the hand for short periods, but does not examine it.

Vision   The baby is very alert; moves the head to gaze around; watches his or her own hands; converges the eyes on a dangling ball; the defensive blink is well developed.

Hearing   The baby quietens to the sound of a rattle, a spoon and cup or the mother's voice; he or she turns the head or eyes towards the source of sound.

Social behaviour   The baby starts to react to familiar situations; enjoys bath and caring routines; responds with pleasure to friendly handling; and reaches out for a toy at about 18 weeks.

Six months

Posture and movement   When lying supine, the baby raises his or her head to look at the feet and plays with them; he or she pulls up to sitting when the hands are grasped, but has only momentary independent sitting; in the sitting position the head is erect and the back straight; when held in a standing position the baby bears weight on his or her feet and may bounce; when held erect and lowered on to floor, the legs spread (parachute reaction); he or she will pass objects from one hand to another.

Vision   He or she is visually insatiable; moves the head and eyes eagerly when his or her attention is attracted; the visual axes should be parallel; squints are abnormal; he or she watches falling toys to their resting place, but forgets them when they fall outside the visual field; watches a rolling ball down to 6 mm diameter at a distance of 3 metres and has quick response to testing of peripheral vision.

Hearing   The baby responds to hearing tests (voice, rattle, cup and spoon, paper and bell) at a distance of 46 cm at ear level.

Speech   He or she laughs, chuckles, squeals in play, uses single and double syllables with pharyngeal (goo, ga-ga), tongue (de, a-da-da, le) and lip movements (ma).

Social behaviour   The baby grasps well and often transfers objects to the mouth; after taking a rattle into a hand he or she enjoys shaking it; he or she is friendly with strangers, though easily upset when approached abruptly.

Nine months

Posture and movement   The baby sits firmly on the floor; leans forward to pick up a toy; and can turn the body to look sideways. He or she moves on the floor by rolling or squirming; tries to crawl, but reciprocal movements are still poorly performed; pulls him or herself to standing momentarily, but soon falls back on to his or her bottom; has purposive, though unsteady, supported walking; forward and lateral protective arm responses; and rapid and accurate hand manipulation; the pincer grasp with finger and thumb is present but clumsy; the baby releases objects by dropping; voluntary placing is not possible.

Vision   The baby is attentive and maintains interest for minutes; watches balls of 3 mm diameter at a distance of 3 m away; fixates mounted balls of 3 mm diameter at 3 m away but it is difficult to hold his or her attention.

Hearing   The baby localizes hearing tests at 1 m from above and below ear level, but not from mid-line.

Speech   He or she exhibits repetitive babbling (dadada, mamama, gaga); understands 'No' and 'Bye-bye'; shouts to attract attention; and waits for a response before shouting again.

Social behaviour   At this stage hand feeding commences; the baby grasps a spoon when fed; arches his or her back when annoyed or irritated; is wary of strangers; may hide his or her face and cling to parent; plays peek-a-boo and imitates hand-clapping; grasps objects offered, but will not return them; and looks for hidden objects.

Twelve months

Posture and movement   At twelve months the baby will sit indefinitely; he or she rises from lying to sitting; crawls on the hands and knees; shuffles on the buttocks; pulls up to standing and lowers him or herself gently by holding on to furniture; cruises sideways along furniture; stands unsupported momentarily; walks with one hand held and may walk alone; may crawl upstairs; points at objects of interest; bangs a cube held in each hand together; and picks up small objects.

Vision   He or she watches rolling and mounted balls down to 3 mm diameter at 3 m away; begins to show an interest in pictures; and looks for and finds toys which roll out of sight.

Hearing   There is an immediate response to hearing tests, but the baby rapidly habituates; he or she comprehends simple commands (e.g. 'give to mummy', 'clap hands').

Speech   Vocalizations contain most vowel and consonant sounds; the baby may have three words; he or she understands several words, e.g. dinner, milk, biscuit, cup, spoon; imitates sounds; and responds to his or her name.

Social behaviour   He or she helps with dressing; mouths objects less; holds a spoon but loses food; places cubes in and out of a container on request; gives toys to adults on request; demonstrates affection to parents and friends; plays clapping games; waves goodbye; and finds toys hidden within sight.

The infant can only acquire the ability to sit, stand and walk when certain postural reflexes appear. The age at which postural reflexes evolve varies to a certain extent, but there is a very clear pattern in the case of normal infants (Paine *et al.*, 1964). At around 3 months of age there is a period of particular inactivity, as many of the primitive responses have disappeared and many of the postural or evoked responses have not yet developed.

Other useful tests

There are a great variety of tests which can be used to examine the nervous system in infancy, but for many of them it is not yet known if they will stand the test of time. Some have already been discussed in the section on neonatal reflexes, and the following have also proved useful.

Positive supporting reaction

A true positive supporting reaction appears at about 6 months of age, but often earlier among children with cerebral diplegia. However, in the first 4 weeks of life, suspending a baby upright with the feet against a flat surface will produce stiffening of the legs but the knees do not extend.

Landau reflex

On ventral suspension after about 6 months of age the neck and back will extend and the legs elevate to some extent. From 8 months to 1 or 2 years of age flexion of the head when the infant is in this position will be followed by flexion of the legs on the trunk.

Parachute responses (protective responses)

These occur on downward, sideways, forward and backward displacement of the body. The first can appear by the fourth month, and is elicited by holding the baby under the arms and rapidly lowering the body towards the couch. The second is often found by the sixth month, the third by the seventh month, and the fourth by the ninth month, but often develop at a later stage. Displacement downwards results in extension of the legs, sideways extension of the arm, and forward and backward extension of both arms.

Tilting or equilibrium reactions

When the body is tilted, by moving the base on which the baby is sitting, these reactions prevent falling. The spine should curve with the concavity towards the higher edge of the base. This appears in the prone position around 5 months, in the supine position at 7 months, in the sitting position at 7–8 months, in the all-fours position from 9 to 12 months, and in the standing position during the second year of life. When there is delayed motor development, stimulation of these responses during physiotherapy seems much more important than any type of standing or walking exercises.

Transillumination of the head

Although not used so often these days, when many neuroradiological tests are relatively non-invasive, it can be useful to perform this test under the age of 1 year, especially if the head seems large or there are obvious anomalies such as spina bifida cystica. It can be used for a year or two longer if hydrocephalus, hydranencephaly or porencephaly are suspected. It must be done in total darkness, allowing time for dark adaptation, with a strong torch fitted with a rubber cap which can make firm contact with the baby's head. There should be only a small halo of light around the edges of the rubber cap. The conditions just mentioned will increase the illumination, and the appearance is most striking in hydranencephaly when the whole head is illuminated. A recent subdural haematoma may reduce the illumination on the affected side.

Examination of the older child

The older the child the more the examination will resemble the adult pattern. It must again be emphasized that the structuring of this is of some importance. It will have to be modified according to age, intelligence and co-operation, and it is important to gain the confidence of the child. Time taken in allaying apprehension by age-appropriate talk and play prior to the start of a more formal examination will be well spent. Other principles stressed by Paine and Oppé (1966) include the importance of deferring procedures likely to cause pain and discomfort until the end of the examination, as well as omission of tests irrelevant to the age of the child. However, unless a system of some kind is followed, serious omissions will occur, and the age of the child should never be used as an excuse for not paying attention to detail. The neurological examination must be based on an understanding of anatomy and physiology, and, when completed, two questions in particular have to be asked (in the following order) if diagnostic errors are to be avoided: (1) Do the findings indicate an involvement of any particular part of the nervous system? (2) What are the possible causes of this? A full examination will often have to be extended over more than one session.

Observation and general examination

Many of the following remarks apply to children of all ages. The appearance of the child will often give important diagnostic clues. Height and weight must be recorded. As in infancy, the way the older child behaves, moves around the room, and plays with toys may tell more than the results of formal tests, both in a psychiatric and neurological assessment.

The skin must be examined for such stigmata as adenoma sebaceum, cafe-au-lait spots, and telangiectasia; and the shape and feel of the body and limbs noted.

Particular attention must be given to the shape of the head and its circumference. Asymmetry of the skull is common and should be interpreted in the context of any other findings. The skull should be measured, even if it is obviously normal, as an assessment of subsequent growth may be of great importance. It is not uncommon to find that mistakes are made if the occipito-frontal circumference is not related to standard chart measurements, and also to the child's height and weight. Palpation of the fontanelles and sutures can suggest changes of intracranial pressure, as can sometimes the production of a 'cracked-pot' sound on percussion, elicited with the head unsupported by bedding. The shape of the neck and spine must be noted, as well as the range of movements.

It can only be mentioned here, and emphasized in the strongest terms, that a neurological examination should not be done in isolation, and that other systems must be tested as well. In the investigation of headaches it is as important to take the blood pressure as it is to examine the optic fundi.

Mental state

Assessment of the state of consciousness may be difficult if its impairment is slight and variable, as in minor forms of epilepsy, when a temporary lack of response can be attributed to deafness or lack of attention. Orientation in place and time must also be assessed. In states of coma from any cause, but particularly after head injury, the Glasgow coma scale is now widely accepted as a most useful method of recording the level of responsiveness; this is modified according to the child's age (Gordon *et al.*, 1983). It is divided into the following sections: eyes opening (spontaneously, to speech, to pain, none); best verbal response (orientated, confused, inappropriate, incomprehensible, none); best motor response (obeying, flexing, extending, none). The scale also helps to distinguish between various conditions such as akinetic mutism and the persistent vegetative state (Teasdale and Jennett, 1974). The scale can be modified for use with very young children, particularly those with limited use of language.

A useful estimate of the child's development and intelligence can often be made, but where there are doubts, or where there is obvious impairment, the use of standardized tests is useful, both as part of the patient's total examination, and as a detailed record of achievements which can be repeated at intervals to measure progress. Less and less importance is being paid to the final figure of the development or intelligence quotient, as this labels the child and lends itself to misleading interpretations. The results of the individual test items, or battery of tests in the case of physically handicapped children, must be analysed. This provides a profile of the child's ability and information on those skills which are wanting and those in which the child is likely to excel. Only in this way can efforts be made to provide the help which a particular child may need.

An assessment of the child's emotional state is always important. Is there evidence of undue anxiety? Is there a reluctance to be separated from the mother? Are there signs of depression? Does the child seem so withdrawn from the environment that it is almost impossible to communicate with him or her?

Emotional lability may be obvious, and this is often associated with an inability to concentrate and an abnormal distractability. Overactive behaviour may be apparent, but care must be taken to relate behaviour to age and intelligence. There is sometimes a tendency to judge children's behaviour by adult standards.

Language function

The diversity of speech and language disorders among children are discussed in

Chapter 6. The nature of a speech defect, for example cleft palate, high tone deafness, a cerebellar dysarthria, may often be discovered by listening to the child talk. It is possible to make a very rough estimate of the level of language development, partly from the history given by the mother and partly from the apparent understanding of requests made to the child and the manner in which the child uses words. The requests may vary from asking the child to name objects to the carrying out of quite complex actions. The analysis of expressive speech varies from the number of different words used to the complexity of sentence structure.

When a defect of speech and language is established the first priority is to attempt to make a medical diagnosis. Is the child suffering from deafness, mental handicap, a developmental speech disorder, structural abnormalities of the organs of articulation, neurological forms of dysarthria, or disorders of voicing; and can the exact causes of such disabilities be established? The diagnosis may indicate the need for various forms of treatment in addition to speech therapy.

The medical diagnosis must be followed by an analysis of the disorder of speech and language, as this helps in determining the prognosis and in planning therapy. Speech therapists are playing an important part in such assessments, and although more standardized tests may be needed, there are already a number of useful methods available, for example the Edinburgh Articulation Test (Anthony *et al.*, 1971) and the Reynell Developmental Language Scales (Reynell, 1969). The assessment of reading and writing difficulties also calls for a team approach, as the causes may vary from truancy from school due to emotional disturbances to specific learning difficulties which can only be analysed by detailed psychometric testing.

Cranial nerves

Reference has already been made to methods of testing vision and hearing in young children, and Sheridan has shown that hearing and vision can be tested accurately from a very early age (Sheridan, 1958, 1969, 1973). If there is resistance by an infant to covering one eye, unilateral blindness should be suspected. In older children it is surprising how accurately visual fields can be charted by confrontation; even with a minimum of co-operation. Most children can be persuaded to fix on the examiner's nose for a few seconds and either state when they first see a moving object brought in from the periphery of the field or reveal that they have seen it by deviation of the eyes or pointing with a finger.

Examination of the optic fundi in the 2–5-year-old who cannot be persuaded to fixate presents problems, and if such an examination is essential a sedative may sometimes have to be given and the pupils dilated with a mydriatic. As already mentioned, it is important to observe the position of the eyes at rest, since, if a squint is present, there may well be paralyses of the ocular muscles. Noting the spontaneous movements of the eyes can confirm this, as well as asking the child to follow a light or an interesting object. The possibility of a squint can be examined by the cover test if the child is able to co-operate. In this test the child is asked to focus on a target, such as a toy or light, and first one and then the other eye is covered, either by the parent's or the examiner's hand or by some opaque material, while a watch is kept on the uncovered eye. If this has been previously squinting it will move to take up fixation of the target when the other eye is covered. If the child cannot co-operate, observation of the position of the reflection of light on the cornea of each eye can be helpful. When the eye is fixing the reflection is central, and when it is not the reflection is deviated from the centre of the pupil. Care must be taken to distinguish epicanthic folds from a convergent squint, and it must be realized that the reflection may be eccentric even in normal eyes.

In paralytic squints the diplopia is most marked in the direction of action of the weak muscle, and only if the elevators or depressors of the eye are involved will the images be tilted. The affected eye is identified when the patient states that covering it causes the outermost image to disappear. The oblique muscles act best as elevators and depressors when the eye is adducted, and the converse is true of the recti. Therefore, for example, in a right superior oblique palsy the maximum separation of the images is on looking downwards and to the left (Gordon, 1969).

Testing the function of the other cranial nerves presents no particular problems. A useful sign of very slight facial palsy is an inability to tuck the eyelashes in on the affected side when screwing up the eyes. It should be remembered that soon after the onset of an acute hemiplegia there may be weakness of the whole of one side of the face, and that when there is unilateral weakness of the tongue this may be protruded towards the hemiparetic side. When testing the tongue muscles, movements can often be encouraged by the use of a lollipop.

Motor system

Muscle power, tone and mass must be systematically examined. Evidence of incoordination or of involuntary movements may have already been noted while watching the child play, and formal testing may not add much useful information, except when the disability is slight or more marked on one side than the other.

The tests of incoordination, such as rapid alternating movements, the finger-nose test, and heel-shin test, may not be sufficient to reveal the subtle perceptual-motor disabilities which so often lead to unusual 'clumsiness' for the child's age in the tasks of everyday life. If these are suspected it is often necessary to use more standardized tests, such as the Frostig Developmental Test of Visual Perception and the Stott Test of Motor Impairment.

Posture can be of considerable help in diagnosis. The adduction and extension of the legs when the child is held in vertical suspension can be the first evidence of cerebral diplegia. The attitude of the unsupported arms with hyperextension, especially of the fingers, can be highly suggestive of athetosis when the involuntary movements are slight. Retraction of the head is a classical (late) sign of meningitis.

The gait can be characteristic of various neurological disabilities: the staggering of a child with a cerebellar lesion; the circumduction of the foot and dragging of the leg on the side of a hemiplegia; the scissors gait of the child with cerebral diplegia; the waddle of the boy with pseudo-hypertrophic muscular dystrophy; and the steppage gait due to foot-drop. Associated movements tend to be suppressed as the child grows older, unless there is a defect of development. Particularly useful tests of persistent synkinesis are the Fog tests (Fig. 1.7). In one, the feet-hands test, the child is asked to walk on the outer side of the feet, when associated movements of the arms appear, particularly supination. In the other, the hand-hand test, the child exerts a certain degree of pressure with the thumb and first finger using spring clips, and the movements of the opposite hand are observed. By 14–16 years of age only a few children will still show these associated movements, and they will be slight (Fog and Fog, 1963). This test can also help to identify a very minimal hemiplegia, with associated movements more marked on the affected side. In fact, asymmetry of the movements is a more helpful finding than their persistence, which usually indicates immaturity of postural control in the older child. Toe walking can occur during early development with no evidence of cerebral palsy, and an early return to complete normality.

Reflexes

Eliciting the tendon jerks and superficial reflexes offers no special difficulties. One of the most common causes of absent tendon jerks is an inability to persuade the child to relax. Reflex abnormalities can help in the localization of a lesion and have the merit of being more objective than many other neurological signs.

Sensory examination

The testing of sensation depends on the co-operation of the child. The responses of the younger child may have to be assessed on a change of facial expression or movement of the stimulated part, when it is touched or pricked. In lesions of the sensory nerve distal to the posterior root ganglion the flare elicited by scratching the skin will be absent. When testing joint position sense it may be possible to persuade the child to imitate the position of the limb, or part of the limb being tested, with the other one; and if the up and down movements of the fingers and toes are carefully demonstrated to the young child they can usually identify the movement with their eyes shut; as long as the examiner gains their confidence. Astereognosis can be assessed in the pre-school child by making a game of it. Interesting objects, e.g. small bits of costume jewellery or material are placed in a 'tunnel' and the child is asked to put his or her hand inside to try to match them with the ones he or she can see. Small toys can also be used, with the promise that if he or she succeeds in identifying them he or she will be made a present of one.

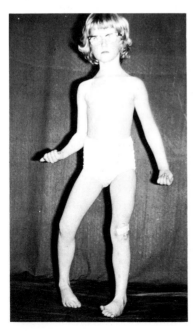

Figure 1.7   Fog test in patient with right hemiplegia.

Autonomic functions

Evidence of autonomic dysfunction is sometimes obvious. Tears may be lacking in the Riley-Day syndrome. Investigation of impaired bladder function often requires special tests such as contrast X-rays or a cystometrogram. The anal sphincter can be examined directly for undue laxity, and at the same time the anal reflex can be elicited by gently pricking the surrounding skin and observing if there is a contraction of the external sphincter.

Special investigations

Reference is made in this book to special tests when these are relevant to the investigation of any particular disease or condition, for example the EEG in the section on epilepsy, the electromyograph in that on myopathies, chromatography in the one on mental retardation, and contrast radiography, computerized tomography (CT) and isotope scanning, and magnetic resonance imaging (MRI) in the chapter on cerebral neoplasms.

Among children who are failing to thrive and develop normally, a number of screening tests on blood and urine should be performed to cover as wide a range of disorders as possible. The laboratory techniques involved may be complex, but this type of investigation causes no risk to the child. Collections of urine and blood over a measured period may cause technical difficulties, but no more than discomfort to the child.

The same cannot be said of lumbar puncture, and any tendency to carry out this test as a routine must be resisted. It is not always possible to be certain that there is no raised intracranial pressure, as signs such as papilloedema are often absent; and then the risks of coning cannot be excluded. In the case of a spinal lesion when there is a possibility that this is due to an extramedullary tumour, an injudicious lumbar puncture may result in impaction of the cord, interruption of its blood supply, and the sudden onset of a paraplegia with retention of urine.

When a subdural haematoma is suspected in an infant with an open fontanelle, or in an older child with separation of the sutures, subdural taps are considered an essential investigation, as well as a therapeutic measure if the diagnosis is correct. However, subdural taps are seldom indicated in the neonatal period as haematoma are rare at this age, and the procedure carries a definite risk of causing haemorrhage (Davies et al., 1972).The technique of subdural tapping is considered in Chapter 10.

References

Amiel-Tison, C. (1968) Neurological evaluation of the maturity of newborn infants. *Archives of Disease in Childhood*, **43**, 89

André-Thomas, S., Chesni. Y. and Saint-Anne Dargassies, S. (1960) *The Neurological Examination of the Infant*, Little Club Clinics No. 1, National Spastics Society, Heinemann, London

Anthony, A., Bogle, D., Ingram, T.T.S. and McIsaac, N.W. (1971) *The Edinburgh Articulation Test*, Livingstone, Edinburgh

Brazelton, T.B. (1973) *Neonatal Behavioural Assessment Scale*, Clinics in Developmental Medicine No. 50. SIMP, Heinemann, London

Brett, M. (1965) The estimation of foetal maturity by the neurological examination of the neonate. In *Gestational Age. Size and Maturity* (eds M. Dasskins, and W.G. MacGregor), Clinics in Developmental Medicine No. 19. SIMP, Heinemann, London

Davies, P.A., Robinson, R.I., Scopes, I.W., Tizard, I.P.M. and Wigglesworth, I.S. (1972) *Medical Care of Newborn Babies*, Clinics in Developmental Medicine Nos. 44/45. SIMP, Heinemann, London

Dubowitz, L.M.S., Dubowitz, V. and Goldberg, C. (1970) Clinical assessment of gestational age in the newborn infant. *Journal of Pediatrics*, **77**, 1

Dubowitz, L. and Dubowitz, V. (1981) *The Neurological Assessment of the Preterm and Full-term Newborn Infant*, Clinics in Developmental Medicine No. 79, Heinemann Medical, London

Dunea, G. (1990) Rounds. *British Medical Journal*, **301**, 547

Egan, D.F. (1990) *Developmental Examination of Infants and Preschool Children*, Clinics in Developmental Medicine No. 112, MacKeith Press, Oxford

Engel, R. and Benson, R.C. (1968) Estimate of conceptional age by evoked response activity. *Biology of the Neonate*, **12**, 201

Farr, V. (1968) Estimation of gestational age by neurological assessment in the first week of life. *Archives of Disease in Childhood*, **43**, 353

Fog, E. and Fog, M. (1963) Cerebral inhibition examined by associated movements. In *Minimal Cerebral Dysfunction* (eds M. Bax and R. MacKeith), Clinics in Developmental Medicine No. 10. SIMP, Heinemann, London

Gesell, A. and Amatruda, C.S. (1947) *Developmental Diagnosis: Normal and Abnormal Child Development. Clinical Methods and Pediatric Applications*, Hoeber, New York

Gordon, N. (1969) Double vision. *Developmental Medicine and Child Neurology*, **11**, 242

Gordon, N., Fois, A., Jacobi, G., Minns, R.A. and Sheshia, S.S. (1983) The management of the comatose child. *Neuropediatrics*, **14**, 1

Illingworth, R.S. (1962) *An Introduction to Developmental Assessment in the First Year*, Little Club Clinics No. 3. SIMP, Heinemann, London

Illingworth, R.S. (1972) *The Development of the Infant and Young Child*, Churchill Livingstone, Edinburgh

Milani-Comparetti, A. and Gidoni, E.A. (1967) Routine developmental examination in normal and retarded children. *Developmental Medicine and Child Neurology*, **9**, 631

Paine, R.S. (1960) Neurologic examination of infants and children. *Pediatric Clinics of North America*, **7**, 471

Paine, R.S., Brazelton, T.B., Donovan, D.E., Drorbaugh, I.E., Hubbell, I.P. and Sears, E.M. (1964) Evolution of postural reflexes in normal infants and in the presence of chronic brain syndromes. *Neurology*, **14**, 1036

Paine, R.S. and Oppé, T.E. (1966) *Neurological Examination of Children*, Clinics in Developmental Medicine, Nos. 20/21. SIMP, Heinemann, London

Peiper, A. (1964) *Cerebral Function in Infancy and Childhood*, Pitman Medical, London

Prechtl, H. (1977) *The Neurological Examination of the Full-term Newborn Infant*, Clinics in Developmental Medicine No. 63, Heinemann Medical, London

Prechtl, H. and Beintema, D. (1964) *The Neurological Examination of the Full-term Newborn Infant*, Clinics in Developmental Medicine No. 12. SIMP, Heinemann, London

Reynell, J. (1969) *Reynell Developmental Language Scales*, National Foundation for Educational Research, Slough

Robinson, R.I. (1966) Assessment of gestational age by neurological examination. *Archives of Disease in Childhood*, **41**, 437

Sheridan, M.D. (1958) Simple clinical hearing tests for very young or mentally retarded children. *British Medical Journal*, **ii**, 999

Sheridan, M.D. (1969) Vision screening procedures for very young or handicapped children. In *Aspects of Developmental and Paediatric Ophthalmology* (eds P. Gardiner, R. MacKeith and V. Smith). Clinics in Developmental Medicine No. 32. SIMP, Heinemann, London

Sheridan, M.D. (1973) The Stycar graded balls vision test. *Developmental Medicine and Child Neurology*, **15**, 423

Sheridan, M.D. (1975) *Children's Developmental Progress from Birth to Five Years;— the Stycar Sequences*, National Foundation for Educational Research, Slough

Sokolov, E.N. (1963) *Perception and Conditioned Reflex*, Pergamon Press, Oxford

Teasdale, G. and Jenett, B. (1974) Assessment of coma and impaired consciousness. *Lancet*, **ii**, 81

Touwen, B. (1976) *Neurological Development in Infancy*, Spastics International Medical Publications. Heinemann Medical, London

2 Some presenting symptoms and signs

This chapter can only be a brief review of a few presenting features of the varied problems of childhood. Each chapter will contain many of these, and too much repetition must be avoided. However, it should be emphasized that children come to the clinic with symptoms and signs, and not with disease entities. It is in this context that experience can sometimes outweigh knowledge, essential as both may be. It will be stressed in a later chapter that perception depends, among other factors, on memory, imagery, attention and concepts; and diagnosis is skilled perception.

The importance of obtaining a careful description of symptoms and the need to question the child as well as the parents cannot be over-emphasized. For example, terms such as 'fits' and 'seizures' are often loosely used, and after a detailed discussion it may become apparent that the child is having temper tantrums and not epilepsy. Also, if a mother is asked about a child's migraine she may deny any prodromal symptoms, but these can be elicited easily from the child by questions phrased in the right manner.

Symptoms

Pain

Pain is a difficult symptom to assess at any age, and in the case of small children it may have to be inferred from associated signs, for example the limp resulting from a painful disorder of the hip joint. The nervous child is more likely to suffer from, and complain of, pain, and under these circumstances a period of careful observation may be more important than a battery of complicated investigations.

The most acceptable theory of pain appreciation at present is the gate theory (Melzack and Wall, 1965). Most of the nerve fibres conducting pain are small, slowly conducting fibres, and there are relatively few large, rapidly conducting fibres. Cells of the substantia gelatinosa of the spinal cord are claimed to act as a control system affecting the afferent pattern before it passes on to the next relay of fibres conducting the impulses to the sensory cortex. Increased activity of the large fibres enhances the inhibitory effect of the substantia gelatinosa on the first central transmission cells in the dorsal horn, whilst increased activity of the small fibres lessens it. If gentle pressure is applied suddenly to the skin, large fibres fire the first central transmission cells and partially close the gate and shorten the barrage generated by these cells. If stimulus intensity is increased the effects of large and small fibres tend to counteract each other, and the output of the transmission cells increases. If the stimulation is prolonged, the large fibres start to adapt with a relative increase of small fibre activity, and the gate opens further with a rise in the output of the transmission cells. This can again be decreased by artificially raising large fibre activity, for example by scratching, which overcomes their adaptation. This may be the main gate, but there may be gates at other levels of the nervous system. Although this is only a hypothesis, there is no doubt that it has played its part in stimulating research (Nathan, 1976), even if certain aspects may be incorrect, for example pain is not invariably the result of stimulation of small non-myelinated fibres, the inhibitory effect of large myelinated fibres cannot always be demonstrated and the role of the substantia gelatinosa in pain is very conjectural. The discovery that the brain can synthesize pentapeptides which produce analgesia may well increase the understanding of the subject. The term endorphin is now used for naturally occurring substances having the properties of opiates, and three effective ones are β-endorphin, leucine enkephalin and methionine enkephalin. They all have other than anti-nociceptive functions. They may also be linked with the apparent effects of acupuncture, as at slow rates of stimulation endorphin appears in the cerebral spinal fluid (Nathan, 1982), and may be the chemical basis for the 'gate theory'. These substances, and an increasing number of neurotransmitters, are being found to have a part in the mechanisms by which painful stimuli are processed in the CNS. It is hoped that this knowledge will lead to more effective treatment.

The distribution of the pain is most helpful in diagnosis. If it is of obvious root distribution this may be the first evidence of a focal lesion such as extra-dural abscess of the spine or a spinal neurofibroma. Neuralgias of any kind are very rare during childhood, but very occasionally pain of atypical distribution can be a symptom of depression.

The quality of pain can be important. When pain is a feature of a focal sensory fit it is hard to describe, as are most sensory epileptic phenomena, because they are distorted sensations. However, one is often left in no doubt that it is a very unpleasant sensation. If the pain is described as severe and long-standing, and yet does not appear to affect the child in any other way, the possibility of a psychogenic origin must be considered. Aching pains in the muscles can be the first sign of weakness, for example such pain can be the first symptom of myasthenia gravis, and perhaps the condition thought to be of rheumatic origin. Muscular aching occurs in hypothyroidism, and shooting and aching pains in the limbs can also be early symptoms of a polyneuritis. Paraesthesia is a more common presenting symptom of peripheral nerve involvement, and, if sympathetically questioned about it, even very young children can describe such sensations.

Headaches

The symptom of headache at any age may be of great importance, but especially so in childhood, if only because tension headaches from which so many people suffer are not so common. The clue to the correct diagnosis is often given by the character and timing of the headaches, and this information is available if time is taken in eliciting the history from the child and mother.

Tension headaches

When the headache is a symptom of anxiety the pain is often described as a feeling of pressure or tightness which increases as the day wears on. The scalp can be tender, even combing the hair being uncomfortable. The symptoms are rarely relieved by analgesics and are more likely to respond to such drugs as diazepam, chlordiazepoxide or chlorpromazine derivatives. However, this is symptomatic treatment, and the main task is to find out the cause of the anxiety and attempt to remove it.

Migraine

Accepting that headaches are relatively uncommon in childhood, one of the most frequent is migraine. Also, in the early years, so-called 'migraine equivalents' quite often take the place of headache; these have sometimes been referred to as the 'periodic syndrome', but this probably contains a number of recurrent conditions. Cyclical vomiting, which may only be associated with headache as age increases, is perhaps more often an early manifestation of migraine. It is suggested that when the vomiting is severe it may be caused by a partial deficiency of ornithine transcarbamylase or other enzymes in the Krebs-Henseleit urea cycle in a heterozygote. As this is a partial lack of the enzyme, the person is able to cope under normal circumstances, but under stress, for example during an infection, hyperammonaemia results. If the diagnosis can be confirmed by finding a significant elevation of the blood ammonia level, it may be possible to prevent the attacks by giving a low protein diet, for instance by using gluten-free products (Russell, 1969). The diagnosis can sometimes only be made for certain by using an ammonium tolerance test, using an oral dose of ammonium chloride (1.75 mg/kg).

A diagnosis of migraine can usually be made by taking a careful history. Although hereditary factors play an important part in causation, it must not be forgotten that the symptoms can sometimes be caused by organic lesions, such as arterio-venous malformations.

It has been suggested that the warning symptoms of a headache may be due to ischaemia. This may result from spasm of certain intracranial arteries. If these are arteries supplying the retina and visual pathways the defects will vary from scotoma to hemianopsia. Transient ischaemia of the occipital cortex will result in the characteristic spectrum of various colours which gradually expands in a zig-zag crescent from a central area, or takes the form of a fortification. Involvement of branches of the middle cerebral artery causes transient dysphasia and unilateral paraesthesia, particularly affecting the face and tongue.

Special diagnostic difficulties can arise when there is spasm of branches of the basilar artery, and great care has to be taken to exclude conditions other than migraine. The vision of both eyes can be affected, and there may be tingling of the hands and feet, diplopia, vertigo and ataxia.

If these aura occur, the pain usually starts as they subside. It is often but not always unilateral, and is maximal in the temporal area. It may be caused by dilation of branches of the external carotid arteries, or by swelling of their walls, and is often of a throbbing nature. The headache is associated with photophobia, nausea and vomiting, and is of the type that is helped by lying down in a darkened room, and if possible going to sleep. The attack can start at any time of day, sometimes awakening the child from sleep. They may be worse under states of stress and anxiety, but occasionally occur at the end of the school week or at the beginning of a holiday, the so-called 'let-down' headache. If the prodromal symptoms are in the territory of the basilar artery the headache is likely to be in the occipital area, and brief impairment of consciousness can occur and even longer periods in which the patient seems to be in a state of sleep. It must again be emphasized that lesions in the posterior fossa must be excluded with particular care. Headache with aura are referred to as classical and those without as common.

In hemiplegic migraine the paralysis lasts for several days and sometimes in consecutive attacks may alternate from one side to the other (*alternating hemiplegia in childhood*). There is often a family history of similar attacks, or at least of severe migraine. Affected children may sometimes develop epilepsy which raises the possibility that the condition is linked to epilepsy as well as to migraine (Sakuragawa, 1992). Treatment is difficult (Hosking, Cavanagh and Wilson, 1978). Haloperidol, and especially flunarazine in alternating hemiplegia, have been used with some success (Caesar and Azou, 1984).

Ophthalmoplegic migraine is another recognized clinical entity, but one which has to be distinguished from other causes of such symptoms, for example cerebral aneurysms, neoplasms or localized inflammatory lesions. The pain is situated in and around the eye and is followed by an ophthalmoplegia of varying degree. When it occurs in childhood it has a greater incidence among boys (Bickerstaff, 1964). It has even been reported in infancy with the sudden onset of a third nerve palsy. It is suggested that normal computerized axial tomography excludes the need for arteriography, but this has yet to be definitely proven. Propanolol can be tried in prophylaxis (Robertson and Schnitzler, 1978).

The alternating constriction and dilation of certain arteries suggests an instability of the autonomic nervous system, probably of cortical origin; and likely to be a secondary phenomenon, although the distribution of the vessels involved cannot be explained. It may also account for the oedema of the arterial wall, causing constriction of the lumen, and the apparent enlargement of the vessel viewed from the outside, as in the superficial branches of the temporal arteries. Presumably there is a chemical cause for this. It may be linked in some way to serotonin, the plasma level of which, after a rise at the start of an attack, falls as the headache progresses (Anthony, Hinterberger and Lancer, 1967). It has been suggested that there may be a primary abnormality of platelet function, with an attack occurring when there is a diminution of platelet-monoamine-oxidases and an increase in platelet aggregation, resulting in a rise in 5-hydroxytryptamine (5-HT) levels, followed by a fall (Harrington, 1978). Although it does not seem to account for all the findings, an alternative hypothesis to the spasm and dilatation of certain vessels has been proposed. The headache is due to stimulation of nociceptive nerve endings in the walls of meningeal vessels which penetrate the outer cortex resulting in localized inhibition or excitation (Blau, 1978). The role of platelet stickiness, and various abnormalities of coagulation, particularly in disorders such as hemiplegic migraine, has still to be elucidated. Vascular and hormonal factors may well be important in the production of certain symptoms, but it is most likely that they depend on an initial *neural mechanism*, which could be at a brain-stem level (Pearce, 1984). Perhaps a mechanism such as Leao's spreading depression, associated with arteriolar spasm, may be involved (Pearce, 1985). Spreading depression could account for many of the symptoms of migraine; and the underlying mechanisms support links between migraine, epilepsy and post-traumatic syndromes (Gordon, 1989). More work is needed to explain all the findings in those who suffer from migraine.

If attacks are occurring frequently it is important to enquire into possible precipitating causes, such as stress caused by difficulties at school, or emotional disturbances within the home. A trial of prophylactic treatment is also justified with drugs such as antihistamines, like promethazine, prochlorperazine, propanolol and pizotifen (Brown, 1977), although their effect is uncertain. Flunarazine, a calcium channel blocker, may be more promising (Sorge *et al.*, 1988). If the EEG shows paroxysmal activity, and there are behaviour disorders, it may be justifiable to try the effect of carbamazepine in an older child. The serotonin antagonist, methysergide, is undoubtedly effective in preventing migraine, but is best avoided before puberty because of its side-effects. Behaviour therapy, employing the technique of auto-hypnosis may be useful.

When the headaches occur at fairly long intervals, and particularly when prodromal symptoms warn of their onset, analgesics such as paracetamol or a chlorpromazine derivative can be given at the start of an attack, especially if the child can lie down for a few hours. If nausea and vomiting are already present it will help to give metoclopromide 5–10 mg 15 minutes before the other drugs. A more specific treatment is the use of ergotamine tartrate, either dissolved under the tongue, or given as a suppository, or by intramuscular injection, although there is a risk of aggravating the vomiting, and it must be given with care. After further research, other serotonin-1 agonists which constrict dural and pial vessels, such as sumatripan, may be found effective at all ages, given intravenously or orally.

Headaches from raised intracranial pressure

Characteristically, such headaches wake the child in the early hours of the morning and are often associated with nausea and vomiting. They tend to wear off during the morning. The pain appears to be due mainly to displacement of the dura and vessels at the base of the brain, and the timing of the attacks may be related to the increased venous pressure within the head, resulting from lying down to sleep. The headache is usually generalized, but, in the presence of posterior fossa tumours, it can be maximal in the occipital region and accompanied by a stiff neck and tilting of the head to one side. Other types of headache and facial pain are rare in childhood but can be referred from the teeth or sinuses. Headaches resulting from refractive errors of the eye do occasionally occur but are rare. Psychogenic headaches will be considered in Chapter 13.

Impairment of vision

If a child does not seem to have adequate vision the ophthalmologist is likely to be the first specialist consulted. However, there are a number of neurological conditions which can present in this way. Neurological syndromes can include cataracts and retinal degeneration in their manifestations. The optic nerves, tracts and radiations can be affected by conditions as varied as demyelinating diseases and cerebral tumours. For example, an acute disseminated encephalomyelitis can present as sudden blindness in a young child. Many of these disorders will be considered in the following text, but in this chapter it is justifiable to consider central blindness in more detail. The possibility of central deafness has been recognized for a long time; the child often being diagnosed as having middle ear deafness but, with increasing age, starting to respond to sound. A similar phenomenon within the sphere of vision has not received the same attention. The term *delayed visual maturation* has been applied to infants who, at the age of 6 weeks or more, show no visual awareness and are unable to fixate or to follow a bright object. This can be due to defects of brain development and can be associated with general retardation or abnormal neurological findings. Illingworth (1980) confirms that the most common cause of delayed visual maturation is mental handicap, and that this, combined with the pale optic disc of the normal young baby, can lead to a wrong diagnosis of blindness. He also confirms that this condition can occur in some apparently normal babies. The findings of initially abnormal visual evoked responses, which soon become normal, suggests a defect of the visual pathways and not of vision itself (Harel, Holtzman and Feinson, 1983). There may be a combination of delayed myelination and delayed dendritic and synaptic formation. This could result from hypoxic-ischaemic brain damage. If vision does seem to develop normally a careful watch must obviously be kept on these children's progress, especially in terms of their ability to learn.

Acquired cortical blindness can follow a number of conditions, such as bacterial meningitis, head injury, cerebral anoxia and hydrocephalus. It can be transient or permanent. In the former case the relevant part of the brain may not be destroyed, or this may be an example of the brain's adaptability in early life (Foley and Gordon, 1985). It can therefore be difficult to give a definite prognosis in these cases, but a period of observation will make a firm opinion possible; and most parents will accept the reasons for uncertainty. The clinical examination of the cortically blind child is well reviewed by Knox (1964). Apart from the obvious need for a careful history, the scheme for examination includes checking following movements of the eyes and head, fixation of a light, opticokinetic nystagmus, response to a threatening gesture, blink reaction and pupil response to a bright light, the range of ocular movements, the response to body rotation, and examination for nystagmus. Responses to non-visual sensory stimuli should also be tested. Clinical examination and neurophysiological tests, including visual evoked responses, can help to resolve the level of a possible lesion, and in predicting recovery. After the recovery of vision these children may well have perceptual difficulties due to the involvement of the parieto-occipital cortex; and a relevant assessment must be done in case remedial teaching is needed.

Weakness

Children often come to the doctor with a complaint from themselves or their parents of floppiness or weakness. Floppiness in infancy will be described in detail in Chapter 7, but it can be emphasized here as well that the most common cause will be cerebral palsy; an early manifestation of mental handicap, and of various forms of cerebral palsy. 'Benign congenital hypotonia' may be a convenient term, but is not a diagnosis. Many floppy children show no abnormalities on investigation, and eventually progress satisfactorily; the condition is presumably a delay in the maturation of the motor system. Some of the children prove to have neuropathies and myopathies of some kind, but these latter conditions are uncommon.

Weakness in infancy can be difficult to assess, especially in the presence of hypotonia, ataxia and lack of balance. The fact that a child cannot stand up may have nothing to do with lack of muscle power but everything to do with a failure of the development of postural reflexes. Much can be learnt from watching the baby in the supine position and noting the spontaneous movements of the arms and legs, and how active these are. The distribution of the weakness is obviously important; for example the unilateral involvement of the frontalis muscle in differentiating an upper from a lower motor neurone facial palsy, and the weakness confined to the motor distribution of a particular peripheral nerve. Whenever possible the most useful grading is by the MRC Scale: $0 = $ no active contraction, $1 = $ visible or palpable contraction without active movement, $2 = $ movement with gravity eliminated, $3 = $ movement against gravity, $4 = $ movement against gravity and resistance and $5 = $ normal power.

Unsteadiness

As will be discussed later in this book, unsteadiness can be of acute or gradual onset and can be due to a variety of diseases and lesions of the nervous system. Careful investigation is required to exclude anything from a cerebellar tumour to a hereditary condition such as ataxia telangiectasia, or an infectious polyneuritis. When the symptoms indicate an acquired condition in a child who was previously developing normally, its significance has to be judged in relation to other symptoms and signs, its mode of onset, and the age of the child. Tests to elucidate its nature can then be planned accordingly.

The position is different when the unsteadiness becomes apparent when the child is learning to walk, and has reached an age when balance is expected to have developed fully. If there is a marked disability the child may well have an ataxic form of cerebral palsy. However, if of slighter degree, the condition may fit better into the syndrome of the 'clumsy child'. From the aetiological point of view it may be a matter of degree, related to the severity, site and timing of the lesion, but labels are an important factor in the attitude towards a child's disability. It may be more helpful to the child to diagnose a perceptuo-motor disability rather than a 'minor' form of cerebral palsy, with the inference that the condition is likely to improve as the child grows older. This will affect the attitude of the parents and teacher to the child, and will encourage a much more optimistic outlook.

Vertigo

Young children can often describe the sensation of vertigo very well. When it is associated with deafness the cause is most likely to be related to a past or present infection of the ear. Vertigo on its own can be a manifestation of focal epilepsy arising in the parietal lobe, in which case the vertigo is not likely to last for more than a few minutes at a time. A careful history for other epileptic manifestations and the EEG may help in the diagnosis. It has already been mentioned that vertigo can occur in basilar migraine; and it has to be distinguished from other types of dizziness, for instance the 'swimmy' feeling in the head which often is the forerunner of a faint. Vertigo can occur after head injury; and when it persists with the head in a certain position it will be due to a lesion of the brain-stem. When it only occurs for a few seconds with the head turned to one or other side, it is most probably due to a lesion of the utricle (Gordon, 1954).

Vestibular neuronitis and Ménière's disease are rare in childhood, and these diagnoses should only be accepted after careful exclusion of other causes. Vestibular neuronitis may include virus infections involving the labyrinth, and the relationship between vestibular neuronitis and benign paroxysmal vertigo is obscure. Benign paroxysmal vertigo is a definite entity in childhood (Basser, 1964). The prognosis is good, and perhaps the main danger is to mistakenly diagnose the attacks as epileptic. Symptomatic treatment of labyrinthine vertigo with cinnarizine or prochlorperazine may help.

Abnormal behaviour

If a child is brought to see the doctor because of a change of behaviour, rather than the persistence of a behaviour pattern, the possible causes are more numerous. They may be purely psychogenic due to anxieties from stresses at home and at school. Young children are obviously very vulnerable to discord in the home, and it may need the help of a skilled social worker to obtain evidence of this. Unhappiness at school can often result from learning difficulties rather than the other way round, and overactivity is rarely due to the hyperkinetic syndrome but more often the result of anxiety or boredom.

An alteration in behaviour and personality is sometimes the first symptom of an organic disease. Epilepsy is suspected more often than proves to be the case. Seizures arising in the temporal lobe are rarely the cause of aggressive outbursts or antisocial behaviour, especially if there are no epileptic phenomena in association. *Petit mal* attacks can be so slight as to escape the notice of even the experienced observer, and then the child can be wrongly accused of inattention and lack of effort at school. Antiepileptic treatment, particularly with barbiturates, can cause behavioural disorders, especially irritability and overactivity.

Certain progressive and serious cerebral diseases present as abnormalities of behaviour. For example, subacute sclerosing panencephalitis may start with altered behaviour, often first noticed at school. Adrenoleucodystrophy is another degenerative cerebral disease that may show psychiatric symptoms before there are any definite neurological abnormalities on examination. In this situation the electroencephalogram may be of help, especially if serial records are carried out, showing deterioration. However, the EEG should not be used as a screening test, and a normal record must not allay clinical suspicions if these are well founded.

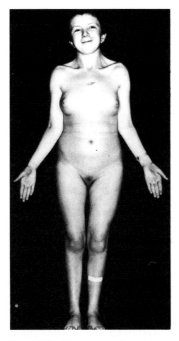
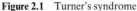
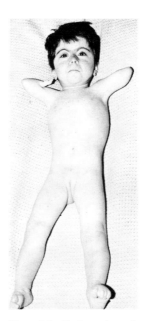

Figure 2.1   Turner's syndrome   **Figure 2.2**   De Lange's syndrome.

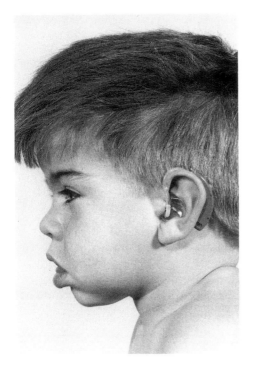

Figure 2.3 Hunter's syndrome.

Signs

Appearance of the child

One look at a child may lead to the correct diagnosis, and if this chance is missed and the doctor becomes absorbed in technical details it may be several weeks and numerous investigations later that the correct answer is found. For example, the penetrating glance may identify the presence of mild hypothyroidism, which can otherwise be easily missed.

The importance of observation of the infant's posture and movements is stressed in the discussion on the clinical examination; but now it is the overall, and, in particular the facial appearance, that is being considered, and some examples will be given. The baby with Down's syndrome and the older child with Turner's syndrome (Fig. 2.1) are obvious instances. The appearance of such chromosome abnormalities is not always easy to identify, especially when it is not a complete syndrome as in mosaicism. There are many syndromes within the field of mental handicap with a characteristic appearance, for example the de Lange syndrome (Fig. 2.2), Hunter's syndrome (Fig. 2.3) and the Rubenstein-Taybi syndrome. Those with a good visual memory will enhance their reputation by recognizing these syndromes, others will need the help of a good reference book (Smith, 1970; Salmon, 1978).

The facial appearance of certain myopathies is typical, especially that of the congenital type of dystrophia myotonica, with drooping eyelids, triangular open mouth, and lack of expression. When this is linked to a waddling gait, the diagnosis may be made before any signs of myotonia are elicited.

The dystrophies of bone and cartilage result in various diagnostic features and syndromes. Premature closure of some of the cranial sutures, combined with exophthalmos, beaked nose and underdevelopment of the maxillae constitutes Crouzon's syndrome. In Apert's syndrome the craniostenosis is associated with syndactyly of the hands and feet. The Seabright-Bantam syndrome (Albright *et al.*, 1942) can be recognized by the mental retardation being associated with short stature and obesity, as well as by a round face, cataracts and brachydactyly. X-ray examination shows abnormalities of the metacarpal and phalangeal bones and epiphyseal deformities. A low calcium and raised phosphate level in the serum may be found, with a normal or raised secretion of parathormone, suggesting an end-organ defect. In that case the term 'pseudo-hypoparathyroidism' is used. When the appearance is not associated with a biochemical disorder it has been called 'pseudo-pseudo-hypoparathyroidism', but it is uncertain if this is a separate entity. This syndrome may be inherited as a sex-linked dominant trait.

The facial bones are severely underdeveloped in the Treacher-Collins syndrome. In addition, the nose is beaked, the ears are malformed, and there is an anti-mongoloid slant to the eyes. Cataracts, colomboma and deafness are also found.

Many of these syndromes are rare, but they must be identified if advances in knowledge are to be made; and, in some instances, genetic advice given.

Failure to thrive

Neurological conditions can often present in the clinic with not just a disorder of development but an obvious impairment of physical health. This can happen before any definite neurological abnormalities appear, particularly in disorders of metabolism. Such conditions will be discussed in later chapters, but it is worth stating as often as possible that time is not on the doctor's side. If treatment is to be effective in preventing damage to the nervous system a diagnosis must be promptly made, and if possible treatment started within a matter of days or weeks after the onset of symptoms. This applies to so many conditions, from chronic undiagnosed infections, even meningitis, to hypothyroidism and enzyme deficiencies such as classical phenylketonuria. It follows that any worries about an infant's progress must lead to a careful assessment and most probably to a number of screening tests to exclude such possibilities. A survey for infections may have to include an examination of the cerebrospinal fluid even in the absence of the classical signs of meningitis, particularly among babies and infants. Not only will the urine have to be tested for abnormal quantities of amino acids, but also for reducing substances. Sometimes X-ray evidence of a delayed bone age can be the first evidence of cretinism, and a plain X-ray of the skull can sometimes, by minimal calcification or slight springing of the sutures, raise the suspicion of a chronic subdural haematoma or other space-occupying lesion. A CT scan can sometimes confirm a diagnosis of tuberose sclerosis.

In a slightly different context, the child taking long-term treatment must be watched carefully for any signs of iatrogenic illness. Rightly, and not before time, medical treatment is being increasingly questioned, as drugs can usually only be taken at the cost of some toxic side-effects. This is well illustrated in the case of anti-epileptic treatment. Over-sedation is highly likely to interfere with learning, and relatively little is known about the long-term effects of these drugs on the child's general health. For example, the folic acid deficiency related to barbiturates and phenytoin therapy may not matter for a few months, but what are the effects on a growing child if it continues for several years? There is no doubt that some children with epilepsy who have been on treatment for years deteriorate gradually in mentality and physique. It is no longer good enough to blame the seizures, for the treatment may well be partly responsible.

Dysarthria

Many children are brought to the doctor because of difficulties of articulation, the parents being naturally worried about the difficulty in understanding what their child is saying, and the effect this will have on his or her relations with other adults and children. In many instances the dysarthria is seen in the context of cerebral palsy, but even a spastic dysarthria can occur in isolation, and is then often referred to as supra-bulbar palsy. Some of the various types of dysarthria can be considered, the choice being their neurological associations and not necessarily their relative importance.

Upper motor neurone lesions

In spastic quadraplegia there is almost always involvement of the muscles of articulation. As with all upper motor neurone lesions there is an impaired range and repertoire of movements and speech is slow and slurred. Tongue and lip movements are restricted, and dribbling of saliva may occur. It is always important to check for associated defects. Even the addition of slight malocclusion or inadequate nasal airway can cause a marked accentuation of the disability, and sometimes the less obvious cause may be the one that can be most successfully treated.

Extrapyramidal disorders

Children with difficulties of articulation due to involuntary movements can be of average, or, very occasionally of above average, intelligence, however much their appearance belies this. Also, the association of high-tone deafness with athetosis has to be borne in mind constantly. Speech will be slow, slurred and irregular. It may constantly be arrested by the movements, and is accompanied by grimacing, aggravated by the efforts to speak. Occasionally, speech is unintelligible.

Cerebellar dysarthria

This type is uncommon in childhood but does occur in such conditions as ataxic cerebral palsy. There is a high incidence of mental handicap and delayed language development among such children, but it is uncertain whether this is due to a focal or generalized cerebral damage. The latter seems more likely, as the syndrome can undoubtedly occur in association with such causes as arrested hydrocephalus.

Lower motor neurone disease

Although it is rare, dysarthria can occur in the type of spinal muscular atrophy associated with bulbar palsy. If there is nuclear agenesis of the lower cranial nerves, pharyngoplasty may help, and an occlusive prosthesis will result in more normal swallowing patterns and less dribbling. Paralysis of the facial nerve can occasionally cause dysarthria, but rarely unless it is bilateral, as sometimes occurs in polyneuritis. It is almost always unilateral in Bell's palsy. This sometimes complicates infections such as herpes zoster and varicella but it may not always be of infectious origin. It is thought to result from inflammation and swelling of the nerve in the Fallopian canal. The weakness is of sudden onset and may be accompanied by pain in the face and behind the ear. The whole side of the face is usually involved, food collects between the gums and cheek, and the eye waters. Taste may be lost over the anterior two-thirds of the tongue if the lesion is proximal to the junction of the chorda tympani with the facial nerve. A search should be made for vesicles in the ear or on the neck which may occur in a herpes zoster infection. Facial palsy can be associated with hypertension, and the blood pressure must be checked. An electromyogram of the facial muscles shows evidence of degeneration after about 10 days. In most children recovery is complete but care must be taken that the eye does not become inflamed (an eye patch is useful). It is uncertain if treatment with steroids is of benefit, which presumably act by reducing the swelling of the nerve within the temporal bone, and so relieving the pressure palsy. In the early stages prednisone can be given for 10–14 days. When recovery is incomplete plastic surgery may be required when the child is older.

Muscular disorders

These are an equally uncommon cause of dysarthria. Myasthenia can result in increasingly unintelligible speech as talking proceeds, and there are two types of muscular dystrophy which affect the muscles of articulation. The facio-scapular-humeral dystrophy has a dominant mode of inheritance and is quite compatible with survival into late adult life. More important is the marked dysarthria that can occur in dystrophia myotonia. This disease usually develops towards the end of childhood or in early adult life. However, as already mentioned there are families in which the affected child is abnormal from birth, and the young infant has difficulty in swallowing and sucking due to facial weakness. Articulation is particularly involved, and these children are often referred to the clinic because of this (Gordon and Hilson, 1967).

Developmental articulatory dyspraxia and language disorders

Persistence of infantile patterns of speech are not uncommon, and do not usually require treatment. Disorders of language development are often associated with defects of spoken speech, which is not surprising as expressive developmental dysphasia is a form of dyspraxia. Very occasionally a child presents with a moderate to severe defect of articulation, usually in the absence of any other physical signs; and in spite of intensive speech therapy the disability can persist. Comprehension is usually adequate, but the child may show other evidence of a disorder of perceptuo-motor function or of language development, for example reading retardation. The term 'developmental articulatory dyspraxia' has been used to describe this apparently isolated difficulty in controlling the movements of lips, tongue and palate in the absence of muscle weakness (Morley and Fox, 1969). The prognosis has to be guarded, as the dysarthria may sometimes continue into adult life; as can a number of other specific developmental disorders. Disorders of language will be considered in Chapter 6.

Cerebral oedema

Cerebral oedema occurs in a wide variety of neurological disorders and will be referred to in the context of status epilepticus and neurosurgical conditions. There are various types of cerebral oedema and the diagnosis of the cause should be as precise as possible if treatment is to be effective. The most common form is *vasogenic* due to increased permeability of the brain capillary endothelial cells, and the white matter is mainly affected. It particularly occurs around local lesions, such as tumours and abscesses. In *cytotoxic* oedema the water accumulates intracellularly and the causes include hypoxia, ischaemia and presumed toxic conditions such as Reye's syndrome. *Hydrostatic* oedema results from increased intravascular pressure when there is a failure of cerebrovascular resistance, with outpouring of water into the extracellular space. Apart from causes such as arterial hypertension, it occurs after prolonged compression of the brain, and may therefore complicate decompression operations. *Hypo-osmotic* oedema has been reported in the syndrome of inappropriate antidiuretic hormone (ADH) secretion when hyponatraemia occurs, and when excessive infusion of intravenous solutions low in sodium are used in the correction of hypernatraemic dehydration. In *interstitial* oedema seen in obstructive hydrocephalus there is an increase in water and sodium content of the periventricular white matter due to movement of the CSF through the ependyma (Miller, 1979).

The advent of computerized axial tomography has greatly assisted diagnosis as the oedema appears as a decrease in density. Intracranial pressure monitoring can help in assessing the progress of the condition. Prevention is obviously important with correction of hypoxia, and excess carbon dioxide, and hyperpyrexia, and if possible maintenance of systolic blood pressure between 110 and 140 mm Hg.

Treatment is often a matter of urgency and is well reviewed by Isler (1986). Fluid intake must be restricted. A continuous sufficient systemic circulation and a continuous sufficient respiration must be maintained. If hypoventilation occurs or the level of consciousness falls the patient should if possible be transferred to an intensive care unit for intubation and artificial hyperventilation. This procedure will include muscular relaxation and sedation with phenobarbitone. Then continuous intracranial pressure monitoring will be needed. The intracranial pressure can be manipulated by hyperventilation, relaxation and sedation. Elevation of body temperature must be prevented with antipyretics. If intracranial pressure is still not controlled various drugs must be tried. Dexamethasone is of proven value in vasogenic oedema but its effect in cytotoxic and other forms of cerebral oedema is uncertain. Hypertonic solutions will have a more dramatic effect. Glucose, sucrose, urea, isosorbide, glycerol and mannitol have been used. A solution of 20 per cent mannitol is the most favoured, and it should be given rapidly, 1 g/kg body weight over about 10 minutes (Miller, 1979). Other forms of treatment include controlled CSF drainage and the use of diuretics, such as acetozolamide and frusemide, which may reduce CSF formation (Fishman, 1978).

Conclusion

These are only some of the infinite variety of ways that disorders and illnesses can present in childhood. This brief review is presented not as an exhaustive list, but as an alternative to the emphasis on diseases. Once suspicions have been raised, the details of a particular condition can be referred to in the most appropriate source of information, but it is the significance of initial symptoms which must provide the clues and alert the observer to the most likely cause.

References

Albright, F., Burnett, C.H., Smith, P.H. and Parson, W. (1942) Pseudo-hypoparathyroidism, an example of 'Seabright-Bantam syndrome'; report of three cases. *Endocrinology*, **30**, 922

Anthony, M., Hinterberger, H. and Lance, I.W. (1967) Plasma serotonin in migraine and stress. *Archives of Neurology*, **16**, 544

Basser, L.S. (1964) Benign paroxysmal vertigo of childhood (a variety of vestibular neuronitis). *Brain*, **87**, 141

Bickerstaff, E.R. (1964) Ophthalmoplegic migraine. *Revue Neurologique*, **110**, 582

Blau, J.M. (1978) Migraine as a vasomotor instability of the meningeal circulation. *Lancet*, **ii**, 1136

Brown, J.K. (1977) Migraine and migraine equivalents in children. *Developmental Medicine and Child Neurology*, **19**, 683

Casaer, P. and Azou, M. (1984) Flunarizine in alternating hemiplegia in childhood. *Lancet*, **ii**, 579

Fishman, R.A. (1978) The pathophysiology and treatment of brain oedema. In *Recent Advances in Clinical Neurology* (eds W.B. Matthews, and G.H. Glasen), Churchill Livingstone, Edinburgh

Foley, J. and Gordon, N. (1985) Recovery from cortical blindness. *Developmental Medicine and Child Neurology*, **27**, 383

Gordon, N. (1954) Post-traumatic vertigo with special reference to positional nystagmus. *Lancet*, **i**, 1216

Gordon, N. (1989) Migraine, epilepsy, post-traumatic syndromes, and spreading depression. *Developmental Medicine and Child Neurology*, **31**, 682

Gordon, N. and Hilson. D. (1967) Myotonic dystrophy: its occurrence in childhood. *British Journal of Clinical Practice*, **21**, 537

Harrington, E. (1978) Migraine: a blood disorder. *Lancet*, **ii**, 501

Harel, S., Holtzman, M. and Feinson, M. (1983) Delayed visual maturation. *Archives of Disease in Childhood*, **58**, 298

Hosking, G.P., Cavanagh, N.P.C. and Wilson, J. (1978) Alternating hemiplegia: complicated migraine of infancy. *Archives of Disease in Childhood*, **53**, 656

Illingworth, R.S. (1980) *The Development of the Infant and Young Child*, 7th Edn, Churchill Livingstone, Edinburgh

Isler, W. (1986) Children with cerebro-vascular disease. In *Neurologically Sick Children: Treatment and Management* (eds N. Gordon, and I. McKinlay), Blackwell Scientific, Oxford

Knox, D.L. (1964) Examination of the cortically blind infant. *American Journal of Ophthalmology*, **58**, 617

Melzack, R. and Wall, I.D (1965) Pain mechanisms: a new theory. *Science*, **150**, 971

Miller, J.D. (1979) The management of cerebral oedema. *British Journal of Hospital Medicine*, **21**, 152

Morley, M.E. and Fox, I. (1969) Disorders of articulation: theory and therapy. *British Journal of Disorders of Communication*, **4**, 151

Nathan, P.W. (1976) The gait-control theory of pain—a critical review. *Brain*, **99**, 123

Nathan, P.W. (1982) Pain. In *Recent Advances in Clinical Neurology* (eds W.B. Matthews, and G.H. Glaser), Churchill Livingstone, Edinburgh

Pearce, J.M.S. (1984) Migraine: a cerebral disorder. *Lancet*, **ii**, 86

Pearce, L.M.S. (1985) Is migraine explained by Leao's spreading depression? *Lancet*, **ii**, 763

Robertson, W.C. and Schnitzler, E.R. (1978) Ophthalmoplegic migraine in infancy. *Pediatrics*, **61**, 886

Russell, A. (1969) A biochemical basis for migraine and cyclical vomiting. In *Enzymopenic Anaemia, Lysosomes and Other Papers*. (eds J.D. Allen, K.S. Holt, J.T. Ireland and R.I. Pollitt), Churchill Livingstone, Edinburgh

Sakuragawa, N. (1992) Alternating hemiplegia in childhood: 23 cases in Japan. *Brain and Development*, **14**, 283

Salmon, M.A. (1978) *Development Defects and Syndromes*, H.M. & M., Aylesbury

Smith, D.W. (1970) *Recognisable Patterns of Human Malformations*. W.B. Saunders, Philadelphia

Sorge, F., De Simone, R., Merano, E. *et al.* (1988) Flunarizine in the prophylaxis of childhood migraine. A double-blind placebo-controlled crossover study. *Cephalagia*, **8**, 1

3 Certain genetically-determined conditions

Neurocutaneous dysplasias

There are a number of disorders in which both the nervous system and the skin are affected. There is strong evidence for a dominant mode of inheritance in most, which suggests a genetically-determined defect of the ectodermal tissue. The overlap between certain abnormalities of the retina and skin also raises the possibility of common aetiological factors.

Neurofibromatosis (von Recklinghausen's disease)

This condition has a dominant mode of inheritance linked to chromosome 17 (Huson, 1989), but a very variable penetrance, and a high mutation rate. Its manifestations may consist of six or more areas of cutaneous pigmentation or café-au-lait spots (Fig. 3.1), or of extensive deformities and tumour formation, with all manner of intermediate variations (Crowe, Schull and Neel, 1956). The number of café-au-lait spots tends to increase as the child grows older, and may be associated with subcutaneous nodules and sometimes with plexiform neuromas. The latter often cause deformities of the affected tissues, especially of the face.

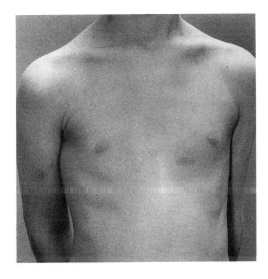

Figure 3.1   Café-au-lait spots.

The disorder sometimes presents with mental retardation and epilepsy, and with various deformities, such as scoliosis, bony overgrowth, and an absent roof to the orbit. The mechanism by which the intelligence is impaired is uncertain. Apart from the neurofibromata on the peripheral nerves, similar tumours may occur on the cranial nerves. If symptoms and signs suggest the possibility of an acoustic neuroma in the cerebello-pontine angle the diagnosis will be supported by the presence of café-au-lait spots on the skin; although these tumours are more common in a separate entity, rare in childhood, known as bilateral acoustic neurofibromatosis, in which there are few or no café-au-lait patches. In the same way, the cutaneous manifestations may help to establish the diagnosis of a glioma of the optic chiasm. Neurofibroma may involve the walls of the larger blood vessels and cause stenosis. These patients are also at risk from other tumours, benign and malignant: pheochromocytomas; ganglioneuromas; meningiomas; glioblastomas; and tumours of the viscera. The cutaneous manifestations will confirm the diagnosis, and treatment can only be directed towards those of the complications which are amenable to surgery.

There is no doubt about the herterogeneity of this condition, and the classical syndrome is now referred to as NF1 with an identified gene; although there is not complete agreement that the presentation with bilateral acoustic neuroma should be referred to as NF2 until other subgroups are identified (Riccaroli, 1987).

Tuberous sclerosis (epiloia) (Bourneville's disease)

Tuberous sclerosis is inherited in the same manner as neurofibromatosis, and a gene linked to the condition has been located on chromosome 9, and a second gene on chromosome 11. In about 70 per cent of affected children it is due to a new mutation. Some aspects of tuberous sclerosis overlap those of neurofibromatosis. The children frequently present in early life with epilepsy, and then there is usually evidence of

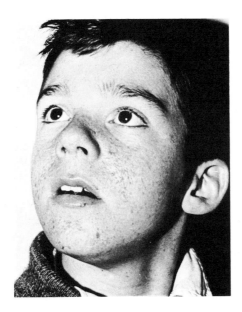

Figure 3.2   Adenoma sebaceum.

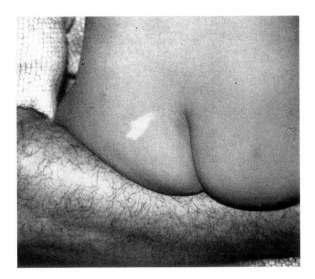

Figure 3.3   Patient with tuberous sclerosis, showing a 'white' spot.

mental retardation as well. This condition should always be considered as a cause of epilepsy in childhood. A significant number of babies with infantile spasms are found to be suffering from this condition in later childhood. The skin lesions of adenoma sebaceum (Fig. 3.2) appear later in childhood, and typically consist of reddish, slightly raised papules in a butterfly distribution over the face. They are not invariably present (Critchley and Earl, 1932). Certain cutaneous lesions appear earlier, particularly white or depigmented spots (Fig. 3.3) which fluoresce under ultraviolet light, and sometimes café-au-lait spots and shagreen patches. These patches are raised, rough areas of skin, mainly over the back. Subungual fibroma should also be looked for on fingers and toes. Other useful diagnostic findings are rectal polyps and increased numbers of dental pits (Lygidakis and Lindenbaum, 1987). There are features common to tuberous sclerosis and neurofibromatosis, such as retinal phakomas. These are seen on ophthalmoscopy as flat, white, roundish masses overlying the blood vessels, and about half the size of the optic disc. There may also be similarities in some of the findings on histological examination of the brain, for example hyaline thickenings in the vessel walls, and abnormal giant cells. There are hard nodules of glial tissue in the brain which may project into the ventricles, giving the typical 'candle guttering' appearance. They may also calcify and reveal themselves on the X-ray or on CT scanning (Fig. 3.4) at an earlier age (Maki *et al.*, 1979). Malignant gliomas may develop, as well as tumours in other organs such as the heart (rhabdomyomata), kidney (angiomyolipoma and carcinoma) and cysts of the kidney and lung. If the cutaneous manifestations are evident the diagnosis presents no difficulties, but this is not always so easy, for instance when tumours occur in the brain with only equivocal signs of the disease. The EEG is often grossly abnormal, especially in the first two years of life. The evolution of the various skin lesions is not related to the course of the epilepsy or the appearance of intracranial calcification (Pampiglione and Moynahan, 1976). CT scanning is essential for diagnosis of suspected patients and their relatives.

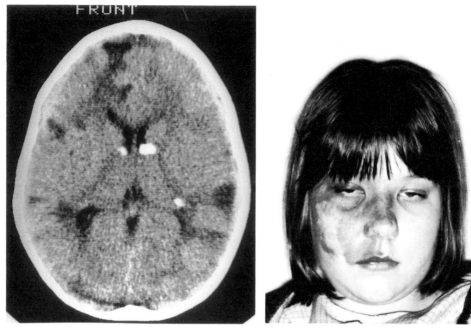

Figure 3.4   CT scan of intracranial calcification in tuberose sclerosis.

Figure 3.5   Sturge-Weber syndrome. Facial appearance.

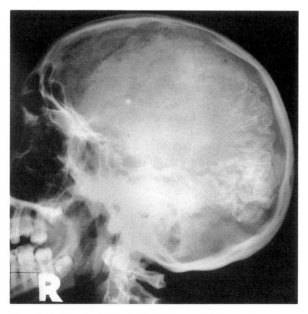

Figure 3.6   Gyral calcification in the Sturge-Weber syndrome.

Treatment can only be symptomatic, medical for the epilepsy, and surgical for the neoplasms, when this is indicated.

Sturge-Weber syndrome (encephalotrigeminal angiomatosis)

The inclusion of the Sturge-Weber syndrome (Fig. 3.5) in the group of neuro-cutaneous dysplasias may be a matter of clinical convenience, as there is no conclusive evidence that it is genetically determined (Pratt, 1967). This syndrome consists of a facial naevus in the distribution of the trigeminal nerve, almost always affecting the first and second divisions on one side, and an angioma of the underlying cortex, usually in the occipital area with calcification of the adjacent brain tissue. There may also be angioma of the choroid of the eye, with increased intraocular pressure and buphthalmus. The cerebral angioma are frequently associated with epilepsy, mental retardation and hemiplegia. The fits are often focal, involving the body on the opposite side to the cerebral lesion. The retardation may be progressive, presumably due to impaired blood supply to the cortex due to shunting of blood through the angioma. This may also be a reason for the laying down of calcium adjacent to the abnormal vessels in the form of 'railway lines', seen on the X-ray of the skull (Fig. 3.6). The diagnosis will be obvious from these signs. If the facial naevus is large it is likely that only cosmetic treatment will be possible. If the epileptic seizures are unresponsive to medical treatment the possibility of removing the affected area of the brain should be considered, although it is still to be proved that surgery can influence the natural course of the disease (Buttler and Schulte, 1975).

Von Hippel-Lindau syndrome

This syndrome consists of the association of angioma of the retina and the cerebellum, and it is thought to be hereditary. Inheritance has been shown to be dominant in many families, with a variable and inconstant appearance of symptoms (Silver, 1954). On examination of the retina, tortuous vessels are seen, sometimes leading to a nodular area (haemangioblastoma) in the periphery of the retina. Haemorrhages, secondary glaucoma and retinal separation can occur, and result in visual failure. The cerebellar lesion is also a haemangioblastoma and will produce the symptoms and signs of any other tumour in this situation.

Tumours and angiomas may occur in other organs, particularly the kidney, liver, spleen and pancreas. Pheochromocytomas are also associated with this syndrome. Irradiation has been used to treat the retinal lesions, and when the presence of a cerebellar tumour has been established it should be removed.

Some syndromes presenting with ataxia and involuntary movements

There are many causes for ataxia in infancy and childhood, and it is not surprising that cells as large and metabolically active as the cerebellar Purkinje cells should be susceptible to a wide variety of influences. When the onset of ataxia is sudden it may be due to viral infections or intoxications with drugs (particularly the anti-epileptic drugs such as phenytoin). Diseases as varied as tumours of the posterior fossa, some of the degenerative cerebral diseases considered in another chapter, and polyneuritis, may present with ataxia, more often with an acute than a chronic onset. When the ataxia is long-standing (ataxic cerebral palsy) the etiology can be equally varied and includes anoxia, hydrocephalus (which has often ceased to progress), congenital malformations of the cerebellum, and the effects of head injury. It is suggested that defects of cholinergic transmission may underlie certain cerebellar movement disorders and that it may be worth trying treatment with choline (4 to 5 g a day, adult dose) (Legg, 1978). In this section various hereditary conditions will be considered in which chronic ataxia is a predominant symptom.

Spino-cerebellar ataxias (Friedreich's ataxia)

These syndromes most often have an autosomal recessive mode of inheritance, although rarely it can be dominant or sex-linked. Friedreich's ataxia is the most common form, inherited in an autosomal recessive fashion. The gene for Friedreich's ataxia has been localized to chromosome 9, making prenatal diagnosis a possibility. Difficulties with walking are first noted during childhood, usually around the age of 7 years, although in some cases the gait seems always to have been unsteady, and a congenital form has been described. The incoordination then affects the arms and eventually all movements. Speech becomes slurred and scanning. There is a reduction of muscle tone and wasting of muscles, sometimes followed by contractures. Loss of position sense, resulting from degeneration of the posterior columns, contributes to the ataxia, and there is also loss of vibration sense, two-point discrimination and stereognosis. The tendon reflexes disappear and the plantar responses become extensor. Other related neurological abnormalities include the rare occurrence of dementia, retinal pigmentation, optic atrophy, progressive external ophthalmoplegia, and nystagmus late in the course of the disease. There are a number of characteristic abnormalities in other systems, particularly deformities of the feet (Fig. 3.7), scoliosis, and cardiac involvement, with progressive heart failure. Electrocardiographic

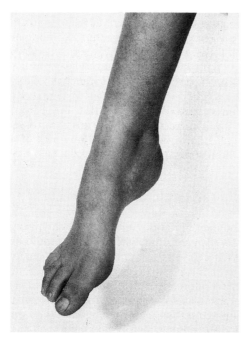

Figure 3.7 Foot of a child with Freidreich's ataxia.

changes include arrythmias and various forms of heart block. Hypertrophic obstructive cardiomyopathy can occur and must be diagnosed and treated. An association with diabetes mellitus has been found (Thoren, 1962).

The diagnosis is made from the clinical picture and the family history, although sporadic cases do occur. Investigations may have to be done to exclude other conditions, such as disseminated sclerosis and focal lesions of the cerebellum and spinal cord. The primary metabolic defect in Friedreich's ataxia may be due to a number of causes: pyruvate dehydrogenase complex deficiency; and mitochondrial malic enzyme deficiency (Stumpf et al., 1982). On histological examination the atrophy affects mainly the long ascending and descending tracts of the spinal cord, the dorsal columns, spino-cerebellar tracts and pyramidal tracts. Loss of Purkinje cells and atrophy of the dentate nucleus and superior cerebellar peduncles have also been found. Orthopaedic treatment can be helpful in a condition which is progressing very slowly.

Other spino-cerebellar ataxias

There is a tendency for the clinical picture to vary slightly from family to family, and there are a number of conditions which merit classification as separate syndromes. *Olivopontocerebellar atrophy* may manifest itself in the second decade, but usually appears in later life. It is more often sporadic than familial. As the name implies, the atrophy chiefly affects the grey matter of the pons. Rigidity and dementia may occur in addition to the cerebellar signs. *Familial spastic paraplegia* seems to contain a number of syndromes, some inherited as a dominant, and some as a recessive, trait (Pratt, 1967). They have been well classified by Harding (1984). The spastic weakness mainly affects the legs and can be associated with cerebellar and extrapyramidal signs and occasionally with dementia. Patients with a hemiplegic distribution have been described (Bickerstaff, 1950). The age of onset is very variable from birth onwards, and the degenerative changes found at autopsy correspond to the clinical findings. Sjögren and Larsson (1957) have described the syndrome of spastic paraplegia associated with mental retardation and ichthyosis, which seems to have a recessive mode of inheritance.

The *Roussy-Lévy syndrome* may form a link between the spino-cerebellar ataxias and peroneal muscular atrophy, examples of all three syndromes having been recorded in one family (Spillane, 1940). Pes cavus and absent reflexes are found from infancy, and as the child grows older there is slight unsteadiness of gait and clumsiness of arm movements, occasionally with wasting of the small hand muscles. The condition is only very slowly progressive. It appears to have a dominant mode of inheritance.

Marinesco-Sjögren syndrome

There are a number of rare syndromes that may occasionally be found among children classified as suffering from cerebral palsy. For example, the Marinesco-Sjögren syndrome is characterized by ataxia and sometimes spasticity, associated with mental retardation and cataracts. The mode of inheritance seems to be autosomal recessive. Crome, Duckett and White Franklin (1963) reported the case of two sisters dying in infancy who showed evidence of delayed development, cataracts, stunted growth and renal tubular necrosis. It was suggested that the finding of renal involvement might be a link between the Marinesco-Sjögren syndrome and Lowe's

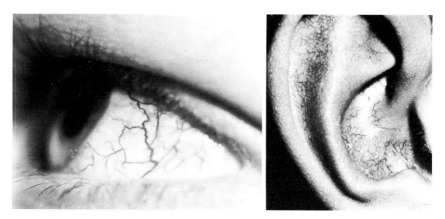

Figure 3.8   Telangiectasia of conjunctiva in a child with ataxia telangiectasia.

Figure 3.9   Telangiectasia of pinna, in a child with ataxia telangiectasia.

oculo-cerebral-renal syndrome. However, the inheritance of the latter is sex-linked recessive. Its chief features are mental retardation, cataracts with or without glaucoma, and renal involvement with a marked amino-aciduria. Renal rickets can also occur.

Ataxia-telangiectasia (Louis-Bar syndrome)

The child with this condition is sometimes late in learning to walk and then develops increasing incoordination affecting all movements. Choreo-athetoid movements appear in association with hypotonia and diminished or absent tendon reflexes. There may be Parkinsonian features, especially lack of facial expression. Other findings include dysarthria, nystagmus and abnormal eye movements. An oculo-motor apraxia is a particularly suggestive finding, with no eye movements to command but with involuntary movements retained. Intelligence is usually within normal limits, but may deteriorate as the child grows older. Telangiectasia is first noticed in the conjunctivae (Fig. 3.8), often before the age of 5 years, although it is not essential for diagnosis at this age. It may also affect the pinnae (Fig. 3.9), the face, and the limb flexures. Although not always present a frequent feature of the syndrome is an undue liability to infections, particularly of the respiratory tract, and there is a relative lack of lymphoid tissue (Boder and Sedgwick, 1963).

The mode of inheritance is recessive, but the mechanism of the cerebellar atrophy is unknown. The clinical diagnosis is supported by the finding of a diminished white cell count and raised erythrocyte sedimentation rate, hypogammaglobinaemia, defects in T lymphocytes, and absent or decreased levels of IgA. The finding of a serum level of alpha-fetoprotein raised above 30 mg/ml may be a useful diagnostic test (Waldmann and McIntire, 1972). An increased spontaneous chromosome breakage rate in lymphocytes and cultured skin fibroblasts has been found, and may be useful in prenatal diagnosis (Shaham *et al.*, 1982). This may be due to defective DNA repair mechanisms, which is no doubt also related to the fact that lymphocytes and fibroblasts from these patients are abnormally sensitive to X-ray and gamma ray irradiation. The association of this syndrome with abnormalities of the thymus, immunological deficiency and malignancy suggests that there may be a disorder in the development or maintenance of a normal immunological system.

A similar syndrome has been described with the same neurological signs but no telangiectasias or other neurological manifestations. The genetic pattern also suggests a recessive autosomal inheritance (Aicardi *et al.*, 1988).

Giant axonal neuropathy

This is a generalized disorder of cytoplasmic intermediate filaments affecting the nervous system in particular. The onset is in the first 7 years of life, with clumsiness, weakness and diminished reflexes, followed by dysarthria, cerebellar and pyramidal tract signs, dementia and sometimes seizures. The hair is often coarse, frizzy or curly. There seems to be an autosomal recessive mode of inheritance. There is no treatment (Ouvrier, 1989).

Lesch-Nyhan syndrome

Children with this syndrome are severely retarded and develop choreoathetosis early in life; later on there is evidence of damage to the cortico-spinal tracts (Hoefnagel *et al.*, 1965). As they grow older they show a characteristic tendency to mutilate themselves, biting their lips and fingers, and their behaviour becomes aggressive. There may be a megaloblastic anaemia and evidence of gout. The serum uric acid level is raised due to a specific enzyme deficiency (hypoxanthine-guanine phosphoribo-syltransferase) (Seegmiller, Rosenbloom and Kelley, 1967), but the exact way in which the brain is damaged is not known. It may be a toxic effect or due to a deficiency of certain metabolites. There seems to be a sex-linked recessive mode of inheritance. Treatment with allopurinol may favourably affect the hyperuricaemia, but seems to have no effect on the neurological complications. This may be due to the fact that allopurinal acts on a more distal part of the uric acid pathway than the site of the enzymatic deficiency in this condition. However, such treatment is justified, as uric acid calculi occur in the kidneys, and urate-staining granules have been found in the brain. During infancy, when the risks of brain damage are greatest, it may be justifiable to give exchange transfusions to supply the missing enzyme in normal erythrocytes (Watts *et al.*, 1974). Extraction of the teeth helps to diminish self-mutilation and it has been suggested that it may be controlled by the oral administration of L-5-hydroxytryptophan in a dose of 1–8 mg per kg body weight per day (Mizuno and Yugari, 1974). However, it certainly does not work in every case, whether it is combined with a peripheral decarboxylase inhibitor (carbidopa 200 mg a day) or not; although it may result in a better sleep pattern and a reduction of daytime irritability and dyskinesis (Anders *et al.*, 1978). It must be stressed that self-mutilation is not uncommon among severely mentally handicapped children, and management with physical restraint and elimination of boredom may be the most effective treatment.

Hepatolenticular degeneration (Wilson's disease)

Signs of liver damage usually appear most frequently during the second decade, to be followed by evidence of brain damage. The condition is inherited as an autosomal recessive trait and is a disorder of copper metabolism, although the exact nature of the disorder is unknown. The gene for Wilson's disease has been mapped to chromosome

13, so the condition is not caused by a primary molecular defect in ceruloplasmin, the gene for which is on chromosome 3. This finding will help in the presymptomatic diagnosis of siblings of affected patients (Frydman *et al.*, 1985). Ceruloplasmin is a globulin to which most of the copper in the plasma is combined, and there may be a defect in this substance. This results in an increased deposition of copper in the liver and brain tissue, but would not account for the finding of increased absorption of copper from the intestine. Another possibility is an abnormality of tissue protein resulting in an excessive uptake of copper (Uzman, 1957). It has been shown that metallothionein from the livers of patients with Wilson's disease may be abnormal, with a copper-binding constant four times as great as that of the protein from control subjects. This would impair transfer of copper to ceruloplasmin; and the accumulation of copper metallothionein in the liver may be hepatotoxic; and when it leaks into the blood stream it could be taken up by other tissues which may then also be damaged (Evans, Dubois and Hambridge, 1973).

The clinical evidence of liver damage can suggest an acute condition such as hepatitis, or a more chronic one, such as cirrhosis. The neurological symptoms may also vary considerably and tend to start after puberty. Intellectual and emotional disturbances may be noted, and the clinical picture tends to be dominated either by tremor or by a Parkinsonian picture. The tremor may be violent and sometimes only present on movement. This, combined with behavioural and emotional disturbances, can lead to a diagnosis of a psychogenic illness. When the findings suggest Parkinsonism there is dysarthria, drooling, oculogyric crises, abnormal postures and generalized rigidity.

A diagnostic sign is the presence of the Kayser-Fleischer copper-containing ring at the margin of the cornea. It is a greenish-brown ring in Descemet's membrane, starting at the top and spreading round the cornea to become complete. In the early stages it may be seen clearly only with a slit lamp. Once suspected, the diagnosis is confirmed by finding a generalized amino-aciduria, an increased excretion of copper in the urine (normal, less than 40 mg/24 h), a low concentration of serum copper (normal, 67–149 mg/100 ml) and a low serum ceruloplasmin level (normal, 20.7–40.2 mg/100 ml.) In very young children the ceruloplasmin level can be low in hepatic dysfunction from other causes. The urine excretion of copper should also be measured after a provocative dose of penicillamine when in Wilson's disease it will rise to 1000–3000 mg/day (Komrower and Sardharwalla, 1978).

Treatment consists of giving a diet low in copper and chelating agents to remove the excess copper. British Anti-Lemisite (BAL) has been largely superseded by penicillamine, and if this is given before the disease is too far advanced the patient can be returned to an active life. The dose of penicillamine should be regulated by measurements of blood and urine copper and is usually 1.5–2.0 g taken daily in two or three doses before meals. Pyridoxine supplements should be given to children, and foods with high copper content should be avoided (Walshe, 1967). Penicillamine may give rise to the nephrotic syndrome, which will necessitate stopping the drug and the trial of some other chelating agent. A possible alternative is triethylene tetramine dihydrochloride (Trientine), 1.8–3 g in divided doses (Walshe, 1973), and recently it has been claimed that Wilson's disease may be treated with oral zinc alone (zinc sulphate 200–300 mg three times daily). This may also be given to patients who do not respond to cupriuretic drugs, such as penicillamine (Hoogenraad, Van Den Hamer and Van Hathum, 1984). Denny-Brown (1964) has suggested that the pseudosclerotic type of Wilson's disease, with tremor as the presenting symptom, tends to respond well to treatment with chelating agents, while the dystonia of the progressive lenticular degeneration form does not. The tremor may, therefore, be due more to the accumulation of copper in the nervous system than the dystonia.

A-β-lipoproteinaemia (Bassen-Kornzweig syndrome)

This is another rare metabolic disorder inherited as an autosomal recessive trait. It presents in infancy with steatorrhoea, and, as the child grows older, weakness, incoordination, and defective vision develop. The malabsorption can lead to secondary vitamin and mineral deficiencies. Mental retardation is rare and so is the occurrence of cardiac complications. The neurological signs are mainly due to a neuropathy, but include ataxia and absent tendon reflexes and extensor plantar responses. Muscle weakness and wasting may be severe, and raise the question of a myopathy, but the presence of marked sensory loss helps to exclude this (Schwartz *et al.*, 1963). The loss of vision is related to a retinopathy affecting the macula and the periphery of the retina. Investigations show an absence of β-lipoprotein on serum electrophoresis, and low levels of cholesterol, phospholipid, and triglyceride. The steatorrhoea appears to be due to a failure of chylomicron formation, but in spite of this there is a fairly adequate absorption of fat, probably through the portal circulation.

Acanthocytosis or thorn cells, red blood cells with spike-like projections, are always present in the Bassen-Kornzweig syndrome, and have been described in another neurological syndrome in which levels of the β-lipoproteins and cholesterol are normal. There is evidence of dyskinesia, particularly affecting the facial muscles, and wasting of the peripheral limb muscles (Critchley *et al.*, 1970).

Treatment of the steatorrhoea is by a low-fat diet, and vitamin supplements should be given, especially vitamins A and E. The latter has a beneficial effect on the neuropathy and retinopathy (Muller, Lloyd and Wolff, 1982). Vitamin E deficiency causing spinocerebellar syndromes may occur in patients with congenital cholestatic jaundice, cystic fibrosis, massive ileal resection, and blind loop syndrome; and vitamin E can produce striking improvement (Brin *et al.*, 1985).

Deficiency of *alpha-lipoprotein (Tangier disease)* is characterized by enlargement of the tonsils, which are of a yellowish colour due to deposition of cholesterol esters. Corneal clouding may occur, and a peripheral neuropathy (Kocen *et al.*, 1967). The latter has not been reported in childhood.

Hartnup's disease

This is a disorder of metabolism of recessive mode of inheritance which may present with ataxia, but quite frequently the condition is asymptomatic (Wilcken *et al.*, 1977). The fully developed syndrome consists of a photosensitive pellagra-like rash (Fig. 3.10), transient cerebellar ataxia, sometimes with pyramidal signs, and occasionally, in older children, personality changes and delayed development. Investigations show a generalized aminoaciduria, hyperindoluria and hypertryptophanuria. The primary abnormality seems to be defective transport of tryptophan, and probably other amino acids, in the small intestine and renal tubules (Wong and Pillai, 1966). The indole metabolites are due to the action of the normal intestinal flora on the unabsorbed tryptophan in the intestine. Large doses of nicotinic acid may help to prevent the photosensitive rash, but the effect on the neurological complications, when these are present, is by no means so certain. Theoretically, it should help if there is a failure to produce nicotinamide from tryptophan, but the neurological symptoms may be due

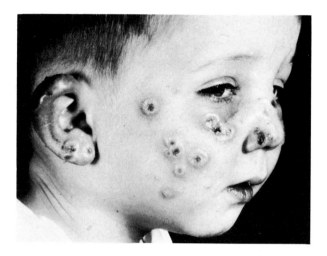

Figure 3.10   Photosensitive rash in Hartnup's disease

to intoxication from excess absorption from the colon of bacterial products of amino acid breakdown (Milne, 1967).

Some hereditary disorders of metabolism

A few of the disorders of metabolism resulting in mental retardation will be mentioned in the Chapters 6 and 11. An increasing number of such conditions have been identified. They are inherited in a recessive manner and include several which, if diagnosed soon enough, can be treated with a special diet to prevent damage to the brain. Among the disorders of amino acid metabolism only a few examples can be given to illustrate the type of problems they present. As more and more of these conditions are discovered, their recognition will become an important part of preventive medicine. To this end, various types of screening programmes have been introduced (Komrower, 1972). The Guthrie test depends on the inhibition of bacterial growth by an amino acid analogue, except when the amino acid is added to the inoculated medium (Guthrie and Susi, 1963). It can be used to identify phenylalanine, tyrosine, histidine, methianine and leucine. Two-dimensional chromatograms of the urine will identify many of these diseases but are ill-suited to large-scale surveys. One-dimensional chromatography of serum obtained from a heel-prick (Scriver, Davies and Culien, 1964) offers an economic means of screening communities for a large number of these metabolic disorders (Komrower, 1970).

An large number of inborn errors of metabolism can be diagnosed antenatally. This is becoming increasingly important as more and more of these conditions can be treated; and, perhaps equally so, in the antenatal diagnosis in pregnancies subsequent to the birth of an affected child in the many that still cannot be treated. Methods used in antenatal diagnosis include fetal liver biopsy, fetal blood sampling, amniocentesis, and chorion villus biopsy. The subject is well reviewed by Cleary and Wraith (1991).

Phenylketonuria

This condition results from a failure to convert phenylalanine to tyrosine due to a deficiency of the enzyme phenylalanine hydroxylase, the gene for which is on chromosome 12. Phenylalanine accumulates, the body tries to get rid of it through alternative metabolic pathways, and there is a deficiency of substances lower down this particular metabolic pathway. Symptoms and signs in disorders of this kind can result for any of these reasons. It is suggested that a raised level of phenylalanine may interfere with the metabolism of myelin, and when this occurs at a stage of rapid brain growth it will lead to brain damage.

The appearance of the child can suggest the diagnosis, as they often, but not always, have pale-coloured hair and blue eyes. Early in infancy it is apparent that development is delayed and this is frequently associated with anorexia, lethargy, epileptic seizures, and evidence of spasticity. The fits can take various forms, for example generalized seizures or myoclonus, sometimes in the form of infantile spasms. If the baby is on a normal protein intake, screening tests on about the sixth day of life should establish the diagnosis before such symptoms arise, or else it may be too late to prevent brain damage. If there is any suspicion that a particular baby may be suffering from phenylketonuria the ferric chloride test can be used. Three to five drops of 10% ferric chloride are added to 1 ml urine and, if positive, a green colour develops immediately. The Phenistix test, in which a special filter paper is applied to the wet nappy is an alternative, but neither of these tests is entirely reliable. If possible, use should be made of either amino acid chromatography or the Guthrie test. Detailed investigations will certainly be needed before treatment is started.

In classical phenylketonuria the blood phenylalanine will be 25 mg per 100 ml or higher, but this group may constitute only about 16% of infants with raised blood phenylalanine levels (Menkes and Eviatar, 1969). Phenylpyruvic, phenylacetic and ortho-hydroxyphenylacetic acids are excreted in the urine, and it is the presence of phenylacetic acid in the sweat which gives rise to the typical musty odour.

In apparently benign hyperphenylalanaemia the blood phenylalanine level will be equally high, but the urine will contain only traces of phenylpyruvic and ortho-hydroxyphenylacetic acids. This means that the ferric chloride test will be negative. In another group there seems to be a temporary phenylalaninaemia. This rarely persists for more than a week or two and the tyrosine level will also be raised. Other children may show a slightly raised blood phenylalanine level on a normal diet and phenylpyruvic and ortho-hydroxyphenylacetic acids are only excreted after a load test, while others only have a raised phenylalanine level on a high protein diet and do not excrete the abnormal acids in the urine. The differential diagnosis is helped by a phenylalanine load test, as only classical phenylketonuria will show a rise of blood phenylalanine much above 20 mg per 100 ml (Blaskovics, Schaeffler and Hack, 1974). The discovery of new types of phenylketonuria supports the view that there are multiple genotypes in phenylketonuria with differing susceptibilities to brain damage from similar degrees of biochemical abnormality, as estimated by the plasma phenylalanine level (Partington, 1978).

When a significantly raised blood level is found in infancy (above 10 mg per 100 ml), whether this is combined with the excretion of the characteristic metabolites in the urine or not, a low-phenylalanine diet must be started. After four months the phenylalanine in the diet can be increased with careful monitoring of the effect, and at the age of one year the daily intake of phenylalanine can be checked before deciding on the need for further strict dieting (Hudson and Clothier, 1975). As it is an essential amino acid, a certain amount of phenylalanine has to be given, approximately 30–40 mg per kg per day in the first year, and then reducing to about 20–25 mg per kg per day (Komrower, 1970). Careful control of the diet is essential so that the phenylalanine level is maintained at about 4–12 mg per 100 ml. There is still controversy about the question of when to stop treatment for classical phenylketonuria, but it becomes increasingly difficult to maintain an older child on a strict diet, and it is perhaps reasonable to consider stopping this after the age of 12 years, although there is a risk that this will result in a deterioration of behaviour and a fall in intellectual progress (Smith *et al.*, 1978). If the diet is stopped the patient should be kept under observation into adult life in case deterioration does occur, and it has to be re-introduced (Thompson *et al.*, 1990). The decision will also have to be reviewed when affected girls reach child-bearing age, as if the level of phenylalanine in the mother's blood is raised the fetus will suffer. The damage may well occur during the first few weeks after conception when the mother may not realize that she is pregnant, so that if such women wish to bear children they should be advised to start a strict low-phenylalanine diet (Smith *et al.*, 1979), but more knowledge is required on the best methods of management (Komrower *et al.*, 1979). Now that more and more girls with metabolic disorders are being treated in early life, and also because it is recognized that even in a condition such as phenylketonuria the affected patient may not be severely retarded, it is essential to screen mothers of retarded children for diseases of this type.

Variants of phenylketonuria have been described (Smith, Clayton and Wolff, 1975) in which the disease is progressive and does not respond to a low phenylalanine diet, and a disorder of biopterin metabolism has been involved. About 1–3% of babies with a positive Guthrie test have been found to suffer from a malignant hyperphenyl-alaninaemia. Hypotonia, especially of the neck and trunk, swallowing difficulties, delayed motor development, or the presence of abnormal movements are suggestive findings. So far all seem to have a deficiency of tetrohydrobiopterin (BH4), which is a co-factor of phenylalanine hydroxalase, tyrosine hydroxalase and tryptophan hydrolase. This results in deficient production of the neurotransmitter products of tyrosine and tryptophan. Treatment with L-dopa and 5-hydroxytryptophan and a low phenylalanine diet has given gratifying results (Danks *et al.*, 1979), and depending on the enzyme at fault there may be a response to alternative treatments such as L-sepiapterin (Niederwieser *et al.*, 1979). Treatment with tetrahydropterins themselves may also be possible (Kaufman *et al.*, 1982).

Basic defects include a lack of dihydropteridine reductase required for the recycling of BH4, and a defective *de novo* synthesis of dihydrobiopterin. In the future the best test to differentiate these types from classical phenylketonuria may be the measuring of the response to a single oral dose of BH4. This will reduce the serum phenylalanine level to normal in these atypical forms, but not in classical phenylketonuria. Kaufman (1985) has recently reviewed the subject and makes the added suggestions of giving a source of tetrahydrofolate, such as N5-formyltetrahydrofolate or N5-methyltetra-hydrofolate in the treatment for the dihydropteridine reductase deficiency, and of giving tetrahydrobiopterin subcutaneously for chronic use when there is a defect in its synthesis (Danks *et al.*, 1979). Now dihydropteridine reductase activity can be established in peripheral leucocytes this will differentiate the two types of disorder.

Homocystinuria

This is a disorder of methionine metabolism characterized by a failure to form cystathionine from homocystine in the presence of serine due to a lack of the enzyme cystathionine synthetase. Children with this disease may be recognized by their fair hair, red cheeks, and dislocated lenses, and by an appearance suggestive of Marfan's syndrome. Kyphoscoliosis and knock-knees are also common, and there may be severe myopia and iridodonesis. In the older child there will be mental retardation, often associated with epileptic seizures, and there is a tendency to vascular thrombosis (Carson *et al.*, 1963). The risk of the latter has to be taken into account when considering operations for ectopia lentis, for instance. Having shown a raised level of homocystine in the urine by means of an amino acid chromatogram, the diagnosis will be confirmed by finding a raised level of methionine and homocystine in the serum. Large doses of pyridoxine may favourably influence the metabolic disorder among some patients (Barber and Spaeth, 1967), while in others a low methionine diet with supplements of cystathionine, serine and cystine may be needed (Komrower *et al.*, 1966).

Histidinaemia

This disorder of metabolism is due to a deficiency of the enzyme histidase, and can be recognized by the urine showing an olive-green colour in the ferric chloride test. It is sometimes associated with mild mental retardation, and has been said to cause a speech defect, but there would appear to be doubts about this, as the evidence is inconclusive (Garvey and Gordon, 1969). Treatment appears to be unjustified.

Maple-syrup-urine disease

In this condition there is a failure of the decarboxylation of certain branched-chain keto-acids. As a result of this the levels of the branched-chain amino-acids leucine, isoleucine and valine are raised in the body fluids, and a derivative of alpha-ketobutyric acid gives to the urine the characteristic smell of maple syrup, particularly after the urine has been allowed to stand for a few hours. The baby, although normal at birth, soon ceases to thrive and becomes apathetic (Menkes, Hurst and Craig, 1954).

Symptoms and signs include cyanosis, increased muscle tone and seizures; hypoglycaemia can occur, perhaps related to the high level of leucine in the blood. Death is likely at an early age if a diagnosis is not made by chromatography, whilst the recognition of the disease offers a chance of treatment with a special diet (Westall, 1967), and certain types are responsive to thiamine by mouth in large doses of up to 100 mg a day. The condition can be diagnosed antenatally. There is another intermittent form of the disease, presumably due to a variation of the enzyme deficiency, in which after developing normally for a few months the child starts to suffer from episodes of ataxia, sometimes associated with irritability and lethargy. These symptoms may be related to intercurrent infection, suggesting that the enzyme system only proves inadequate under conditions of stress (Dancis, Hutzler and Rokkones, 1967).

Organic acidurias and other disorders of amino acid metabolism

Among the increasing number of metabolic disorders that are being discovered are some which cause recurrent episodes, often precipitated by infections or other stresses; and the symptoms may include vomiting, lethargy, convulsions and coma due to intermittent metabolic acidosis. These disorders include such conditions as propionic acidaemia and methylmalonic aciduria. Proprionic acidaemia can be found in association with hyperglycinaemia (ketotic hyperglycinaemia) due to a defect of proprionyl-co-A carboxylase (Nyham, Ando and Rasmussen, 1972). These conditions can cause death of the affected infant early in life, or produce life-threatening attacks of acidosis from time to time. If the response to an infection seems to be more severe than expected, the differential diagnosis should include the possibility of this type of disease. The acidosis may respond to intravenous bicarbonate, but sometimes peritoneal dialysis has to be considered. The diagnosis of the particular type of organic aciduria can often be made by gas chromatographic examination of the urine.

Similar clinical findings can occur in subacute necrotizing encephalomyelopathy (Leigh's syndrome) considered in another chapter, and in other examples of the heterogeneous group of congenital lactic acidoses.

Such illnesses can also be associated with a raised level of ammonia in the blood, as in lysine intolerance and hyperammonaemia. Long-term treatment is possible in some of these diseases, for example by giving a low protein diet in hyperammonaemia (Levin and Russell, 1967), or a protein-restricted diet and vitamin B12 (1 mg intramuscularly per day) to some children with methylmalonic aciduria (Rosenberg, Lilljeqvist and Hsia, 1968), and biotin (5 mg twice a day) to some with propionic acidaemia (Raine, 1975).

Organic acidurias presenting in the neonatal period still have a poor prognosis. Their management has been reviewed by Saudubray et al. (1984), and antenatal diagnosis has been reviewed by Cleary and Wraith (1991).

Non-ketotic hyperglycinaemia

If hyperglycinaemia is unassociated with elevated levels of glycine in the cerebrospinal fluid there will be no neurological disturbances, but if the level of glycine in the cerebrospinal fluid is elevated there will be hypotonia, lethargy, myoclonus and respiratory disturbances starting a few days after birth (glycine encephalopathy). Development is severely retarded and fits of various kinds continue, including infantile spasms. The EEG shows periodic bursts of spikes against a flat background, involving into a hypsarrhythmic pattern. Early death is common and the characteristic finding at autopsy is spongiosis of the myelinated pathways (Dalla Bernadina et al., 1979). Treatment has been tried with sodium benzoate to reduce glycine concentration and with strychnine to antagonize glycine, but their effectiveness is unproven (Arneson et al., 1979). This is probably the most frequent of the genetic diseases of neurotransmitters.

Galactosaemia

Disorders of carbohydrate metabolism can also be inherited in an autosomal recessive manner. Galactosaemia results from a deficiency or absence of the enzyme galactose-1-phosphate uridyl transferase, although the condition does not always take a classical form. The clinical features consist of a failure to thrive and vomiting, followed by jaundice, enlargement of the liver and spleen, cataracts, and mental retardation. The hepatomegaly results from cirrhosis (Komrower et al., 1966). Sometimes the disease may have an acute onset in the first 48 hours of life with severe jaundice and signs of an encephalopathy, and may be fatal if the correct diagnosis is not made. The urine will give a positive Benedict's test, and will also show a proteinuria and a generalized amino-aciduria. The diagnosis can be confirmed by the estimation of the enzyme activity in the red blood cells (Beutler and Baluda, 1966). If an early diagnosis can be made it may be possible to prevent damage to the brain, liver and eyes which is otherwise likely to occur. The baby is put on a lactose-free diet, but this will have no effect on lesions already established, and may not entirely prevent an interference with cerebral development (Komrower and Lee, 1970).

Fructose intolerance

A deficiency of fructose-1-phosphate aldolase causes hypoglycaemia due to an overproduction of insulin. Vomiting, drowsiness and coma start when fructose is introduced into the baby's diet. If the condition is unrecognized the child will fail to grow normally, the liver and spleen will enlarge and death may occur (Nordmann, Schapira and Dreyfus, 1969). The diagnosis is confirmed by finding a low blood glucose, and a raised blood fructose and fructosuria when fructose-containing food is eaten. Fructose must be eliminated from the diet, although in adult life small amounts may be tolerated.

Among other hereditary disorders of carbohydrate metabolism, certain examples involving glycogen metabolism are considered in Chapter 7, and examples affecting mucopolysaccharide metabolism in chapter 11. Hereditary diseases of fat metabolism and leucodystrophies are also considered in Chapter 11.

Kinky (steely) hair syndrome (Menkes' syndrome)

This syndrome is characterized by slow growth and progressive cerebral degeneration, with death before the age of 3 years (Menkes et al., 1962). The infants have stubbly white hair (pili torti) (Figs. 3.11 and 3.12) and scaly skin. The mental retardation becomes severe and is accompanied by episodes of hypothermia, convulsions, and bony changes such as widening of the metaphyses and the formation of lateral spurs. Hydronephrosis, hydroureter and bladder diverticula, presumably due to disturbed innervation have been reported (Wheeler and Roberts, 1976). There is widespread

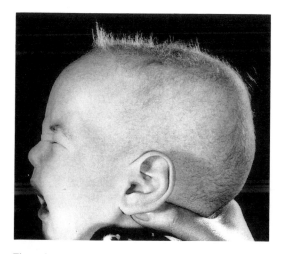

Figure 3.11   Child with Menkes' syndrome, showing kinky or steely hair.

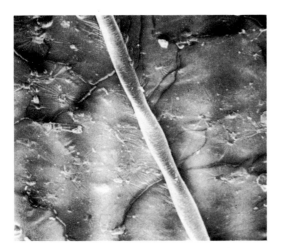

Figure 3.12   Hair from patient with Menkes' syndrome (scanning electron microscopy × 100).

arterial tortuosity and variation in the lumen, with loss of elastin in the walls of the arteries and the veins. The cerebral pathology may be the result of vascular lesions, as well as being due to the metabolic disorder. Inheritance is sex-linked recessive, and has been reported only in boys.

Although this condition may be more common than first thought, the real excuse for emphasizing it is the possibility of effective treatment in the future. Investigations have shown that the levels of serum copper and ceruloplasmin are low, and that the reason for this is a defect in absorption of copper from the gut and possibly of its utilization. There may be a defect in the binding between copper and metallothione within the mucosal cells. It is therefore reasonable to try the effect of copper given parentally or in large doses by mouth, as some absorption does occur (Danks *et al.*, 1972; Grover and Scrutton, 1975). It appears that treatment must be started within a few days of birth to be effective, as placental transport of copper may be defective. Also, some of these infants are born prematurely, before the main part of the copper stores have been transferred to the fetus. However, if there is any defect in copper utilization the response is likely to be limited or ineffective (Daish *et al.*, 1978). There may be a possibility of treatment with copper histinate.

Acute intermittent porphyria

Among the genetically-determined disorders of prophyrin metabolism intermittent symptoms occur in acute intermittent porphyria, hereditary coproporphyria and variegate porphyria, and are therefore of particular interest to the neurologist. The first of these is the most common and is characterized by attacks of intestinal colic associated with episodes of muscle weakness and mental disturbances. It does not usually manifest itself until adult life, but has been reported among young children (Kreimer-Birnbaum and Bannerman, 1975). It must certainly be considered when an adolescent suddenly develops such symptoms, particularly when there is a suggestion that they have been precipitated by barbiturates, sulphonamides and certain other drugs. The abdominal colic may be accompanied by nausea, vomiting, constipation or diarrhoea. The weakness affecting the limbs is often associated with acute pain and later by wasting, and this neuropathy has been considered in Chapter 7. The cerebral symptoms include insomnia, depression, delirium, convulsions and coma. It is important to consider the diagnosis of acute porphyria in cases of unexplained refractory epilepsy, especially when there appears to be an improvement on withdrawing drugs (Houston *et al.*, 1977). Hypertension, paroxysmal or sustained, may occur. In the type of porphyria cutanea tarda found to be widespread in South Africa (variegate porphyria) there is, in addition to the abdominal and nervous symptoms, a fragility of the skin and often an intolerance to sunlight (Dean, 1960). Photosensitivity also occurs in hereditary coproporphyria.

The characteristic finding in acute intermittent porphyria is the grossly excessive excretion of delta aminolaevulinic acid and porphobilinogen in the urine, constantly in acute intermittent porphyria and during attacks in the other two types considered. This excess in some, but not all, patients with acute intermittent porphyria may be due to a decreased activity of porphobilinogen deaminase in the erythrocytes (Goldberg, 1985). In hereditary coproporphyria and porphyria cutanea tarda there may be an increase in faecal porphyrin between the attacks and also of porphyrin-peptide conjugates; and in variegate porphyria coproporphyrin and uroporphyrin are also found in the urine between attacks. The diagnosis of acute intermittent porphyria can be confirmed by assaying red cell uroporphyrinogen synthetase (Kreimer-Birnbaum and Bannerman, 1975). If the patient succumbs to an acute attack of weakness the *post mortem* examination shows demyelination in both the central nervous system and the peripheral nerves. The disease is transmitted by a dominant inheritance, and its occurrence has been claimed in members of the British royal family (Macalpine, Hunter and Rimington, 1968).

Because of the relapsing nature of the illness, the effects of treatment are difficult to judge, but encouraging results have been reported with adenosine-5-mono-phosphoric acid (Gajdos and Gajdos-Torok, 1961). The theoretical basis for this treatment is the possibility that increased synthesis of porphyrins can result in defective synthesis of adenine and guanine. Carbohydrate infusions, carbohydrate loading with fructose (400 mg/day), and large doses of pyridoxine have been given, and intravenous haematin can be used in prophylaxis and treatment (4 mg/kg) (Pierach and Watson, 1978; McColl *et al.*, 1979). Supportive measures, sometimes including assisted ventilation, are of importance. Seizures may best be treated with bromides, as barbiturates, clonazepam and sodium valproate are all porphyrinogenic (Bankowski *et al.*, 1980). If all else fails intravenous magnesium can be tried (Sadeh *et al.*, 1991). When asymptomatic, the patient's urine should be tested quantitatively for porphobilinogen and faecal porphyrins measured. Families need to be screened so that affected members can be warned against taking drugs that can precipitate an acute attack. In acute intermittent porphyria the activity of porphobilinogen-deaminase can be estimated, and those with variegate porphyria and hereditary coproporphyria are initially screened by measurement of faecal porphyrins.

Hereditary optic atrophies

Optic atrophy may be inherited in a number of ways (Pratt, 1967). There is a dominant form of inheritance, but in Leber's optic atrophy, although once thought to be transmitted as a sex-linked recessive, the maternal inheritance can be explained by the mitochondrial origin of the disease due to a mutation in mitochondrial DNA (Singh, Lott and Wallace, 1989; Yoneda, Tsuji and Yamauchi, 1989). Alternative modes of transmission may have to be considered, such as cytoplasmic transfer of an agent, possibly viral.

In the dominant transmitted form the visual defect starts in early life with a small scotoma between the blind spot and the point of fixation. The loss of vision progresses only very slowly. Leber's optic atrophy may become apparent at any age from infancy to adult life. There is a rapid loss of vision over a period of weeks or months, and subsequent deterioration may be very slow. The optic discs are sometimes swollen in the early stages and then become pale and atrophied. Visual evoked potentials confirm the loss of nerve fibres with demyelination. A number of other conditions, such as epilepsy, mental retardation and signs of upper motor neurone degeneration can be associated with the optic atrophy.

There is evidence that in various types of optic atrophy there may be an inborn metabolic error of cyanide detoxication which causes different clinical pictures according to the particular enzyme involved. In families known to be at risk prophylactic measures such as advice against smoking and the early treatment of visual failure with hydroxocobalamin are important (Wilson, Linnell and Matthews, 1971). Optic atrophy can be found in neurological diseases of genetic type such as globoid cell leucodystrophy (Krabbe's disease). In Behr's syndrome the optic atrophy is associated with ataxia, spasticity, posterior column sensory loss, peripheral neuropathy and mental retardation. It is probably inherited as an autosomal recessive trait (Landrigan, Berenberg and Bresnan, 1973).

Genetic counselling

When a child is found to have a recessive, dominant, or sex-linked disease the parents are entitled to know the risks to further children that may be born to the family. Blyth and Carter (1969) stress that a prerequisite for genetic counselling is in almost all cases a precise diagnosis. If the condition shows regular dominance, there being almost always some clinical manifestation in those heterozygous for the affected gene, the risk to the children is one in two. The children of unaffected members of the family are not at risk. When normal parents have an affected child it probably means that a fresh mutation is involved and the risk to other children of these parents is small. Conditions inherited in this manner may show variable penetrance, as in neurofibromatosis; they may become manifest at different ages; and they may exhibit irregular dominance so that there can be the skipping of a generation.

When diseases are inherited in an autosomal recessive manner the heterozygotes are normal and those affected are homozygous. There is a one in four risk of further children developing this disease, and a one in two risk of their being carriers, although even in a condition of high heterozygote frequency the chances of marrying another heterozygote are very slight, except, of course, among cousins.

When the inheritance of a disease is sex-linked recessive the mother is heterozygous; there is a one in two risk of her daughters being similarly affected and a one in two risk of her sons carrying the mutant gene on their only X chromosome and suffering from the disease. If a male relative of the mother is affected she is likely to be a heterozygote, but otherwise it is possible that the boy's condition is the result of a fresh mutation (Blyth and Carter, 1969). In that case the risk to further sons is considerably reduced (Carter, 1978).

In many conditions the risks are not clear-cut, and it is realized that there is an interplay of genetic and environmental factors, for example the approximate one in 20 risk of another child being born with spina bifida cystica once one has been born into a family and between a one in four and one in ten risk after there have been two or more such children (Carter and Roberts, 1967). Such multifactorial risks are calculated on surveys carried out among large numbers of the population and the risks are usually less than one in 20, although they may vary from one area to another. Such a low risk may not be thought sufficient to advise limitation of the family, but this may greatly depend on individual circumstances and on attitudes to antenatal diagnosis (when this is possible); with abortion of affected fetuses. Some parents faced with the care of a handicapped child will not consider having more children whatever the risk; others may feel that with one handicapped child in the family there is a particular need for normal children.

The paediatric neurologist must certainly have a working knowledge of genetics and be able to give some advice to parents, particularly when children are affected by diseases inherited in a relatively simple way as in a Mandelian dominant, recessive, and sex-linked recessive manner. However the subject of genetics is becoming increasingly complex and in most cases a clinical geneticist should be consulted. This will increasingly be the case in the future with all the possibilities of diagnosis, especially pre-natal diagnosis, and the use of recombinant DNA techniques in identifying certain diseases (Rosenberg, 1984). Research with DNA probes has already advanced the knowledge of conditions such as Duchenne muscular dystrophy, and opens up exciting possibilities, not only of diagnosis, but also of treatment.

References

Aicardi, J., Barbosa, C., Andermann, E. *et al.* (1988) Ataxia-ocular motor apraxia: a syndrome mimicking ataxia telangiectasia. *Annals of Neurology*, **24**, 497

Anders, Th.F., Cann, H.M., Ciaranello, J.D. *et al.* (1978) Further observations on the use of 5-hydroxytrypophan in a child with Lesch-Nyhan syndrome. *Neuropädiatrie*, **9**, 157

Arneson, D., Ch'ien, L.T., Chance, P. and Wimlroy, R.S. (1979) Strychnine therapy in non-ketotic hyperglycinemia. *Paediatrics*, **63**, 369

Barber, G W. and Spaeth, L. (1967) Pyridoxine therapy in homocystinuria. *Lancet*, **i**, 337

Beutler, E. and Baluda, M.C. (1966) Improved method for measuring galactose-1-phosphate uridyl transferase activity of erythrocytes. *Clinica Chimica Acta*, **13**, 369

Bickerstaff, E.R. (1950) Hereditary spastic paraplegia. *Journal of Neurology, Neurosurgery and Psychiatry*, **13**, 134

Blaskovics, M.E., Schaeffler, G.E. and Hack, S. (1974) Phenylalaninaemia: differential diagnosis. *Archives of Disease in Childhood*, **49**, 835

Blyth, H. and Carter, C. (1969) A guide to genetic prognosis in paediatrics. *Developmental Medicine and Child Neurology*, Suppl. 18

Boder, E. and Sedgwick, R.P. (1963) Ataxia telangiectasia. A review of 101 cases. In *Cerebellum, Posture and Cerebral Palsy* (ed. G. Walsh), Little Club Clinics in Developmental Medicine No. 8. SIMP, William Heinemann, London

Bonkowski, M.L., Sinclair, P.R., Emery, S. *et al.* (1980) Seizure management in acute hepatic porphyria: risks of valproate and clonazepam. *Neurology*, **30**, 588

Brin, M.F., Fetell, M.R., Green, P.H.A. *et al.* (1985) Blind loop syndrome, vitamin E malabsorption and spinocerebellar degeneration. *Neurology*, **35**, 338

Buttler, G. and Schulte, F.J. (1975) Zur operativen Behandlung des Sturge-Weber-Syndromes. *Neuropädiatrie*, **6**, 135

Carson, N.A.J., Cusworth, C.E., Dent, C.E. *et al.* (1963) Homocystinuria: a new inborn error of metabolism associated with mental deficiency. *Archives of Disease in Childhood*, **38**, 425

Carter, C.O. (1978) Genetic counselling. *British Journal of Hospital Medicine*, **19**, 557

Carter, C.O. and Roberts, J.A.F. (1967) The risk of recurrence after two children with central nervous system malformations. *Lancet*, **i**, 306

Cleary, M.A. and Wraith, J.E. (1991) Antenatal diagnosis of inborn errors of metabolism. *Archives of Disease in Childhood*, **66**, 816

Critchley, E.M.R., Nicholson, J.T., Betts, J.J. and Weatherall, D.J. (1970) Acanthocytosis, normolipoproteinaemia and multiple tics. *Postgraduate Medical Journal*, **46**, 698

Critchley, M. and Earl, C.J.C. (1932) Tuberose sclerosis and allied conditions. *Brain*, **55**, 311

Crome, L.. Duckett, S. and White Franklin, A. (1963) Congenital cataracts. renal tubular necrosis and encephalopathy in two sisters. *Archives of Disease in Children*, **38**, 505

Crowe, F.W., Schull, W.J. and Neel, J.V. (1956) *Multiple Neurofibromatosis*, Charles C. Thomas, Springfield, Illinois

Daish, P., Wheeler, E.M., Roberts, P.F. and Jones, R.D. (1978) Menkes' syndrome. Report of a patient treated from 21 days of age with parentral copper. *Archives of Disease in Childhood*, **53**, 956

Dalla Bernadina, B., Aicardi, J., Goutieres, F. and Plouin, P. (1979) Glycine encephalopathy. *Neuropädiatrie*, **10**, 209

Dancis, J., Hutzler, J. and Rokkones, T. (1967) Intermittent branched chain ketonuria. Variant of maple-sugar-urine disease. *New England Journal of Medicine*, **276**, 84

Danks, D.M., Campbell, E., Stevens, B.J. *et al.* (1972) Menkes' kinky hair syndrome. An inherited defect in copper absorption with widespread effects. *Pediatrics*, **50**, 188

Danks, D.M., Cotton, R.G.H. and Schlesinger, P. (1979) Diagnosis of malignant hyperphenylalininaemia. *Archives of Disease in Childhood*, **54**, 329

Dean, G. (1960) Routine testing for porphyria variegata. *South African Medical Journal*, **34**, 745

Denny-Brown, D. (1964) Hepatolenticular degeneration (Wilson's disease). Two different components. *New England Journal of Medicine*, **270**, 1149

Evans, G.W., Dubois, R.S. and Hambidge, K.M. (1973) Wilson's disease: identification of an abnormal copper-binding protein. *Science*, **181**, 1175

Frydman, M., Bonné-Tamir, B., Farrer, L.A., *et al.* (1985) Assignment of the gene for Wilson's disease to chromosome 13: linkage to the esterase D locus. *Proceedings of the National Academy of Science USA*, **82**, 1892

Gajdos, A. and Gajdos-Torok, M. (1961) The therapeutic effect of adenosine-5-monophosphoric acid in porphyria. *Lancet*, **ii**, 175

Garvey, A.M. and Gordon, N. (1969) Histidinaemia and speech disorders. *British Journal of Disorders of Communication*, **4**, 146

Goldberg, A. (1985) Molecular genetics of acute intermittent porphyria. *British Medical Journal*, **291**, 499

Grover, W.D. and Scrutton, M.C. (1975) Copper infusion therapy in trichopoliodystrophy. *Journal of Pediatrics*, **86**, 216

Guthrie, R. and Susi, A. (1963) A simple phenylalanine method for detecting phenylketonuria in large populations of newborn infants. *Pediatrics*, **32**, 338

Harding, A.E. (1984) *The Hereditary Ataxias and Related Disorders*, Churchill Livingstone, Edinburgh

Hoefnagel, D., Andrew, E.D., Mireault, N.G. and Berndt. W.O. (1965) Hereditary choreoathetosis. self-mutilation and hyperuricaemia in young males. *New England Journal of Medicine*, **273**, 130

Hoogenraad, T.U., Van Den Hamer, C.J.A. and Van Hathum, J. (1984) Effective treatment of Wilson's disease with oral zinc sulphate: two case reports. *British Medical Journal*, **289**, 273

Houston, A.B., Brodie, M.J., Moore, M.R. *et al.* (1977) Hereditary coproporphyria and epilepsy. *Archives of Disease in Childhood*, **52**, 646

Hudson, F.A. and Clothier, C. (1975) Phenylalaninaemia. *Archives of Disease in Childhood*, **50**, 576

Huson, S.M. (1989) Recent developments in the diagnosis of neurofibromatosis. *Archives of Disease in Childhood*, **64**, 745

Kaufman, S. (1985) Hyperphenylalaninaemia caused by defects in biopterin metabolism. *Journal of Inherited Metabolic Disease*, **8**, Suppl. 1.,20

Kaufman, S., Kapatos, G., McInnes, R.R. *et al.* (1982) Use of terahydropterins in the treatment of hyperphenylalaninaemia due to defective synthesis of tetrahydrobiopterin. Evidence that tetrahydropterins peripherally administered enter the brain. *Paediatrics*, **70**, 376

Kocen, R.S., Lloyd, J.K., Lascelles, P.T., Fosbrooke, A.S. and Williams, D. (1967) Familial a-lipoprotein deficiency (Tangier disease) with neurological abnormalities. *Lancet*, **i**, 1341

Komrower, G.M. (1970) Screening methods relating to inborn errors of metabolism. In *Modern Trends in Pediatrics* (ed. J. Apley), Butterworth, London

Komrower, G.M. (1972) Community screening programmes for metabolic disorders. *Developmental Medicine and Child Neurology*, **14**, 397

Komrower, G.M. and Lee, D.H. (1970) Long-term follow-up of galactosaemia. *Archives of Disease in Childhood*, **45**, 367

Komrower, G.M. and Sardharwalla, I.B. (1978) Detection, diagnosis and management of inborn errors of metabolism. *Medicine*, 3rd Series, 79

Komrower, G.M., Schwarz, V., Holzel, A. and Golberg, L. (1956) A clinical and biochemical study of galactosaemia: a possible explanation of the biochemical lesion. *Archives of Disease in Childhood*, **31**, 254

Komrower, G.M., Lambert, A.M., Cusworth, D.C. and Westall, R.G. (1966) Dietary treatment of homocystinuria. *Archives of Disease in Childhood*, **11**, 666

Komrower, G.M., Sardharwalla, I.B., Coutts, J.M.J. and Ingham, D. (1979) Management of maternal phenylketonuria: an emergency clinical problem. *British Medical Journal*, **i**, 1383

Kreimer-Birnbaum, M. and Bannerman, R.M. (1975) Acute intermittent porphyria in childhood: a neglected diagnosis. *Archives of Disease in Childhood*, **50**, 494

Landrigan, P.J., Berenberg, W. and Bresnan, M. (1973) Behr's syndrome: familial optic atrophy, spastic diplegia and ataxia. *Developmental Medicine and Child Neurology*, **15**, 41

Legg, N.J. (1978) Oral choline in cerebellar ataxia. *British Medical Journal*, **ii**, 1403

Levin, B. and Russell, A. (1967) Treatment of hyperammonemia. *American Journal of Diseases of Children*, **113**, 142

Lygidakis, N.A. and Lindenbaum, R.H. (1987) Pitted enamel hypoplasia in tuberous sclerosis patients and first degree relatives. *Clinical Genetics*, **32**, 216-221

Macalpine, I., Hunter, R. and Rimington, C. (1968) Porphyria in the royal houses of Stuart, Hanover and Prussia. A follow-up study of George III's illness. *British Medical Journal*, **i**, 7

Maki, Y., Enomoto, T., Maruyama, H. and Maekawa, K. (1979) Computed tomography in tuberous sclerosis—with special reference to relation between clinical manifestation and C.T. findings. *Brain and Development*, **1**, 38

McColl, K.E.L., Thomson, G.T., Moore, M.R. and Goldberg, A. (1979) Haematin therapy and leucocyte aminolaevulinic-acid-synthase activity in prolonged attacks of acute porphyria. *Lancet*, **i**, 133

Menkes, J.H., Hurst, P.L. and Craig, J.M. (1954) A new syndrome: progressive familial infantile cerebral dysfunction associated with unusual urinary substance. *Pediatrics*, **14**, 462

Menkes, J.H. and Eviatar, L. (1969) Biochemical methods in the diagnosis of neurological disorders. In *Recent Advances in Neurology* (ed. F. Plum), Blackwell Scientific, Oxford

Menkes, J.H., Alter, M., Steigleder, G.K., Weakley, D.R. and Sung, J.H. (1962) A sex-linked recessive disorder with retardation of growth, peculiar hair, and focal cerebral and cerebellar degeneration. *Pediatrics*, **29**, 764

Milne, M.D. (1967) Hereditary abnormalities of intestinal absorption. *British Medical Bulletin*, **23**, 279

Mizuno, T. and Yugari, Y. (1974) Self-mutilation in Lesch-Nyhan syndrome. *Lancet*, **i**, 761

Muller, D.P.R., Lloyd, J.K. and Wolff, O.H. (1982) Vitamin E and neurological function. *Archives of Disease in Childhood*, **57**, 800

Niederwieser, A., Curtins, H.Ch., Bettoni, O.I. *et al.* (1979) Atypical phenylketonuria caused by 7, 8-dihydrobiopterin synthetase deficiency. *Lancet*, **i**, 131

Nordmann, Y., Schapira, F. and Dreyfus, J.C. (1969) A structurally modified liver aldolase in fructose intolerance: immunological and kinetic evidence. In *Enzymopenic Anaemias, Lysosomes and Other Papers* (ed. J.D. Allen, K.S. Holt, J.T. Ireland and R.J. Pollitt), Churchill Livingstone, Edinburgh

Nyhan, W.A., Ando, T. and Rasmussen, K. (1972) Ketotic hyperglycinaemia. In *Organic Acidurias* (ed. J. Stern, and C. Toothill), Churchill Livingstone, Edinburgh

Ouvrier, R. A. (1989) Giant axonal neuropathy—a review. *Brain and Development*, **11**, 207

Pampiglione, G. and Moynahan, E.J. (1976) Tuberous sclerosis syndrome: clinical and EEG studies in 100 children. *Journal of Neurology, Neurosurgery and Psychiatry*, **39**, 666

Partington, M.W. (1978) Long term studies of untreated phenylketonuria II: the plasma phenylalanine level. *Neuropädiatrie*, **9**, 255

Pierach, C.A. and Watson, C.J. (1978) Treatment of acute hepatic porphyria. *Lancet*, **i**, 1361

Pratt, R.T.C. (1967) *The Genetics of Neurological Disorders*, Oxford University Press, Oxford

Raine, D.N. (1975) *The Treatment of Inherited Metabolic Disease*, Medical and Technical Publishing, Lancaster

Riccaroli, V. M. (1987) Neurofibromatosis. In *Neurocutaneous Diseases* (ed. M.R. Gomez), Butterworth, Boston and London

Rosenberg, R.N. (1984) Molecular genetics; recombinant DNA techniques, and genetic neurological disease. *Annals of Neurology*, **15**, 511

Rosenberg, L.E., Lilljeqvist, A.C. and Hsia, Y.E. (1968) Methylmalonic aciduria: an inborn error leading to metabolic acidosis, long-chain ketonuria and intermittent hyperglycinemia. *New England Journal of Medicine*, **278**, 1319

Sadeh, M., Blatt, I., Martonovitz, G. and Karni, A. (1991) Treatment of porphyric convulsions with magnesium sulphate. *Epilepsia*, **32**, 712–715

Saudubray, J.M., Ogier, H., Charpontier, C. *et al.* (1984) Neonatal management of organic acidurias. Clinical update. *Journal of Inherited Metabolic Disease*, **7**, Suppl. 1., 2

Schwartz, J.F., Rowland, L.P., Eder, H. *et al.* (1963) Bassen-Kornzweig syndrome: deficiency of serum lipoprotein. A neuromuscular disorder resembling Friedreich's ataxia, associated with steatorrhea, acanthocytosis, retinitis pigmentosa. and a disorder of lipid metabolism. *Archives of Neurology*, **8**, 108

Scriver, C.R., Davies, E., Cullen, A.M. (1964) Application of a simple micro-method to the screening of plasma for a variety of aminoacidopathies. *Lancet*, **ii**, 230

Seegmiller, J.E., Rosenbloom, F.M. and Kelley, W.N. (1967) Enzyme defect associated with a sex-linked human neurological disorder and excessive purine synthesis. *Science*, **155**, 1682

Shaham, M., Voss, R., Becker, Y. *et al.* (1982) Prenatal diagnosis of ataxia telangiectasia. *Journal of Pediatrics*, **100**, 134

Silver, M.L. (1954) Hereditary vascular tumours of the nervous system. *Journal of the American Medical Association*, **156**, 1053

Sjögren, T. and Larsson. T. (1957) Oligophrenia in combination with congenital ichthyosis and spastic disorders. A clinical and genetic study. *Acta Psychiatrica Scandinavica*, Suppl. 113

Smith, I., Clayton, B.E. and Wolff, O.H. (1975) New variant of phenylketonuria with progressive neurological illness unresponsive to phenylalanine restriction. *Lancet*, **i**, 1108

Smith, I., Lobascher, M.E., Stevenson, J.E. *et al.* (1978) Effect of stopping low-phenylalanine diet on intellectual progress of children with phenylketonuria *British Medical Journal*, **ii**, 723

Smith, I., Macartny, F.J., Erdohazi, M. *et al.* (1979) Fetal damage despite low-phenylalanine diet after conception in phenylketonuric women. *Lancet*, **i**, 17

Spillane, J.D. (1940) Familial pes cavus and absent tendon-jerks: its relationship with Friedreich's disease and peroneal muscular atrophy. *Brain*, **63**, 275

Stumpf, D.A., Parks, J.K., Egusen, L.A. and Haas, R. (1982) Friedreich's ataxia III. Mitochondrial malic enzyme deficiency. *Neurology*, **32**, 221

Thompson, A.J., Smith, I., Brenton, D. *et al.* (1990) Neurological deterioration in young adults with phenylketonuria. *Lancet*, **336**, 602–605

Thoren, C. (1962) Diabetes mellitus in Friedreich's ataxia. *Acta Paediatrica Scandinavica*, **51**, Suppl. 135, 239

Uzman, L.L. (1957) Studies on the mechanism of copper deposition in Wilson's disease. *Archives of Neurology and Psychiatry*, **77**, 164

Waldmann, T.A. and McIntire, K.R. (1972) Serum alpha-fetoprotein levels in patients with ataxia telangiectasia. *Lancet*, **ii**, 1112

Walshe, J.M. (1967) The physiology of copper in man and its relation to Wilson's disease. *Brain*, **90**, 149

Walshe, J.M. (1973) Copper chelation in patients with Wilson's disease. *Quarterly Journal of Medicine*, **NS XLII**, 441

Watts, R.W.E., McKeran, R.O., Brown, E. *et al.* (1974) Clinical and biochemical studies on treatment of Lesch-Nyhan syndrome. *Archives of Disease in Childhood*, **49**, 693

Westall, R.G. (1967) Dietary treatment of maple sugar urine disease. *American Journal of Diseases of Children*, **113**, 58

Wheeler, E.M. and Roberts, P.F. (1976) Menkes' steely hair syndrome. *Archives of Disease in Childhood*, **51**, 269

Wilcken, B., Yu, J.S. and Bronn, D.A. (1977) Natural history of Hartnup's disease. *Archives of Disease in Childhood*, **52**, 38

Wilson, J., Linnell, J.C. and Matthews, D.M. (1971) Plasma-cobalamins in neuro-ophthalmological diseases. *Lancet*, **i**, 259

Wong, P.W.K. and Pillai, P.M. (1966) Clinical and biochemical observations in two cases of Hartnup's disease. *Archives of Disease in Childhood*, **41**, 383

Yoneda, M., Tsuji, S., Yamauchi, T. *et al.* (1989) Mitochondrial DNA mutation in family with Leber's hereditary optic atrophy. *Lancet*, **i**, 1076

4 Developmental abnormalities of the brain and spinal cord

Abnormalities at birth due to faults in the early growth and development of the body are many and varied, and can affect every system. Some of those which involve the nervous system, either directly or indirectly, will be considered in this chapter.

Babies born with malformed nervous systems are at considerable risk of dying in the early months of life. Many causes of death in early life are now preventable, but because so few causes of malformations are known, little progress has been made in reducing their incidence. Improvement in methods of prenatal identification, and the offer of abortion may hold out a hope of rectifying this situation.

Some of the known causes are considered in Chapter 5, as CNS malformations are often associated with mental retardation; obvious examples are chromosome abnormalities. There may be extra chromosomes, such as autosomal trisomies: D trisomy 13 (Patau's syndrome), E trisomy 16–18 (Edward's syndrome) and G trisomy 21 (Down's syndrome), are all characterized by severe and multiple disabilities. Deletions or additions of the sex chromosomes will also cause abnormalities, as in Turner's syndrome (XO) and Klinefelter's (XXY) syndrome.

Infections during pregnancy are a well recognized cause of physical and mental defects. Syphilis, rubella, cytomegalovirus disease and toxoplasmosis can all damage the developing fetus. There are also toxic causes, particularly the drugs taken by the mother during pregnancy; thalidomide and cytotoxic agents are classical examples.

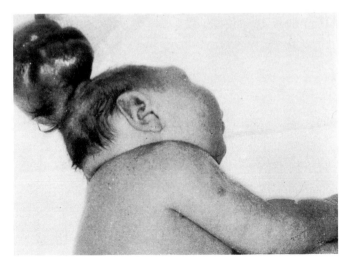

Figure 4.1 Anencephaly and meningoencephalocele.

Deficiency of folic acid may occur in mothers on anti-epileptic drugs, and folate deficiency is five times more common among mothers of malformed babies than among those with normal babies (Hibbard and Smithells, 1965).

Malnutrition, if severe, will affect the development of the fetal nervous system (Dobbing, 1970). Animal experiments have shown the effects of vitamin deficiency in causing conditions such as anencephaly and hydrocephalus, and it is suggested that hypovitaminosis A, caused by prediabetes or hypothyroidism, may be one of the prenatal causes of malformations in the human newborn (Hoet, Commas and Hoet, 1960). Malformations are frequently associated with hydramnios, with diseases such as maternal diabetes, and with cytopathic agents such as excessive irradiation. Various deformities, such as microcephaly, spina bifida, blindness, cleft palate and micromelia, have been associated with too frequent X-ray exposure during pregnancy.

The number of disorders due to one particular aetiology may often be quite small, and this may prevent the recognition of environmental causes: a nationwide register of these conditions would make this possible.

Abnormalities of cranial development

Anencephaly

Anencephaly results from failure of the anterior neural tube to close (Fig. 4.1). It affects females four times as frequently as males, and is the most common severe malformation found among stillbirths (Norman, 1971). There is a familial incidence, particularly among Celtic races, suggesting that genetic factors play a part in the aetiology. However, environmental influences must also be important, and account perhaps for findings such as the seasonal incidence. Whatever the cause, it must act very early in pregnancy, probably at about the third or fourth week. Hydramnios is often associated with this condition, and the diagnosis can then be confirmed by X-ray examination. Failure to palpate the head in utero may suggest anencephaly, and prenatal diagnosis is possible by finding a raised level of maternal plasma alpha-fetoprotein (Brock et al., 1974), and by ultrasound. If not stillborn, the baby will usually die within a few hours of birth. Genetic advice is obviously important, as the risk of another child being born with anencephaly or spina bifida can be as high as 1 in 20 (Smithells, 1963).

Hydranencephaly

In hydranencephaly the cerebral cortex is destroyed but the meninges remain intact. In the first few weeks of life the baby's appearance can be normal, and his or her behaviour may give rise to no particular concern. Soon after the neonatal period the development of the baby is noted to be retarded; the head may enlarge unduly rapidly (Fig. 4.2) and the baby becomes increasingly irritable. Evidence of spasticity appears, seizures may occur, and a swinging temperature due to poor temperature control is a very suggestive finding. Transillumination of the head confirms the diagnosis; the whole cranium will light up, only the vessels showing as dark lines over the surface of the enormously dilated ventricles (Fig. 4.3). The EEG is flat and featureless. The child may sometimes survive for several years.

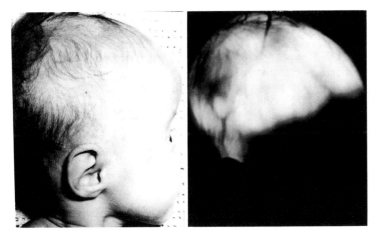

Figure 4.2   Child with hydranencephaly showing enlargement of head.

Figure 4.3   Transillumination of the head of the child in Figure 4.2.

It is suggested that the condition may be caused by a number of noxious agents acting towards the end of the second month of inter-uterine life. The most favoured theory is an obstruction of the internal carotid arteries and an infarction of the brain which is subsequently absorbed, but why this should occur is a mystery. In animals, hydranencephaly can be caused by virus infections (Osburn *et al.*, 1971).

Holoprosencephaly

This defect is due to failure of the primary cerebral vesicle to cleave and expand bilaterally, and it involves associated midline facial defects. There may be a single large ventricular cavity. The thalamus remains undivided, the inferior frontal and temporal regions are often absent, and the remainder of the cortex is rudimentary, with only the primary motor and sensory cortex present (Volpe, 1987). There are various other associated anomalies including microphalmia, and facial mal-formations. The latter may be very severe with a single median eye and small displaced nose; but they can be absent.

Usually the cause is unknown, but it can be associated with chromosomal anomalies, especially trisomy 13–15, and there can be a familial incidence with various forms of inheritance. If born alive, those babies severely affected do not survive for long. Those with lesser degrees of deformity will suffer from mental retardation and cerebral palsy. The diagnosis can be confirmed by ultrasound or CT scanning.

Lissencephaly, with few or any gyri, is another condition associated with gross anomalies and severe handicaps.

Porencephaly

Although in certain instances porencephalic cysts may have the same aetiology as hydranencephaly, it seems better to keep porencephalic cysts in a separate category as they are likely to be due to a number of different causes. Some will result from lack of development of the brain, and some from destruction of brain tissue, usually for unknown reasons. Occasionally these cysts can follow vascular lesions and repeated tapping of the lateral ventricles. The cysts may or may not communicate with the ventricles, and may communicate intermittently or by a valve-like mechanism.

The clinical findings will be diverse, depending on the extent and site of the lesion, and are in no way pathognomonic. The presence of porencephalic cysts is occasionally detected by transillumination of the skull in infancy; it is confirmed by CT scan or by MRI. These investigations will also help to identify other less obvious anomalies of the brain, such as pachygyria and micropolygyria, which may also be present.

Megalencephaly

Occasionally, abnormal enlargement of the head can be due to an excessive brain mass and not to hydrocephalus of any kind, and this can cause considerable diagnostic difficulties. This may occur in such diseases as Gm_2 gangliosidosis and Alexander's disease, and sometimes there is an association with conditions such as neurofibromatosis and tuberous sclerosis. However, there are a few children whose brains are enlarged for no obvious reason. There is often a delay in development and epilepsy, but the former is usually not severe (De Myer, 1972), and many of these children are not handicapped in any way. There is a familial incidence in probably more than 50% of cases, with a male to female ratio of 4 to 1 (Day and Schutt, 1979). The head circumference is large at birth, and in 80% of these children there is an above normal rate of head growth in the first 4 months after birth and in a further 12% in late infancy (Lorber and Priestly, 1981).

There may be a generalized overgrowth of all neural elements, with abnormal organization of both grey and white matter. Also additional anomalies are frequent. A CT scan will help to settle the diagnosis, and if there is any doubt about the role of hydrocephalus perfusion studies can be used, providing cerebrospinal fluid formation rates, volume of distribution and measurement of absorption at various pressures (Bresnan and Lorenzo, 1975).

Microcephaly

Microcephaly is defined as a head cicumference more than two standard deviations below the mean for age and sex (Fig. 4.4). Many of the causes of severe mental retardation are associated with a small head, both acquired and genetic. Rarely it can occur in families with an autosomal recessive mode of inheritance. Some children have relative microcephaly, a head proportionately small for length and weight. When examined during childhood they can have normal intelligence (Brennan, Funk and Frothingham, 1985).

Agenesis of the corpus callosum

The corpus callosum may be completely or partially absent, and this defect can be associated with a lipoma or cyst between the hemispheres. The corpus callosum develops between the 12th and 22nd week of gestation, and some unknown factor must operate during this time. It is seen in 13/15 (D) trisomy syndrome, and has been reported to be inherited as a sex-linked, recessive characteristic (Menkes, Phillipart and Clark, 1964). The possibility of maldevelopment of certain fibre tracts on a

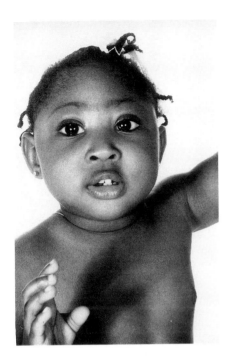

Figure 4.4   Child with microcephaly.

genetic basis raises interesting possibilities when considering the genetics of specific learning disorders.

The absence of the corpus callosum can be demonstrated by CT scanning, when the ventricles are seen to be widely separated and the third ventricle elevated. It is associated with a variety of symptoms and signs, such as epilepsy, mental retardation, hemiplegia, quadriplegia, disorders of language development, and hydrocephalus. The presence of these symptoms and especially of epilepsy seems to depend not so much on the absence of the corpus callosum as on associated cerebral anomalies.

Aicardi syndrome

This syndrome has only been reported in girls. It has been suggested that it may result from a mutation of a dominant gene on the X chromosome, and that this is lethal in the male (Dennis and Bower, 1972). The clinical features are infantile spasms and severe mental handicap. On examination there is usually a characteristic chorio-retinopathy, with lacunae which look like holes rather than deposits. There may be vertebral anomalies. The EEG shows the chaotic features of hypsarrhythmia, but these occur independently on the two sides, and CT scanning shows varying defects of the corpus callosum.

Hydrocephalus

Hydrocephalus in childhood (Fig. 4.5), apart from its association with spina bifida cystica, can result from overproduction of cerebrospinal fluid, obstruction to its flow, or interference with its absorption. It is also divided into communicating and non-

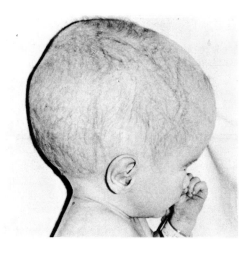

Figure 4.5 Hydrocephalus.

communicating hydrocephalus, depending on whether the fluid is able to leave the fourth ventricle and reach the subarachnoid spaces.

Overproduction of cerebrospinal fluid occurs from the presence of a choroid plexus papilloma, and is the probable cause of some instances of acute hydrocephalus seen in meningeal infections, lead encephalopathy and occasionally complicating steroid therapy. It may also occur during other infections, for example those of the upper respiratory tract, and this may upset a previously stable situation of arrested hydrocephalus. Apart from such rare lesions there is a possibility that this mechanism may play some part in causing the hydrocephalus complicating spina bifida cystica (Drummond and Donaldson, 1974).

Defective absorption of the cerebrospinal fluid will result from such causes as obstruction within the arachnoid villi, and possibly due to interference with lymphatic drainage. Pressure will then be high within the subarachnoid space as well as within the ventricles, and therefore the latter will be small. Obstruction of the vessels within the villi can occur after meningitis and subarachnoid haemorrhage, and may be the cause of the raised intracranial pressure that occasionally complicates the Guillain-Barré syndrome. It has been suggested that the high protein level in the fluid leads to its precipitation within the villi (Morley and Reynolds, 1966). Venous sinus obstruction may occur in association with middle-ear infection (otitic hydrocephalus), dehydration and hypercoagulable states, but in order to cause hydrocephalus it may be that the thrombosis must spread beyond the sagittal sinus, as this cause has not been proven by experimental studies. Such obstruction may also occur after head injuries, and even spontaneously to account for some instances of benign intracranial hypertension. Apart from these rare disorders, hydrocephalus results from obstruction to the pathways of cerebrospinal fluid flow at the points of narrowing. These are sites within the aqueduct, at the roof of the fourth ventricle, around the tentorial opening, and within the basal cisterns.

The symptoms and signs will vary according to the age of the patient and the severity of the block. Excessive enlargement of the head may be almost imperceptible. Unless hydrocephalus is suspected and careful measurements taken, and plotted on standard occipito-frontal circumference growth charts, the diagnosis may be missed. When the pressure rises more rapidly in infancy the baby will become irritable with a high-pitched cry and may start to vomit. In addition to enlargement of the head the fontanelle will bulge, the scalp veins will dilate, and the sutures will separate. The latter can often be felt on palpation of the head. Tapping the skull with the head unsupported sometimes elicits a 'cracked-pot' sound, but this tends to be an unreliable finding. In the absence of treatment the forehead will become unduly prominent and the eyes will be displaced downwards, leading to the setting-sun sign (Fig. 1.4), in which the lower lid covers part of the iris and the sclera is visible around the upper rim. In the older child enlargement of the head may not be so obvious, but signs of intracranial pressure will tend to dominate the clinical picture. Papilloedema will occur more readily, and this can be followed by optic atrophy and rapid visual failure. Nystagmus is often an early sign of failing vision in young children. At any age a progressive hydrocephalus may lead to spasticity and ataxia. From time to time the hydrocephalus will become arrested, and this often seems to occur when the obstruction is at the level of the aqueduct. Such a block is most likely to compress the structures, particularly the cerebellum, within the posterior fossa, with resulting ataxia. Arrested hydrocephalus may be associated with the hypotonic and the ataxic forms of cerebral palsy. Also it can cause clumsiness resulting in difficulties in learning motor skills (Lonton, 1979). However the term 'arrested' may not be acceptable only on the basis of regular measurements of the head circumference. It is important to assess the state of the ventricular system to make sure that this is not gradually enlarging, and this can now be done by serial scans (computerized axial tomography). Also, the term 'normal pressure hydrocephalus' is no longer acceptable, as in these cases the pressure may be normal for long periods, but continuous monitoring can show episodic fluctuations. In many instances the abnormalities are due to defects of cerebrospinal fluid absorption (Lorenzo, Bresnan and Barlow, 1974). The slow ventricular dilatation can be associated with dementia and other neurological abnormalities including ataxia and incontinence, and sometimes improvement results from shunting operations (Gordon, 1977).

The appearance of the child will usually suggest the diagnosis, but bilateral subdural haematomata will have to be excluded (particularly in the older infant), as well as the possibility that the hydrocephalus is caused by a cerebral tumour, especially a medulloblastoma in the posterior fossa. Plain X-rays of the skull may show bone thinning, with craniolacunae, separation of the sutures with irregular margins, and increased convolutional markings. The latter finding does not necessarily indicate raised intracranial pressure. Intracranial calcification suggests the possibility of toxoplasmosis or cytomegalovirus infection which can cause obstruction to the cerebrospinal fluid flow.

Computerized axial tomography has revolutionized the management of hydrocephalus. Particularly in infancy it will help to differentiate between hydro-cephalus and subdural haematoma and may preclude the need for subdural taps. It will also identify megalencephaly as the cause of the enlarging head (Ellison, 1978). More recently, ultrasound sector scanning has been shown to have certain advantages in the diagnosis of hydrocephalus in infancy (Strassburg, Weber and Sauer, 1981). The rare possibility of a subarachnoid haemorrhage or infection may justify examination of the cerebrospinal fluid.

If additional information is required, or computerized axial tomography is not available, and an abnormal increase of head size indicates progressive hydrocephalus the neurosurgeon's first procedure is likely to be ventriculography, often with a contrast medium such as 'Myodil', to establish the site of the cerebrospinal fluid block. Intracranial pressure monitoring can help in management, not only in the initial assessment and in deciding on the type of valve needed, but in the follow up after operation when questions of lengthening the shunt, removing it, or checking for blockage arise (Minns, 1977). Radioisotopic examination will sometimes allow investigation of the hydrodynamics of cerebrospinal fluid flow over a period of 24 hours, which can be useful in outlining pooling and rate of absorption.

Stenosis of the aqueduct of Sylvius

Malformations of the aqueduct of Sylvius may be associated with the Arnold-Chiari malformation and spina bifida cystica, and may also be caused by a block to cerebrospinal fluid flow at a more caudal level. The hydrocephalus causes downward migration and flattening of the tentorium with lateral and vertical squeezing of the midbrain (Williams, 1971). Thus the aqueduct is kinked and compressed (Shellshear and Emery, 1975), and a secondary cause of obstruction is therefore added. A number of small ventral channels usually end blindly, whilst a large dorsal one connects the third and fourth ventricles. The ependyma is unaffected. Occasionally the block is due to over-growth of the subependymal glia, and it is then difficult to be sure if this is due to true neoplasia. Some cases are due to single gene defects which show sex-linked recessive inheritance, and then the primary defect may be a communicating hydrocephalus leading usually to aqueduct stenosis (Landrieu et al., 1979). Post-meningitic adhesions can also obstruct the flow of cerebrospinal fluid through the aqueduct, and the aqueduct can be kinked and not malformed; and the interference to the flow of cerebrospinal fluid can be intermittent.

The hydrocephalus, due to obstruction of the aqueduct, can be very slowly progressive or may arrest spontaneously. The diagnosis can be suggested by the presence of a shallow posterior fossa on the lateral X-ray film of the skull. Ataxia and dyskinesia are often the presenting symptoms in older children.

Atresia of the foramina of Magendie and Luschka

Blockage of these foramina prevents the cerebrospinal fluid gaining entry into the basal cisterns. The Dandy-Walker syndrome is often associated with this finding; and this malformation may be due to pre-natal atresia of the foramina, resulting in gross dilatation of the fourth ventricle and a small cerebellum. However, there are doubts about this always being the case. It can be genetically determined and shows recessive inheritance. Gardner (1965) has suggested that such a block sets in train processes which result in syringomyelia and spina bifida cystica with associated hydrocephalus. The foramina can also be obstructed by adhesions resulting from meningitis or haemorrhage and the most common cause of intracranial haemorrhage in infancy is birth injury. Lorber and Bhat (1974) have emphasized that the prognosis can be improved by early diagnosis and treatment. The cerebellum is likely to be atrophied, especially the vermis, and a prominent occiput is a characteristic finding. Apart from dilatation of the fourth ventricle the Dandy-Walker malformation is a term used to include isolated cysts of the posterior fossa.

Arnold-Chiari malformation

It is convenient to consider the Arnold-Chiari malformation in this section even though it does not always cause hydrocephalus. It is a defect of the hindbrain, with kinking of the medulla oblongata (Chiari malformation), and of the cerebellum, with a tongue of cerebellar tissue protruding through the foramen magnum (Arnold malformation). The surrounding meninges are often congested and become thickened in time. It complicates nearly all cases of myelomeningocele, but only occasionally occurs on its own. There is a close association with other CNS deformities, particularly aqueduct stenosis, and also with anomalies of the vertebrae and ribs. It used to be thought that this deformity was caused by traction from below, when the lower end of the spinal cord was fixed and could not retract upwards with growth. This theory is no longer in favour, and a more likely explanation seems to be pressure from above, e.g. from smallness of the posterior fossa resulting from a low tentorium due to the presence of a hydrocephalic forebrain in fetal life (Gardner, 1977), or overgrowth of the tissues of the hindbrain (Barry, Patton and Stewart, 1957), or from overproduction of cerebrospinal fluid (Caviness, 1976), or obstruction of the foramina in the roof of the fourth ventricle forcing the cerebellar contents through the foramen magnum, although pressure differentials are probably not the only explanation and there may well be teratogenic influences (Williams, 1977a). A spina bifida cystica may initially lower the spinal pressure before removal, when it will rise. However, a partial obstruction at the foramen magnum can allow fluid to flow upwards more easily than downwards due to a valvular mechanism and the effect of coughing and straining; and then the hydrocephalus will progress. Similar mechanisms may account for some instances of aqueduct stenosis (Williams, 1975). When occurring in isolation, the malformation can present with the symptoms and signs of cerebellar and upper cervical cord compression.

The tentorial opening

Obstruction can also occur at this level, e.g. after meningitis or haemorrhage, and cause a form of communicating hydrocephalus.

Treatment of hydrocephalus

Once the site of the block has been established, treatment will be directed towards producing a by-pass. In rare instances, and usually only as a temporary measure, isosorbide can be given in a dose of 2g/kg four times a day (Lorber, 1975). The main indications for this treatment are uncomplicated infantile hydrocephalus with a cerebral mantle of 20 mm or more, and in those infants with spina bifida whose cerebral mantle is between 15 and 25 mm, especially if the treatment is started within a few days of the closure of the spinal lesion. Careful biochemical monitoring will be needed to prevent complications such as hypernatraemic dehydration and diarrhoea. Repeated lumbar punctures can sometimes be effective in the transient post-haemorrhagic hydrocephalus in premature infants

In the case of aqueduct stenosis, the Torkildsen operation will drain the cerebrospinal fluid from the lateral ventricles via a tube under the scalp to the basal cisterns. When the block is distal to the aqueduct, and the basal cisterns cannot be used, the cerebrospinal fluid has to be drained into the vascular system or into another body cavity. In young infants the Spitz-Holter or the Pudenz-Heyer valve is used, first of all on the right side. The proximal catheter is inserted into a lateral ventricle through a burr-hole. The valve is secured below the pericranium at a site above and behind the ear to avoid trauma to the skin when the child lies on that side of the head. The distal 'Silastic' catheter is threaded subcutaneously through the external jugular vein into the right auricle, or into the peritoneum. Early operation should be considered whenever there is evidence of raised intracranial pressure, whatever the thickness of the cerebral mantle, so as to avoid gross head enlargement.

Although complications are common they should never detract from the very real value these procedures have in reducing mortality and morbidity. Both the proximal and the distal catheters can become partially or completely obstructed; this can be detected by finding that the valve fails to empty on firm pressure, empties slowly, or takes a long time to refill. Sudden blockage may result in a rapid rise of intracranial pressure, with drowsiness and vomiting, and sometimes the sudden onset of blindness (Keen, 1973). Blockage must always be regarded as an emergency requiring external drainage and other measures to reduce the pressure. The hydrocephalus can remain arrested despite a non-functioning valve, and revision is only indicated if there are signs of raised intracranial pressure. The tubing occasionally separates from the valve. Fracturing of the catheters has not been a problem since the introduction of 'Silastic' tubing.

Infection of the drainage system is a serious hazard and can be associated with meningitis, ventriculitis and septicaemia. Failure to thrive should always raise a suspicion of a shunt infection. A variety of organisms can be found, but often it is caused by staphylococcus epidermidis (albus). Injection of antibiotics into the valve has been used but usually the valve has to be removed, the infection treated, including the use of intraventricular antibiotics such as gentamycin and cloxacillin, and a new valve subsequently inserted. Under these circumstances it is not uncommon to find an endocarditis which can cause multiple embolization and pyaemic abscesses which make vigorous treatment with appropriate antibiotics essential. A high cerebrospinal fluid protein may result in recurrent blockage of the drainage system, and is one of the occasions when repeated ventricular taps are necessary to control the hydrocephalus until a new valve can be inserted.

Occasionally, cerebrospinal fluid will leak around the valve and produce a cystic swelling, making replacement of the drainage system necessary. It is also important to prevent too rapid drainage of cerebrospinal fluid and collapse of the brain, as this can result in rupture of the bridging vessels and the production of subdural haematoma. Upward 'coning' of the brain-stem may occur, with pallor, sweating, and cardiac arrhythmias or respiratory arrest. Milder manifestations are fairly common and often transient. They respond to nursing head down with ample fluid intake.

If the intracranial pressure is very high at the time the diagnosis is made, these procedures may have to be postponed while this is reduced by tapping the ventricles, preferably by continuous external drainage with a hydrostatic 'blow-off' pressure of 80–100 mm of cerebrospinal fluid.

Meningoencephaloceles

When the neural tube fails to close at the cranial end, the meninges may bulge through a defect in the back of the skull or in the cervical spine, and may contain neural tissue (Fig. 4.6). Very occasionally the defect is in the roof of the nose or in the wall of the orbit.

Associated neurological abnormalities include epilepsy, mental defect and cerebral palsy, and damage to the occipital lobes can result in central blindness.

Transillumination will identify any solid tissue within the sac, and X-ray of the skull shows a bony defect. Early operation is indicated in view of the possible rupture of the sac and to inspect associated cerebral abnormalities. In the case of cranial meningoceles the results are likely to be satisfactory. If a large encephalocele is present it is a

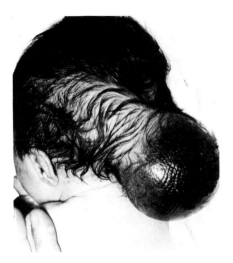

Figure 4.6   Cranial meningoencephalocele.

different story, as the cerebral tissue cannot be replaced within the skull and has to be removed. Death may occur from hydrocephalus or meningitis, and, if the child survives, mental retardation is common.

Abnormalities of spinal canal development

Spina bifida cystica

The anomaly can vary from a spina bifida occulta to a complete absence of the vertebral arches and protrusion of the meninges and neural tissues.

Spina bifida occulta

This is a common finding on routine X-ray of the spine, and its relationship to severer anomalies is obscure. Occasionally there are associated abnormalities such as a tuft of hair (Fig. 4.7), a naevus, or a lipoma (Fig. 4.8) overlying the defect. There is also the possibility of an underlying deformity affecting the spinal cord, such as the bands and spurs found in diastematomyelia. Neurological symptoms or signs, if marked or progressive, indicate the need for further investigations, including CT and myelography. Indications for laminectomy include progressive foot deformities, incontinence, myelographic evidence of abnormality, or a low situation of the conus medullaris (James and Lassman, 1972).

Meningocele

The term meningocele is used for cases in which a cystic swelling occurs along the spinal axis, most often over the lumbar or sacral region. It is usually covered by skin, although this may be thin, and the sac has a blue appearance. Nervous tissue is not involved unless damaged, for instance by infection.

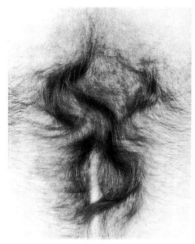

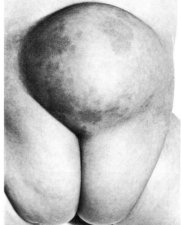

Figure 4.7   Hairy patch and spina bifida.   **Figure 4.8**   Lipoma and spina bifida.

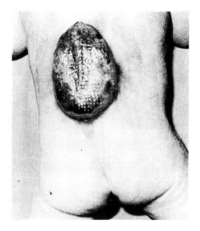

Figure 4.9   Meningomyelocele.

Meningomyelocele

In this form of spinal dysraphism there is always an associated abnormality of the spinal cord. It is most frequently seen in the lumbar region, but also occurs in the cervical and thoracic spine (Fig. 4.9). The appearance varies greatly from one case to the next. The lesion often consists of a slightly raised but flat ridge of tissue representing the neural plate; this may be open or enveloped with a thin, transparent membrane which at times contains blood vessels. There is often a lipomatous mass, and tufts of hair may be seen on the surrounding skin.

More rarely, the lesion is partially or completely covered with skin. Palpation and transillumination may reveal the nerve roots and blood vessels within the sac, and this helps to differentiate it from the uncomplicated meningocele. Abnormalities of the underlying vertebral bodies are easily felt. The covering membrane breaks easily, thus allowing the cerebrospinal fluid to leak out and infection to gain access to the spinal canal.

The lesions are commonly multiple, and the most obvious cutaneous lesion may not reflect the most serious spinal abnormality. The whole skull and spine should be X-rayed in the assessment of any case. Hemivertebrae and fused or absent ribs are often detected.

Neurological findings

The level of the spinal lesion is indicated by the neurological findings, and it is of obvious importance to establish this before decisions are taken on treatment and management. Stark and Baker (1967) have described the different clinical pictures that may be found. There may be complete loss of function below a certain segmental level; a gap in cord function with flaccid paralysis extending over many segments and isolated cord function distally; a gap so narrow that the findings are those of complete cord transection; and incomplete transection so the child has spastic paraplegia with some voluntary movement. Occasionally, only half of a split cord is involved in the meningomyelocele.

If there is a complete flaccid paralysis below the L4 segment the action of the tibialis anterior will be unopposed by the peronei and there will be marked inversion of the feet. When a gap in cord function exists there may be a flaccid paraplegia below T12, except for spasticity and reflex activity in the peronei and extensor hallucis longus innervated from L5, Sl; and the feet will be everted.

When one or both lower limbs are normal or show only a mild pyramidal lesion the children usually have efficient bladder emptying. Most of those with some voluntary function in S2 to S4 segments on at least one side have an active detrusor, but an ideal automatic reflex bladder is rare. If there is neither voluntary movement nor reflex activity below S1 there is rarely any detrusor activity (Stark, 1971).

The neurological signs are incompatible with the suggestion that the paraplegia is due to a lower motor neurone lesion caused by a failure of cord development, but nerve roots are often damaged. Lendon (1969) has shown that in the absence of secondary damage, the neurone count of the affected cord may be normal. The paraplegia may be due to trauma, resulting from pressure on the neural plate where it joins the normal cord from the upper edge of the bony deformity during or shortly after birth, and in most instances there is probably a combination of upper and lower motor lesions.

Associated problems

Hydrocephalus

It has already been emphasized that meningomyeloceles are frequently associated with hydrocephalus. The head may be large at birth, but it is more usual for the hydrocephalus to be confined to ventricular dilation at this stage and for the skull enlargement to become obvious some days or weeks after birth. This may be due in part to the effects of intra-uterine pressure. Palpation of the head reveals the craniolacunae and the irregular margins of the sutures.

The hydrocephalus has usually been attributed to the Arnold-Chiari malformations and aqueduct stenosis, but this may not be the entire explanation. Later on, infection

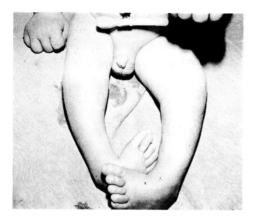

Figure 4.10   Talipes equinovarus with spina bifida.

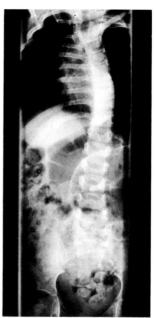

Figure 4.11   Scoliosis with cervical spina bifida.

may play a part in adding to the obstruction of the cerebrospinal fluid flow, as well as overproduction of cerebrospinal fluid (Drummond and Donaldson, 1974).

The presence of some degree of hydrocephalus in most children with spina bifida is undoubtedly the reason for the high incidence of perceptuo-motor disabilities affecting arm and hand movements, and of other learning difficulties.

The skeletal system

Many children with meningomyeloceles have obvious skeletal deformities at birth. Talipes equinovarus (Fig. 4.10) is the most common and needs early correction. Dislocated hips should be tested for early, and appropriate orthopaedic management commenced. The spine can show kyphosis, scoliosis (Fig. 4.11), or even gibbus formation at an early age; and deformities of the cervical vertebrae producing a short neck are occasionally seen.

Many skeletal deformities, such as hip and knee contractures, as well as a variety of foot deformities, are due to unopposed muscular activity of normally innervated or spastic muscle against a weak or completely flaccid antagonist.

The renal tract

Malformations of the renal tract occur in about 20% of children with spina bifida cystica. When the hydrocephalus has been controlled then problems related to renal and bladder function pose the greatest threat to survival and health. It follows that a careful assessment of bladder function should be carried out by three months of age in all treated cases of spina bifida. Cystometrograms, intravenous pyelograms and micturating cystometrograms delineate patterns of bladder function; and regular urine culture identifies infection. Much renal damage by hydronephrosis and risk of pyelonephritis with septicaemia can be anticipated and avoided.

Incidence and aetiology of spina bifida cystica

The incidence of spina bifida cystica varies widely, ranging in the UK from one in 250 births in South Wales to one in 500 births in East Anglia. There is a pronounced excess of affected females (Carter, 1974). Seasonal variations have also been noted, with an increase due to conceptions in the winter months. The malformation is determined by the fourth week of gestation and is most probably due to an interaction of genetic and environmental factors; for example hyperthermia during pregnancy has come under suspicion. The possibility of prevention of neural tube defects by periconceptional vitamin supplementation is recommended (Smithells et al., 1980, 1981, 1983), or the giving of folic acid supplements to mothers who have had an affected fetus (Laurence et al., 1981). The latter policy has been supported by a recent study by the Medical Research Council (1991). If one baby in a family has been born with this deformity, there is a 1 in 20 risk of other babies being similarly affected, and after two such babies have been born, the risk rises to one in six (Carter and Roberts, 1967). It has been suggested that residual trophoblastic material, either from a previous miscarriage or a co-twin, may interact unfavourably with another fetus to produce spina bifida and anencephaly (Clarke et al., 1975). A possible clinical application of this theory is the advisability of dilatation and curettage after miscarriage and infertility (Field and Kerr, 1976). Others have claimed that miscarriages are another manifestation of an underlying disorder rather than a cause of anencephaly and spina bifida (Laurence and Roberts, 1977). It is possible that these dysraphic states are in some cases anyhow the result of distension of the central canal resulting from blockage of the cerebrospinal fluid pathways in the posterior fossa (Gardner, 1977), a mechanism which will be considered in the aetiology of syringomyelia. It is evident that spina bifida can develop as the result of reopening of the neural tube, but under other circumstances the neural tube may fail to close. The incidence of this condition is undoubtedly declining, due to such factors as improved maternal nutrition, prenatal diagnosis for high risk pregnancies, maternal alpha-protein screening, and ultrasound screening of pregnancies and selective termination (Laurence, 1989). Also the incidence may have been dropping due to unknown non-medical reasons, so that there is a possibility that it may rise again in spite of the above measures; which is an excuse for considering the condition in such detail.

Prenatal diagnosis

Many of the present management difficulties would be resolved by diagnosis in early pregnancy and abortion. So far this is rarely possible for a first case in a family, but estimation of the amniotic fluid alpha-fetoprotein ensures that such early diagnosis is increasingly possible (Allan et al., 1973). The detection rate for cases of anencephaly and open spina bifida is more than 90% (Weld and Cuckle, 1979). Such an investigation is justifiable if a child with spina bifida cystica has already been born into a family, but obviously cannot be used as a screening test in all pregnancies. So far the estimation of maternal plasma alpha-fetoprotein has only proved sufficiently reliable to identify some affected fetuses, but methods may well be improved (Ferguson-Smith et al., 1978). It may be reasonable to restrict amniocentesis to the 2% of singleton pregnancies with the highest maternal serum alpha-fetoprotein.

New techniques, such as the use of high resolution diagnostic ultrasound, combined with measurements of alpha-fetoprotein in maternal serum (Persson *et al.*, 1983), will increase the accuracy of the prenatal screening for neural tube defects, which will be of greater importance as the prevalence of the defects falls. Other examples are the morphology of rapidly adhering amniotic fluid cells (Gosden and Brock, 1977), the proportion of amniotic alphafetoprotein that binds with conanavallin A (Smith *et al.*, 1979), and the use of qualitative electrophoresis of acetylcholinesterase in amniotic fluid combined with amniotic alpha-fetoprotein estimations, which yields more information than either test used alone (Harris and Read, 1981). Macrophage counts of the amniotic fluid can help in the presence of equivocal findings, although false positive results can occur (Sutherland, 1975). Direct visualization of the fetus by fetoscopy may be used in certain cases in spite of the risks involved (Harris, 1980).

Management

The policy of operating on all babies with spina bifida cystica as soon after birth as possible is, in the author's opinion, largely unacceptable, now that the degree of suffering this policy imposes on some children and their families is appreciated. It has been shown that by establishing careful criteria of selection the quality of life for the survivors is greatly improved (Lorber, 1971, 1972; Keys Smith and Durham Smith, 1973). The contra-indications to active treatment are gross paralysis of the legs with no innervation below L3, lesions extending above the fourth lumbar vertebra, severe kyphosis and scoliosis, grossly enlarged head with a maximal circumference of 2 cm or more above the 90th percentile for birth weight, intracerebral birth injury, and other gross congenital defects (Lorber, 1973). After closure in the newborn period, the occurrence of meningitis or ventriculitis in a baby who already has a severe handicap is also a contra-indication to active treatment. Social factors, such as rejection by the parents and single parent families, must also be considered.

Those babies who are not operated upon should, in the author's opinion, be given normal nursing care and be fed on demand. Apart from this, treatment is confined to analgesics; oxygen, tube feeding, antibiotics and resuscitation are not given. In Lorber's (1973) follow-up study all 25 untreated infants died within nine months. If the baby does survive in good condition for over six months, necessary treatment for hydrocephalus and renal and orthopaedic complications can then be reconsidered.

In forming a judgement on selection one is bound to be influenced by the quality of life of the survivors. Exactly what these children and their families may have to endure has been well shown in studies by social workers (Freeston, 1971; Walker, Thomas and Russell, 1971; Woodburn, 1973). The need for parental support cannot be over-stressed, and much thought needs to be given to how they are best helped. All must be given time to explore their own reactions to their handicapped child and the situation that is created for the family. Feelings of guilt need discussion, and genetic advice should be given. It is important to arrange educational placement early, and many children are ready to participate in a nursery school setting soon after 2 years of age.

Surgical treatment

If it is decided that the baby is to have an operation, this should be done as soon as possible to prevent infection ascending the spinal canal and producing meningitis and ventriculitis. There are a variety of procedures involving mobilization and rotation of skin flaps depending on the size and site of the defect. When this is large, lateral relieving incisions can be made in the loins which will prevent sloughing at the suture line and will themselves rapidly epithelialize. A close watch will have to be kept for developing hydrocephalus, and the necessary tests and treatment must be carried out.

Treatment of associated problems

Careful splinting can help weak or deformed legs, but should not impair mobility or increase discomfort. When the paraplegia is severe, a 'clicking' brace with firm platforms under the shoes allows these children to assume the erect posture and attain some slight mobility. Teaching and training in ambulation are of the utmost importance.

Urinary incontinence is a major social disadvantage which calls for great ingenuity in management. Penile urinals can be used for boys, but even with care they can leak. No satisfactory collecting urinal is available for girls, and repeated catheterization may be contra-indicated because of the considerable risk of introducing infection. Indwelling 'Silastic' catheters obviate the need for many diversions (Rickwood and Zachery, 1977), and in view of the fact that a significant number of children ultimately become continent of urine early urinary diversion, even in the presence of a neurological deficit, is not indicated for incontinence alone, but only if there is a progressive deterioration of renal function (Brereton, Zachary and Lister, 1977). Among older children who remain incontinent, ileo-cutaneous ureterostomies with suitable collecting bags have resulted in a major transformation. As soon as urinary obstruction is identified this must be relieved by appropriate treatment. When spastic sphincters with poor detrusor activity or high emptying pressures are found, pudendal neurectomy or sphincterotomy can convert the distended bladder with overflow to a continuously emptying bladder. Ureterostomies may be needed if the ureters are very dilated, and ileal diversions considered when the ureters are more normal but the bladder muscle is ineffective. In a recent review of the management of the neuropathic bladder it is suggested that clean intermittent catheterization and drug therapy (e.g. propanthaline or ephedrine) should be the treatment of choice (Borzyskowski, 1984). An up to date review of treatment, including the management of the neuropathic bladder, has been given by Minns (1986) and a review of surgical management by Guthkelch (1986).

A patulous anus often results in repeated faecal incontinence and its attendant social problems. Faecal retention and impaction can also cause difficulties. The latter need judicious management with mild aperients, suppositories and an occasional enema. Where some anal sphincter tone is present and rectal sensation is absent, some conscious effort towards bowel emptying is necessary, and training must be directed towards that end.

Sensory deficits are widespread in these children; trophic ulceration occurs easily, either by self-injury when playing, by ill-fitting shoes or appliances, or from burns from hot-water bottles. Circulatory disturbances are common, and the lower extremities are often very cold, despite being plethoric. The use of sheepskin rugs and woollen socks can be used in prevention and treatment of vascular lesions. Counselling of adolescents and their families on sexual functions will be needed (Comarr, 1977).

Dermal sinuses and dermoids

Dermal sinuses can occur at any level, but are most often seen in the lumbo-sacral and occipital regions. When the sinus grows hair it is often referred to as a 'pilonidal sinus'. Occasionally they are associated with dermoids and lipoma. If the sinus communicates with the subarachnoid space there is a grave risk of infection spreading inwards and causing meningitis. They should therefore be removed along with any associated dermoid.

Syringomyelia

This condition is characteristically a disease of early adult life, although the onset of symptoms and signs can occur during the second decade. The characteristic clinical findings are well known, with dissociated sensory loss affecting the upper limbs, wasting of the hand muscles, and long tract signs. In childhood, kyphoscoliosis is prominent and often rapidly progressive, and a flaccid or spastic paraplegia an early symptom. The pathogenesis has not yet been fully elicited, and it is unlikely that this will be the same in all cases. Gardner (1965) believed that the primary lesion was a block to cerebrospinal fluid flow resulting from a failure of permeation of the roof of the fourth ventricle, or other interference with the cerebrospinal fluid pathways around the foramen magnum causing diversion of the fluid down the central canal of the cord. This would result in hydromyelia, and when the ependyma ruptured, syringomyelia. Williams (1977b) doubts that syringomyelia is due to downward pulsation or hydrostatic pressure. Two valve-like mechanisms may play a part in the enlargement of the cavity. If the foramen magnum is obstructed from above, as in the Arnold-Chiari malformation, by adhesions following infections or haemorrhage in the newborn, or by occipital moulding and descent of the cerebellar tonsil through the foramen magnum resulting from difficult labour, the cerebrospinal fluid in the subarachnoid space can more easily enter the cranium than it can leave it. It may therefore be diverted into the central canal and any cavities that communicate with it. At the junction of the syrinx and the central canal the tissues may also form a valve which can interfere with the exit and entry of fluid (Williams, 1972). If there is no communication between the syrinx and the ventricular system presumably the condition cannot be explained by a hydrodynamic theory. In these cases the frequent association with spinal cord tumours suggests a faulty development of embryonic spongioblasts transforming either to gliosis with subsequent disruption of tissue, or to neoplasia (Eggers and Hamer, 1979). Another possibility is that cavitation of the cord results from ischaemia, particularly at the interface between areas of the cord supplied by the anterior and posterior syrinx arteries (Sherk et al., 1984).

X-ray examination of the skull may show evidence of basilar impression, enlargement of the posterior fossa and of the foramen magnum, a Klippel-Feil deformity of the cervical spine and widening of the intraspinal canal. Myelography does not invariably show enlargement of the cord as the cyst can remain collapsed during the examination. Supine myelography is essential to demonstrate the abnormalities at the level of the cisterna magna resulting from the Arnold-Chiari malformation. Air myelography can confirm an obstruction at the foramen magnum and sometimes narrowing of the upper part of the cervical cord. Techniques have been developed for punctures of the cyst and for delineating its extent by myelocystography (Williams, 1970). Magnetic resonance imaging, when generally available, may well be the investigation of the future.

The pathogenesis of syringomyelia is still the subject of a great deal of conjecture, but the ideas have stimulated the development of more effective treatment for the condition. For example, an artificial cisterna magna is formed and the obstruction to the flow of cerebrospinal fluid through the foramen magnum is removed. Where the presence of arachnoiditis makes this procedure impossible, by-pass operations, or posterior fossa decompression, may be tried. In the case of non-communicating hydromyelia a decompressive laminectomy with hydromyelostomy is indicated. More recently the insertion of shunts has been developed (Suzuki *et al.*, 1985).

Diastematomyelia

The division of the spinal cord into two can also result from hydromyelia (Gardner, 1977) and nothing can be done as far as the anomaly itself is concerned. Bone, cartilage or fibrous tissue may pass between the two parts of the cord and produce two vertebral canals (James and Lassman, 1972). It used to be thought that this prevented the differential growth between the spinal cord and vertebral column and caused progressive symptoms and signs as the child grew older, but this explanation can no longer be accepted as the process is almost complete by a few months of age. Guthkelch (1974) suggests that deterioration may occur from mild trauma and traction at the level of the spur during repeated head and neck flexion in the growing child, and he recommends early operation, except when there is an associated myelocele. It must be stressed to the family that the progressive signs will respond to surgery but not those associated with the neuronal and mesodermal hypoplasia which have been prenatally determined. These usually consist of deformity and dwarfing of one leg below the knee. Overlying the anomaly may be a tuft of hair, a dimple or a naevus. X-rays of the spine usually confirm the diagnosis, and myelography outlines the extent of the lesion (Fig. 4.12). If the septum and bands are removed there is every chance of preventing further progression of any motor and sensory or sphincter disturbances that may be present.

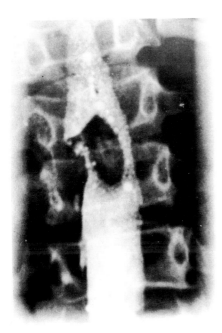

Figure 4.12   Diastematomyelia: a myelogram outlining a filling defect caused by a bony spur.

Klippel-Feil syndrome

This syndrome consists of fusion of one or more cervical vertebrae, a reduction in the number of the vertebrae (some remaining as hemivertebrae), and fusion and deformities of the ribs. As a result, the neck is short and there is a low hair-line; movements of the neck are also restricted. Sometimes involuntary movements can occur. The deformity may be associated with syringomyelia and other anomalies, and occasionally with deafness.

Agenesis of cranial nerve nuclei

Sometimes it is difficult to be sure if the signs are due to absence of the cranial nerve nuclei or of the muscles themselves. The third, fourth and sixth nerves may be affected with congenital ptosis, unreacting pupils and ocular palsies. The Marcus Gunn phenomenon occurs when opening of the jaw causes elevation of the drooping eyelid. In congenital sixth nerve palsy, attempts to adduct the other eye cause retraction of the bulb of the affected eye (Duane's syndrome). Congenital facial palsy or Mobius' syndrome has to be differentiated from injury to the facial nerves at birth. Agenesis of the vagus and hypoglossal nuclei can occur, and it is important to recognize this and consider radical treatment such as pharyngoplasty and occlusive protheses to try to improve the speech defect (Ingram, 1969).

References

Allan, L.D., Ferguson-Smith, M.A., Donald, I. *et al.* (1973) Amniotic fluid alpha-fetoprotein in the antenatal diagnosis of spina bifida. *Lancet*, **ii**, 522

Barry, A., Patton, B.M. and Stewart, B.H. (1957) Possible factors in the development of the Arnold-Chiari malformation. *Journal of Neurosurgery*, **14**, 285

Borzyskowski, M. (1984) Management of neuropathic bladder in childhood. *Developmental Medicine and Child Neurology*, **26**, 401

Brennan, T.L., Funk, S.G. and Frothingham, T.E. (1985) Disproportionate intra-uterine head growth and developmental outcome. *Developmental Medicine and Child Neurology*, **27**, 746

Brereton, R.J., Zachary, R.B. and Lister, J. (1977) Urinary continence in open myelomeningocele. *Archives of Disease in Childhood*, **52**, 703

Bresnan M.J. and Lorenzo, A.V. (1975) Cerebrospinal fluid dynamics in megalencephaly. *Developmental Medicine and Child Neurology*, **17**, Suppl. 35, 51

Brock, D.J.H., Bolton, A.E. and Scimgeon, J.B. (1974) Prenatal diagnosis of spina bifida and anencephaly through maternal plasma alpha-fetoprotein measurement. *Lancet*, **ii**, 767

Carter, C.O. (1974) Clues to the aetiology of neural tube malformations. *Developmental Medicine and Child Neurology*, **16**, 3

Carter, C.O. and Roberts, I.A.F. (1967) The risk of recurrence after two children with central nervous system malformations. *Lancet*, **i**, 306

Caviness, V.S. (1976) The Chiari malformations of the posterior fossa and their relation to hydrocephalus. *Developmental Medicine and Child Neurology*, **18**, 103

Cheng, D.W., Chang, L.F. and Bairnson, T.A. (1957) Gross observations on developing abnormal embryos induced by maternal vitamin E deficiency. *Anatomical Record*, **129**, 167

Clarke, C.A., Hobson, D., McKendrick, O.M. *et al.* (1975) Spina bifida and anencephaly: miscarriage as possible cause. *British Medical Journal*, **4**, 743

Comarr, A.E. (1977) Neurological disturbances of sexual function among patients with myelodysplasia. In *Myelomeningocele* (ed. R.L. McLaurin), Grune & Stratton, New York

Day, R.E. and Schutt, W.H. (1979) Normal children with large heads—benign familial megalencephaly. *Archives of Disease in Childhood*, **54**, 512

De Myer, W. (1972) Megalencephaly in children. *Neurology*, **22**, 634

Dennis, I. and Bower, B.D. (1972) The Aicardi syndrome. *Developmental Medicine and Child Neurology*, **14**, 382

Dobbing, J. (1970) Undernutrition and the developing brain. The relevance of animal models to the human problem. *American Journal of Diseases of Children*, **20**, 411

Drummond, M.B. and Donaldson, A.A. (1974) Air, myodil and conray studies in the hydrocephalus of myelomeningocele. *Developmental Medicine and Child Neurology*, Suppl. 32, 131

Eggers, Ch. and Hamer, J. (1979) Hydrosyringomyelia in childhood. Clinical aspects, pathogenesis and therapy. *Neuropädiatrie*, **10**, 87

Ellison, P.H. (1978) Re-evaluation of the approach to an enlarging head in infancy. *Developmental Medicine and Child Neurology*, **20**, 738

Ferguson-Smith, M.A., Rawlinson, H.A., May, H.M. *et al.* (1978) Avoidance of anencephalic and spina bifida births by maternal serum alphafetoprotein screening. *Lancet*, **i**, 1330

Freeston, B.M. (1971) An enquiry into the effect of a spina bifida child upon family life. *Developmental Medicine and Child Neurology*, **13**, 456

Field, B. and Kerr, C. (1976) Aetiology of anencephaly and spina bifida. *British Medical Journal*, **ii**, 107

Gardner, W.J. (1965) Hydrodynamic mechanisms of syringomyelia: its relationship to myelocele. *Journal of Neurology, Neurosurgery and Psychiatry*, **28**, 247

Gardner, W.J. (1977) Etiology and pathogenesis of the development of myelomeningocele. In *Myelomeningocele* (ed. R.L. McLaurin), Grune and Statton, New York

Gordon, N. (1977) Normal pressure hydrocephalus and arrested hydrocephalus. *Developmental Medicine and Child Neurology*, **19**, 540

Gosden, G.M. and Brock, D.J.H. (1977) Morphology of rapidly adhering amniotic-fluid cells as an aid to the diagnosis of neural tube defects. *Lancet*, **i**, 919

Guthkelch, A.N. (1974) Diastematomyelia with median septum. *Brain*, **97**, 729

Guthkelch, A.N. (1986) Aspects of surgical management of myelomeningocele: a review. *Developmental Medicine and Child Neurology*, **28**, 525

Harris, R. (1980) Maternal serum alphafetoprotein pregnancy and the prevention of birth defects. *British Medical Journal*, **i**, 1199

Harris, R. and Read, A.P. (1981) New uncertainties in prenatal screening for neural tube defect. *British Medical Journal*, **i**, 1416

Hamby, W.B., Krauss, R.F. and Beswick, W.F. (1950) Hydranencephaly: a clinical diagnosis. *Pediatrics*, **6**, 371

Hibbard, E.D. and Smithells, R.W. (1965) Folic acid metabolism and human embryopathy. *Lancet*, **i**, 1254

Hoet, J.P., Commas, A. and Hoet, J.J. (1960) Causes of congenital malformations: a role of prediabetes and hypothyroidism. In *Ciba Foundation Symposium on Congenital Malformations* (eds. G.E.W. Wolstenholme and C.M. O'Connor), Churchill Livingstone, London

Ingram, T.T.S. (1969) Disorders of speech in childhood. *British Journal of Hospital Medicine*, **4**, 1608

James, C.C.M. and Lassman, L.P. (1972) *Spinal Dysraphism*, Butterworths, London

Keen, J.H. (1973) Blindness in children with myelomeningocele and hydrocephalus. *Developmental Medicine and Child Neurology*, Suppl. 29, 112

Keys Smith, G. and Durham Smith, E. (1973) Selection for treatment in spina bifida cystica. *British Medical Journal*, **iv**, 189

Landrieu, P., Ninane, J., Ferrière, G. and Lyon, G. (1979) Aqueductal stenosis in X-linked hydrocephalus: a secondary phenomenon? *Developmental Medicine and Child Neurology*, **21**, 637

Laurence, K.M. (1989) A declining incidence of neural tube defects in the UK. *Zeitschrift fur Kinderchirurgie*, **44**, Suppl. 1, 51

Laurence, K.M. and Roberts, C.R. (1977) Spina bifida and anencephaly: are miscarriages a possible cause? *British Medical Journal*, **ii**, 361

Laurence, K.M., James, N., Miller. *et al.* (1981) Double blind randomised controlled trial of folate treatment before conception to prevent recurrence of neural-tube defects. *British Medical Journal*, **i**, 1509

Lendon, R.G. (1969) Neuron population in the lumbosacral cord of myelomeningocele children. *Developmental Medicine and Child Neurology*, Suppl. 20, 82

Lonton, A.P. (1979) The relationship between intellectual skills and the computerised axial tomograms of children with spina bifida and hydrocephalus. *Kinderchirurgie*, **28**, 368

Lorber, J. (1971) Results of treatment of myelomeningocele. *Developmental Medicine and Child Neurology*, **13**, 279

Lorber, J. (1972) Spina bifida cystica. Results of treatment of 270 consecutive cases with criteria for selection for the future. *Archives of Disease in Childhood*, **47**, 854

Lorber, J. (1973) Early results of selective treatment of spina bifida cystica. *British Medical Journal*, **iv**, 201

Lorber, J. (1975) Isosorbide in treatment of infantile hydrocephalus. *Archives of Disease in Childhood*, **50**, 431

Lorber, J. and Bhat, U.S. (1974) Posthaemorrhagic hydrocephalus: diagnosis, differential diagnosis, treatment, and long-term results. *Archives of Disease in Childhood*, **49**, 751

Lorber, J. and Priestley, B.L. (1981) Children with large heads: a practical approach to diagnosis in 557 children with special reference to 109 children with megancephaly. *Developmental Medicine and Child Neurology*, **23**, 494

Lorenzo, A.V., Bresnan, M.J. and Barlow, C.F. (1974) Cerebrospinal fluid absorption deficit in normal pressure hydrocephalus. *Archives of Neurology*, **30**, 387

Medical Research Council (1991) Prevention of neural tube defects: results of the Medical Research Council Vitamin Study. *Lancet*, **338**, 131

Menkes, J.H., Phillipart, M. and Clark, D.B. (1964) Hereditary partial agenesis of the corpus callosum: biochemical and pathological studies. *Archives of Neurology*, **11**, 198

Minns, R.A. (1977) Clinical application of ventricular pressure monitoring in children. *Z. Kinderchir.*, **22**, 430

Minns, R.A. (1986) Children with spina bifida and hydrocephalus. In *Neurologically Handicapped Children: Treatment and Management* and In *Neurologically Sick Children: Treatment and Management* (eds. N. Gordon and I. McKinley), Blackwell Scientific, Oxford

Morley, I.B. and Reynolds, E.H. (1966) Papilloedema and the Landry-Guillain-Barré syndrome. *Brain*, **89**, 205

Norman, A.P. (1971) *Congenital Abnormalities in Infancy*, 2nd edn, Blackwell Scientific, Oxford

Osburn, B.I., Silverstein, A.M., Prendergast, R.A. *et al.* (1971) Experimental viral-induced congenital encephalopathies. 1. Pathology of hydranencephaly and porencephaly caused by blue tongue vaccine virus. *Laboratory Investigation*, **25**, 197

Persson, P.H., Kullander, S., Gennser, G. *et al.* (1983) Screening for fetal malformations using ultrasound and measurements of a-fetoprotein in maternal serum. *British Medical Journal*, **i**, 747

Rickwood, A.M.K. and Zachary, R.B. (1977) Urinary incontinence. *British Medical Journal*, **ii**, 891

Shellshear, I. and Emery, J.L. (1975) The tectum and the aqueduct of sylvius in hydrocephalus unassociated with myelomeningocele. *Developmental Medicine and Child Neurology*, **7**, Suppl. 35, 26

Sherk, H.H., Pasquariello, P.S., Rorke, L.B. and Schut, L. (1984) The pathogenesis of progressive cavitation of the spinal cord. *Developmental Medicine and Child Neurology*, **24**, 514

Smith, A.D., Wald, N.J., Cuckle, H.W. *et al.* (1979) Amniotic-fluid acetylcholinesterase as a possible diagnostic test for neural-tube defects in early pregnancy. *Lancet*, **i**, 685

Smith, C.J., Lelleher, P.C., Belanger, L. and Dallaire, L. (1979) Reactivity of amniotic fluid alpha-fetoprotein with conanavallin A in the diagnosis of neural tube defects. *British Medical Journal*, **i**, 920

Smithells, R.W. (1963) *The Early Diagnosis of Congenital Abnormalities*. Cassell, London

Smithells, R.W., Sheppard, S., Schorah, C.J. *et al.* (1980) Possible prevention of neural-tube defects by periconceptional vitamin supplementation. *Lancet*, **i**, 339

Smithells, R.W., Sheppard, S., Schorah, C.J. *et al.* (1981) Apparent prevention of neural tube defects by periconceptual vitamin supplementation. *Archives of Disease in Childhood*, **56**, 911

Smithells, R.W., Seller, M.J., Harris, R. *et al.* (1983) Further experience of vitamin supplementation for prevention of neural tube defect recurrences. *Lancet*, **i**, 1027

Stark, G.D. (1971) Prediction of urinary continence in myelomeningocele. *Developmental Medicine and Child Neurology*, **13**, 388

Stark, G.D. and Baker, G.C.W. (1967) The neurological involvement of the lower limbs in myelomeningocele. *Developmental Medicine and Child Neurology*, **9**, 732

Strassburg, H.M., Weber, S. and Sauer, M. (1981) Diagnosing hydrocephalus in infants by ultrasound sector scanning through the open fontanelles. *Neuropediatrics*, **12**, 254

Sutherland. G.R. (1975) Antenatal misdiagnosis of spina bifida. *Lancet*, **ii**, 280

Suzuki, M., Davis, C., Lindsay, S. and Genitili, F. (1985) Syringoperitoneal shunt for treatment of cord cavitation. *Journal of Neurology, Neurosurgery and Psychiatry*, **48**, 620

Volpe, J.J. (1987) *Neurology of the Newborn*, 2nd edn, W.B. Saunders, Philadelphia

Walker, I.H., Thomas, M. and Russell, I.T. (1971) Spina bifida-and the parents. *Developmental Medicine and Child Neurology*, **13**, 462

Weld, N.J. and Cuckle, H.S. (1979) Amniotic fluid alpha-fetoprotein measurements in antinatal diagnosis of anencephaly and open spina bifida in early pregnancy. *Lancet*, **ii**, 651

Williams, B. (1970) Current concepts of syringomyelia. *British Journal of Hospital Medicine*, **8**, 331

Williams, B. (1971) Further thoughts on the valvular action of the Arnold-Chiari malformation. *Developmental Medicine and Child Neurology*, **25**, 105

Williams, B. (1972) Pathogenesis in syringomyelia. *Lancet*, **ii**, 969

Williams, B. (1975) Cerebrospinal fluid pressure-gradients in spina bifida cystica, with special reference to the Arnold-Chiari malformation and aqueductal stenosis. *Developmental Medicine and Child Neurology*, Suppl. No. 35, 138

Williams, B. (1977a) On the pathogenesis of the Chiari malformation. *Z. Kinderchir.*, **22**, 533

Williams, B. (1977b) Difficult labour as a cause of communicating hydrocephalus. *Lancet*, **ii**, 51

Woodburn, M. F. (1973) *Social Implications of Spina Bifida*, Scottish Spina Bifida Association, Edinburgh

5 Disorders of mental development

Relatively little is known about the exact relationship between the anatomical structure of the brain and its intellectual function. Some children with obvious brain damage, e.g. the hydrocephalic child or the child severely disabled by dyskinetic cerebral palsy, may be of above average intelligence. Also, the pattern of development rarely proceeds at an equal rate in all its aspects, and this applies to those of below average intelligence as much as to the intellectually brilliant. The genius is notoriously deficient in some aspects of life, and the idiot may or may not be excessively clumsy. Obviously, with severe mental handicap, such variations will be much less apparent against the overall background of retardation, but they must be taken into account when planning help, for such a child is unlikely to find ways of overcoming or circumventing particular difficulties unless he or she is shown how to do so. The more intelligent child has a chance of discovering his or her own remedies.

Genetic and acquired factors can interfere with the growth of the brain and can lead to mental and physical handicap. They may also be associated in varying degrees with the less obvious conditions, such as clumsiness and dyslexia, and to disorders such as epilepsy and hyperkinesis. Accepting that the brain is a very adaptable organ in early life, if its structure is interfered with in this way it can never entirely compensate for failure of development or destruction of tissue. Much can be done to help these children, but some degree of handicap will remain. In view of this, a major medical contribution must be in the field of prevention, and for this to be effective the causes must be known. This chapter will therefore be concerned mainly with the more frequent aetiological factors, and, to avoid repetition, much of what is said will apply to defects of mental and physical development and specific disorders of learning. This does not necessarily mean a spectrum of clinical findings from whatever the cause may be. Apart from the severity of the lesion, its timing may be of equal importance. If there is no obvious cause it may well be best to use terms such as minimal cerebral dysfunction, or, in other words, the brain is not working very well for no known reason. However, it is of importance to always seek a cause, so that even if treatment is not possible, steps can be taken to prevent the disability in other children.

Aetiology

Learning begins in infancy. The baby is gaining experience from the day of birth and probably *in utero* as well, and the mother is the first to estimate the progress that results. There are a number of syndromes, such as Down's syndrome, which identify mental retardation from an early age, but often the parents only gradually suspect this possibility. This may be due to such factors as a lack of response to the environment, delayed motor development, or later on to lack of speech. Such abnormalities are not always due to mental retardation, and assessment may have to be continued over a period of time before any reliable opinion can be given.

An increasing number of causes are being discovered and the subject is no longer a matter of complacency, but early diagnosis is urgent if appropriate treatment is to be given in time. Aetiology can be considered under three headings: prenatal, perinatal and postnatal, but these must be viewed against the background of the child's environment. In some instances the causes differ from those resulting in cerebral palsy. About two thirds of all cases with severe mental retardation may be the result of very early acting prenatal factors, which is not surprising when it is realized that most neurons have appeared by mid pregnancy. In order to reduce the number of those with unclassified mental retardation it is necessary to study all possible aetiologies which may operate during the first trimester of pregnancy, such as viral infections, irradiation and metabolic disorders.

Social factors

Many of the aetiological factors to be discussed will cause severe mental retardation, while environmental influences tend to play a more important part among children assessed as moderately handicapped. Lack of opportunity and of stimulation, poverty, inadequate nutrition, and disturbed parent-child relationships are among the factors which lead to retarded development. The exact effects of malnutrition, before and shortly after birth, and of emotional deprivation in early life have yet to be established, but they cannot be ignored (Davis, 1970). Such deprived children will tend to predominate in schools for educationally subnormal children, while in those for severely mentally handicapped children there is likely to be a more even distribution of children from all social classes. This may make it difficult for some parents to accept the benefits of a good special school for their child, especially when a disability is of moderate degree, and many of the children may be admitted to the school more because of behavioural than learning disorders.

Prenatal causes

The most important prenatal causes of mental handicap include intra-uterine anoxia, failure of fetal nutrition and infections, but some of the conditions to be considered are genetically determined. Almost all of these are transmitted by a recessive mode of inheritance. If the chance of subsequent children being affected is as high as 25% and the condition is known to result in disability, the parents must be told. Many will consider the risks too great, and genetic counselling is undoubtedly an important means of preventing mental retardation and other handicaps. Some malformations of the brain are genetically determined, although the mode of inheritance is not always clear.

Chromosome abnormalities

The various syndromes associated with chromosome abnormalities cannot be considered in detail. Also, apart from rare examples, for instance being able to give genetic advice in the case of translocated Down's syndrome, knowledge of the subject has yet to make a major contribution to the prevention and treatment of mental handicap. Further research may well provide fundamental knowledge and understanding of these syndromes so that their identification is not just an exercise of the collector's instinct. Also, new 'banding' techniques will aid in the identification of individual chromosomes. Trisomies are associated with severe disabilities. Babies with trisomy 13–15 or D-trisomy (Patau's syndrome) are severely retarded and usually do not survive more than a year or two, and the same applies to trisomy 17–18 or E-trisomy (Edward's syndrome).

Down's syndrome

Down's syndrome or mongolism, 21 trisomy or G-trisomy (Fig. 5.1) is easy enough to recognize by the typical facial appearance and other characteristics, including hypotonia, congenital heart disease, duodenal atresia, abnormal palmar and plantar creases, and Brushfield spots. Atlantoaxial instability and abnormalities of the odontoid may be a problem and lead to spinal cord damage. This should be taken into account, especially among those taking part in sports (Elliot, Moreton and Whitelaw, 1988), but X-ray examination is of limited value. The mental retardation is usually severe, but there are definite exceptions to this. There is a relationship between 21 trisomy and maternal age. When the mother is over 35 years of age the increased risk is in the order of 2%, and rises with age thereafter. The screening of all mothers over the age of 35 years, by chorionic villus sampling at 10 weeks' gestation or by amniocentesis at about 16 weeks, and examination of fetal cells is increasingly accepted as a justifiable means of preventing the birth of children with Down's syndrome. The former carries a higher risk of stimulating a miscarriage. An association has also been found between low levels of alpha-fetoprotein in the serum in the second trimester and fetal trisomies 18 and 21 (Brock, 1984); and the use of this estimation, and of the serum concentration of unconjugated oestriol and serum human gonadotrophin, and of maternal age can be used in the second trimester as an effective alternative to amniocentesis, especially for those under the age of 35 years

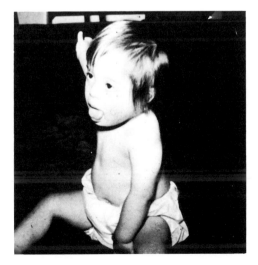

Figure 5.1 Down's syndrome.

when more invasive techniques are not justifiable (Ruta and Leece, 1988; Ward *et al.*, 1988).

Other chromosome disorders

Occasionally, the extra chromosome is attached to another one, particularly in the 13–15 or D group. Then the condition may be inherited instead of occurring in the usual random fashion. In D-G interchange with maternal transmission the recurrence rate is about 10–15% for a woman and 2–3% for a man. Rarely a parent is found to have both of the 21 chromosomes joined together, in which case all offspring will have Down's syndrome.

Deletions of chromosomes may result in severe mental retardation associated with various physical deformities, for instance partial deletion of one of the short arms of the 4–5 group in the cri-du-chat syndrome. Ring chromosome 18 is also associated with severe retardation. In syndromes associated with abnormalities of the sex chromosomes there tends to be a relationship between the severity of mental handicap and the number of extra X chromosomes, but there are exceptions to this. For further details of this subject the reader is referred to Zellweger and Simpson (1977). Recently, attention has been paid to fragile sites on the long arm of the X chromosome, and an association between this anomoly and X-linked mental retardation (Turner and Opitz, 1980). Female carriers may also be mildly retarded (Berry, 1981). Fragile X-linked mental retardation is now the second most frequent cause of mental retardation in males after Down's syndrome, and there are reasonable grounds for screening all mentally retarded individuals for this condition (Turner *et al.*, 1986). Other findings include abnormal facies, macro-orchidism and autistic-like behaviour. The trait may behave as an X-linked dominant gene with uncertainty how the phenotype/genotype interaction takes place (Jordan, 1987). It may soon be possible with new techniques to identify carrier status in mothers in the absence of fragile X expression. Treatment with folate has been tried, but the response is unconfirmed.

Nutrition and anoxia

The nutrition of the developing fetus must be of importance. Research suggests that maternal malnutrition from mid-pregnancy to delivery and defective nutrition of the infant to the end of the second year of life during the main spurt of brain growth will have a lasting effect on the development of the brain (Dobbing, 1970). The fetus can be starved *in utero* by causes other than the mother's lack of food. If, for example, there is placental insufficiency from some cause or other the fetus will not be provided with adequate nutrition during a vital period of development and will be born 'small-for-dates'. It has certainly been shown that babies who are very light for dates have a poorer attainment than those with a short gestation. In other words, it is better to be born too soon than too small (Neligan *et al.*, 1976), although this may be less true now with modern methods of management. As has been pointed out, severe mental retardation is more likely to result from disorders in the first half of gestation when the neurons are developing, rather than during the main spurt of brain growth mainly due to the development of the glial cells and their axons and dendrites.

Vascular lesions in the placenta, for example complicating toxaemia of pregnancy, can also lead to fetal anoxia. If this causes circulatory failure, venous thrombosis and infarction may occur. If this happens in the earlier weeks of the last trimester the damage will tend to be located in the periventricular areas of the cerebrum (Towbin,

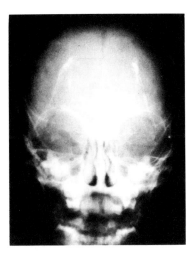

Figure 5.2   Calcification in the walls of the ventricles in cytomegalic inclusion disease.

1969). Among babies born with a weight of 2000 g or less, Drillien (1967) found that a third were handicapped, and that in a quarter of these there was evidence that the cause was related to inter-uterine hypoxia. In both malnutrition and hypoxia the degree of damage will vary from severe to slight and result in disabilities ranging from gross mental retardation, through different types of cerebral palsy to clumsy children with specific learning difficulties.

Infections

Maternal infections during pregnancy can result in considerable risks to the fetus, and these will be considered again in Chapter 10. Rubella is well known as a cause of mental retardation, and of microcephaly, cataract, deafness, congenital heart disease and other conditions. It has been found that cytomegalic inclusion disease can damage the fetal brain, as can toxoplasmosis. Both these infections may produce a clinical picture soon after birth which is not unlike haemorrhagic disease of the newborn, with jaundice, haemorrhages and hepatosplenomegaly. X-ray of the skull may show intra-cerebral calcification (Fig. 5.2). It has been estimated that infection with cytomegalovirus may account for about 10% of mentally retarded children with microcephaly, and that rubella and toxoplasmosis are responsible for about 2–3% of all cases of mental deficiency (Stern *et at.*, 1969; Peckham *et al.*, 1983). Congenital syphilis is now very uncommon, but it seems possible that there are a number of other inter-uterine infections, particularly of virus origin, which will no doubt prove to be of aetiological significance. Much can be done to prevent inter-uterine infections, and with the use of rubella immunization it should be possible to eradicate this particular risk. Other preventative measures include giving gamma-globulin to pregnant women who are rubella contacts, the trial of a cytomegalovirus vaccine in adolescence (Elek and Stern, 1974), and possibly treating mothers infected with toxoplasmosis in the latter part of pregnancy (Thalhammer, 1973). Both spiramycin and a mixture of sulphadiazine and pyrimethamine have been used in the treatment of toxoplasmosis.

Toxic causes

The toxic effects of drugs during pregnancy is another field in which there is much to learn. Anticonvulsant drugs given to expectant mothers may adversely affect the fetus, and the role of folic acid deficiency resulting from taking these drugs has still to be determined. Hibbard and Smithells (1965) have shown that the mothers of malformed babies are five times more likely to demonstrate defective folate metabolism than the mothers of normal babies. So the possibility of folic acid deficiency must be considered when any woman on treatment with anticonvulsant drugs becomes pregnant. In the case of anencephaly and spina bifida doubts have been cast on the role of folic acid deficiency (Emery, 1977), but there seems to be no doubt that mothers taking sodium valproate during pregnancy have a greater risk of having babies with spina bifida (Lammer, Sever and Oakley, 1987).

The most common malformations reported among babies born of mothers on anti-epileptic treatment, particularly barbiturates and phenytoin, are facial clefts and congenital heart disease. Rarely such babies have presented sufficiently characteristic appearances to suggest a syndrome. The fetal phenytoin syndrome is characterized by defective growth and mental development. Limb defects include hypoplasia of the phalanges and nails, finger-like thumbs and variations in palmar creases and dermatoglyphics. The craniofacial appearances show a broad low nasal bridge, epicanthic folds, short upturned nose, hyperteleorism, ptosis, strabismus, low set ears, wide mouth with prominent lips, and variations in head size and shape (Hanson and Smith, 1975).

It is of interest that similar syndromes have been reported when mothers have been taking troxidone during pregnancy (Zackai et al., 1975), paramethadione (German, Kowal and Ehlers, 1970), and phenobarbitone (Seip, 1976). In fetal alcohol syndrome the children born to mothers with chronic alcoholism show growth deficiency, developmental delay, microcephaly, short palpabral fissures, epicanthic folds, ptosis, maxillary hypoplasia, cleft palate, micrognathia, joint anomalies, altered palmar creases, small nails, and sometimes cardiac lesions, abnormal external genitalia and hirsutism (Hanson, Jones and Smith, 1976). Admittedly there may be many medical influences affecting children born of alcoholic mothers, but direct ethanol poisoning is the most obvious possibility (Jones et al., 1973).

All these various syndromes have features in common (retarded development, abnormal facies, particularly a wide mouth, and defects of the hands and fingers). As they are abnormal at birth there must be a disorder of embryogenesis or of fetal development. Such features as abnormal palmar creases and the type of cerebral deformity (Jones and Smith, 1973) suggests that the damage occurs before the 80th day of gestation. It is tempting to think that the syndromes may not be specific to a particular drug but the result of a variety of toxins acting at a particular point of time during pregnancy. Perhaps in the present state of our ignorance the best policy is to eschew all drugs during pregnancy unless they are absolutely necessary.

Kernicterus

Kernicterus is included in this section because the diagnosis of the most common causes of this should be made before birth. An excellent example of the success of medical research in preventing brain damage is the story of haemolytic disease of the newborn (erythroblastosis fetalis), which used to cause so many instances of basal ganglia lesions, but which has now become a rare disease. Antenatal care now ensures that babies at risk are identified, and exchange transfusion is carried out when indicated. The advances, resulting from the research into the effects of anti-D gamma globulin, may prevent the disease altogether. If women at risk are given 5 ml of anti-D gamma globulin within 48 hours of delivery there is evidence that this will protect them against Rh-immunization and their children against rhesus haemolytic disease (Clarke, 1967).

Other prenatal causes

Although many premature babies develop normally, there is no doubt that the lower the birth-weight the more risks there are of damage to the brain, which stresses the importance of preventative measures, such as improving the mother's health before and during pregnancy, the interval between pregnancies, parity, maternal age and the early recognition and treatment of toxaemia. There are many other possible prenatal factors, such as radiation of the mother's pelvis, trauma and maternal ill-health, and one must be constantly looking out for conditions that can be added to the list. Hagberg (1975) has shown that prenatal factors constitute the majority of undiagnosed causes of brain damage.

Perinatal causes

Anoxia and birth injury

Some years ago there was no doubt that anoxia and trauma at birth often caused damage to the brain, but with the present antenatal care and obstetrical services that are available such complications are far less likely to occur. Birth trauma can result from separation of the squamous and lateral parts of the occipital bone which will not be recognized unless carefully looked for. This can cause lesions of the cerebellum and brain-stem which are potentially lethal. They can be prevented by Caesarean section if there is any suspicion of disproportion, and in breech delivery by avoidance of excessive pressure on the suboccipital region (Wigglesworth and Husemeyer, 1977). It is always difficult to predict the effect of anoxia at birth, and it is probably a combination of various factors (e.g. jaundice, hypoglycaemia, impaired temperature regulation, cardiac failure) which determines the degree of cerebral injury. Also, in small for date babies events during pregnancy are likely to be the most important ones as something must have gone wrong in the early stages causing failure to thrive as well as predisposing the baby to further troubles during birth. Complications at birth, however, cannot be ignored and may be severe enough to cause cerebral damage. Seizures may be the best predictor of brain damage after anoxia but these can be due to other factors. The ability of the baby to withstand the effects of anoxia is mainly due to the use of anaerobic glycolysis which is possible at this time of life as long as there is not a deficiency of glycogen as a result of malnutrition. The influence of social class operating before birth must also be taken into account.

The possible association is most often a retrospective one, the only obvious, significant event in the past history of a mentally handicapped child being an abnormal birth. This may suggest the cause of the child's condition, but it can rarely be proved for certain, and the obstetrician can easily be unfairly blamed for difficulties occurring during labour if it not realized that the real causes of these are often very complex and involve a number of prenatal factors as well as genetic and social ones (Illingworth 1979). The damage occurring from anoxia at term will predominate in the cortical regions and grey matter of the brain-stem, as these are now the most actively growing areas of the brain. The blood gas changes will cause a breakdown of the blood-brain barrier, with cerebral oedema leading to secondary cerebral ischaemia (Pape and Wigglesworth, 1979). The treatment of cerebral oedema has been considered in Chapter 2.

Intraventricular haemorrhage (IVH)

In the newborn period IVH occurs almost exclusively among premature infants. It is an important cause of perinatal deaths, and of severe physical and mental disabilities. Seizures, which occur at the time of bleeding, resemble decerebrate posturing (Tsiantos *et al.*, 1974). The overall incidence of the condition as estimated by Fredrick and Butler (1970) is 1.1 per 1000 live births. The highest incidence of IVH (176.1 per 1000 live births) occurs among infants born before 28 weeks' gestation. There is an association between IVH and maternal infection, pre-eclampsia, hyaline membrane disease, and retarded birth-weight for gestational age; and a disproportionate number of male infants are affected. With the use of computerized axial tomography it has been shown that the incidence of IVH in surviving infants whose birth-weight is less than 1500 g is much greater than reported and that the majority of these haemorrhages are clinically silent (Papile *et al.*, 1978). These findings have been confirmed with real-time ultrasound studies which is now the investigation of choice as it is much less disturbing to the infant and can be repeated at regular intervals (Levene, Wigglesworth and Dubowitz, 1981). However, the possible links between these haemorrhages and handicaps such as specific learning disorders in later life must await the results of further long-term follow-up studies.

The site of bleeding is usually in the subependymal tissue matrix of the lateral ventricles (germinal layer haemorrhage). If blood leaks into the lateral ventricles it may accumulate in the cisterna magna and it may block the normal flow of cerebrospinal fluid and lead to hydrocephalus (Larroche, 1972). Any damage to the matrix will result in neuronal cell deficiencies among survivors.

It is generally agreed that asphyxia is an important factor in the pathogenesis of IVH, particularly in view of the association between IVH and hyaline membrane disease (Leech and Kohnen, 1974). Hypoxia associated with hypercapnia can cause an increase in cerebral blood flow, cerebral vasodilatation and a rise in venous pressure, and this may cause rupture of the capillaries or terminal veins, possibly in relation to an area of infarction. Raised arterial pressure may also be a factor, although perhaps not so important as cerebral blood flow; and this can be prevented by treatment of epileptic seizures and apnoea, a minimum of handling, and by the use of diazepam and chlorpromazine (Lou, Lassen and Früs-Hanson, 1979). The role of raised venous pressure is open to doubt; and it is suggested that haemorrhage may occur in the presence of normal arterial and central venous pressure as a result of ischaemic damage to capillary walls. Hypotension following asphyxia will be greatest in the subependymal layer due to the anatomy of the arterial supply and, after restoration of normal pressure, flow to the subependymal layer will be disproportionately increased due to loss of autoregulation in the ischaemic area; and this may result in haemorrhage through the ependymal layer and into the ventricles (Robinson, 1979). From 30 weeks' gestation onwards another possible cause of an excessive pressure gradient between blood-vessel lumen and the surrounding brain tissue, with resultant haemorrhage, is decreased tissue pressure due to loss of water content (de Courten and Robinowicz, 1981).

It has also been suggested that IVH can be caused by excessive administration of sodium bicarbonate solution (Simmons *et al.*, 1974). It may be that the infusion of solutions which are hyperosmolar compared with plasma, and which will therefore cause loss of tissue fluid through the umbilical vein, have a toxic effect on immature blood vessels, or cause a sudden rise in central venous pressure; but alkali therapy is probably not to blame (Anderson *et al.*, 1976). Other contributory conditions may include abnormalities in haemostasis, with either disseminated intravascular coagulation or a fall in vitamin K dependent factors, and continuous inflating pressure, particularly airway pressure (CPAP).

Any measures designed to avoid prenatal or postnatal asphyxia may reduce the occurrence of IVH, and careful attention must be given to the volume of buffer-containing solution infused. Trials in which clotting factors were replaced by giving plasma or fresh blood have given conflicting results (Hambleton and Appleyard, 1973).

Neonatal hypoglycaemia

Neonatal hypoglycaemia occurs most often in babies that are small-for-dates, born in a starved condition and depleted of liver glycogen reserves. Pathological studies on babies dying from anoxia and hypoglycaemia in the first week of life have shown a different distribution of cerebral lesions, the damage being more selective and less severe in the former. This may be due to the fact that the heart in early life has a better store of glycogen than the brain and is able to utilize substrates other than glucose for its energy. Therefore the heart is not so susceptible to hypoglycaemia, and babies will tend to die from anoxia before severe brain damage occurs, but not from hypoglycaemia. Also, focal lesions due to circulatory failure are more likely to occur from anoxia than hypoglycaemia (Anderson, Miner and Strich, 1967).

Several conditions are associated with neonatal hypoglycaemia; haemolytic disease of the newborn, hypothermia, respiratory distress syndrome and birth injury, and babies born of diabetic mothers are particularly at risk. Symptoms due to hypoglycaemia will usually be resolved by glucose infusion, but occasionally other measures such as giving hydrocortisone are needed. Prompt treatment of the hypoglycaemia, particularly if this is started before symptoms arise, is likely to prevent brain damage, but the prognosis will have to be guarded if there is a suggestion of birth injury.

Neonatal seizures

As the problems of neonatal seizures are detailed in Chapter 9 it need only be emphasized here that, whatever the cause of these fits may be, their treatment is a matter of urgency if brain damage is to be avoided. If there is any delay in obtaining the results of investigations it may be necessary to treat possible metabolic disorders, such as hypoglycaemia, hypomagnasaemia and hypocalcaemia to see if a response is obtained.

Infections

Meningitis and septicaemia occurring in the first few days of life must be diagnosed and treated immediately if brain damage is to be avoided, and these diseases will be considered again in Chapter 10. Their presence is often not obvious but has to be suspected from signs such as refusal of feeds, weight loss, vomiting and cyanotic attacks. A screening programme must then be carried out to exclude the various possible sites of infection, and this must include examination of the cerebrospinal fluid. Details of these programmes will be found in Chapter 10.

Postnatal causes

Infections

Various infections can cause brain damage post-natally. Viral infections such as measles may be complicated by encephalitis, and the younger the child the more serious it is likely to be. The diagnosis of such diseases will become more important as more antiviral agents are discovered. Herpes simplex encephalitis, with its pre-dilection for the temporal lobes, may benefit from treatment with cytaribine (Marshall, 1967), and more recently with the less toxic acyclovir (Whitley *et al.*, 1977). This treatment can be combined with steroids in an effort to prevent damage from the inflammatory reaction, as well as from the direct invasion of the virus. When there is a possibility that the 'encephalitis' is an allergic response to the virus infection, resulting in demyelination, treatment with steroids may prevent further brain damage.

In the case of bacterial infections, causing meningitis or cerebral abscess, early diagnosis and appropriate treatment is essential if complete recovery is to occur. Pus in the meninges can cause thrombosis of the blood vessels supplying the brain, and pus within the brain acts as a space-occupying lesion, as well as being a constant threat to spreading infection which destroys the cerebral tissues.

Trauma and toxic agents

In this day and age accidents are unfortunately a common cause of injury to the brain. The number of children injured on the roads shows no sign of decreasing, but this is surely a field in which there could be more effective prevention (Jackson, 1978). Non-accidental injury (battered babies) will be discussed in another chapter, but may well be an important cause of physical and mental handicap, quite apart from the number who die. The frequency of this problem has been underestimated in the past (Oliver, 1975). Poisoning has also become an increased risk, with the advent of many new drugs and chemical agents. Acute lead poisoning can cause a severe encephalopathy which may be fatal, but the role of chronic lead poisoning as a significant cause of mental retardation remains unproven (Gordon, King and Mackay, 1967). In a recent review of research findings Rutter (1980) concludes that the evidence suggests that raised blood lead levels above 40 µg per 100 ml may cause slight cognitive impairment and less certainly may increase the risk of behavioural difficulties. However, there is no doubt that mentally handicapped children are especially at risk from lead poisoning. They are more apt to crawl around the floor, put things in their mouths, and suffer from pica. If a serum lead level of above 40 µg per 100 ml is found this must raise suspicions, but a single estimation is of limited value, and serial tests may have to be done before a definite diagnosis of persistent lead poisoning can be made and treatment started. Apart from the possible causal effects of lead, the question of secondary poisoning among handicapped children is worth considering in the presence of such symptoms as irritability, aggressive outbursts and failure to thrive. The treatment of questionable symptomatic children with increased lead absorption is controversial. Removal of lead from the child's environment is mandatory and nutritional deficits and iron deficiency must be corrected. Short courses of chelation treatment can be given in the chronic situation if there are a number of signs of excessive lead ingestion, and in acute lead poisoning parenteral edathomil calcium disodium and BAL (dimercaprol) are given, with oral D-penicillamine as a secondary agent if long-term treatment is warranted (Chisolm and Barltrop, 1979). Many poisons taken accidentally by children can cause damage and death, and deliberate poisoning must not be forgotten (Munchausen by proxy) (Meadows, 1989).

Epilepsy (and other causes)

The complications of epilepsy will be discussed in another section, particularly the dangers of status epilepticus. If this is not treated as a matter of urgency some degree of brain damage or increase of existing damage will be an almost inevitable result.

Disorders due to abnormal amino acid metabolism

Most metabolic disorders have a recessive mode of inheritance; they can affect protein, fat and carbohydrate metabolism, and a few examples will be given. Disorders of this kind occur in only a small percentage of mentally retarded children, but they do include a number of conditions which, if diagnosed and treated early in life, can be compatible with normal or near normal development. Phenylketonuria is the best known example of the disorders of amino acid metabolism, and in the classical form a diet low in phenylalanine does influence the course of the disease. Not all infants who are found to have phenylketonuria have the typical disorder of phenylalanine metabolism; with stigmata such as fair hair, blue eyes, eczema, and broad, widely-spaced incisor teeth, associated with severe mental retardation. Some of the variations seen in specific metabolic disorders result from genetic heterogenicity. A particular gene mutation may result in a reduction in the level of an enzyme in several different ways. The protein may be altered so that the ability to bind with the co-enzyme is affected, or the stability of the enzyme may be changed, or the abnormal synthesis of the enzyme results in defective catalytic properties. If each parent is carrying a different mutation, some of their children will be heterozygous for the gene which codes for the amino acid sequence of a polypeptide chain in the enzyme (Harris, 1970). This can apply to the enzyme phenylalanine hydroxylase, and at least three heterozygous phenotypes have been distinguished (Gutler and Hanson, 1977); but varying types of phenylketonuria can also result from deficiency of different enzymes in this particular metabolic pathway (Smith, Clayton and Wolff, 1975)(see Chapter 3.)

Phenylketonuria is a fairly rare disorder, but there are now an increasing number of conditions such as homocystinuria and maple-syrup-urine disease which can be treated by special diets (Westall, 1963, Komrower et at., 1966). Homocystinuria has a striking clinical picture, with skeletal lesions resembling Marfan's syndrome or arachnodactyly, fair hair, highly coloured cheeks, dislocated lenses and a tendency to vascular thrombosis, as well as convulsions and mental retardation. Maple-syrup-urine disease is identified by the characteristic smell of the urine, particularly after it has been left standing for a few hours. The number of disorders of this kind that are now recognized makes screening surveys of infants a more practical proposition.

As more of these conditions are recognized and become amenable to treatment, additional problems will arise. For example, a careful check will have to be kept on phenylketonuric mothers, and it may be necessary to think in terms of planned pregnancies with dietary restrictions. Starting a strict dietary regime when the woman is trying to get pregnant is the alternative, but this is not very practicable, and, if the patient defaults, damage to the fetus is likely to occur early on, before the pregnancy has been confirmed (Yu and O'Halloran, 1970). Mothers of mentally handicapped children should be screened for phenylketonuria and other possible metabolic disorders.

Metabolic disorders due to abnormal carbohydrates and lipids

Disorders of carbohydrate metabolism are not so frequent as amino acid disorders, but occasionally present similar situations. Galactosaemia is due to an inability to metabolize galactose from lactose due to a deficiency of phosphogalactose uridyl transferase (Komrower, 1969). If the diagnosis is not made early in life and lactose excluded from the diet, the liver will suffer damage, cataracts are likely to develop, and in most cases there will be severe mental retardation. Disorders of mucopoly-saccharide metabolism cause different types of gargoylism, most of which are associated with mental backwardness (Gordon and Thursby-Pelham, 1969). The diagnosis is suggested by the unusual appearance of the children; and the differentiation of the various syndromes is made on both clinical and biochemical grounds. The estimation of excess urinary excretion of the glycosaminoglycans is helpful in making the diagnosis (Manley and Williams, 1969), and the deficiency of specific enzymes can be identified in cultured fibroblasts (Neufeld and Muenzer, 1989). The lipidoses are a depressing group of genetically-determined conditions which lead to progressive deterioration and for which there is limited treatment. Because of their progressive nature they will be considered in Chapter 11.

Other metabolic and endocrine causes

Other metabolic disorders, e.g. *idiopathic infantile hypercalcaemia (Williams' syndrome)* (Fig. 5.3), can be associated with mental handicap. In the first few months of life the infant ceases to thrive. Vomiting, wasting and constipation appear; and these symptoms are often associated with dehydration. The condition gradually

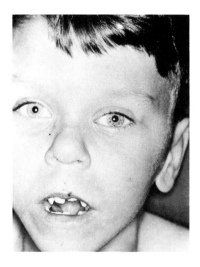

Figure 5.3   idiopathic infantile hypercalcaemia.

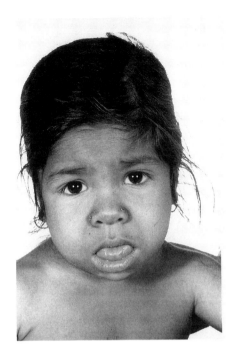

Figure 5.4   Child with cretinism.

improves, and if not recognized at this early age the child may present later on with mental retardation. They have 'elfin-like' facies and there can be an associated infundibular aortic stenosis. A stellate pattern identified in photographs of the iris can be a useful finding (Holmström *et al.*, 1990). By that time the calcium level in the serum is likely to be normal (Schlesinger, Butler and Black, 1956). Behavioural and social difficulties may persist into adult life (Udwin, 1990). It is suggested that the initial condition may be related to an intake of vitamin D which is excessive for individual tolerance, or, possibly, a deficiency of thyrocalcitonin causes an impairment of the normal inhibition of bone resorption in response to hypercalcaemia (Forbes *et al.*, 1972). If there is hypercalcaemia a low calcium diet should be given, and occasionally cortisone to reduce calcium absorption.

Cretinism (Fig. 5.4) will lead to mental retardation, although if treatment with thyroxine can be started in the first three months of life the child has a chance of reaching a level of average intelligence. However, even if replacement therapy is started very early in life, the child is likely to suffer from a variety of disabilities, such as clumsiness and other learning disorders, speech and language difficulties and abnormal behaviour; which are probably due to abnormalities of axonal and dendritic connections rather than loss of cell numbers (Macfaul *et al.*, 1978). It seems that neonatal hypothyroidism is much more common than had been thought. Screening programmes, using neonatal dried blood or cord blood for estimation of T4 (thyroxine), THS (thyrotropin) and T3U (tri-iodothyronine resin) uptake have shown an incidence of thyroid abnormalities of 1 per 3000 births, about twice that in retrospective studies (Walfish *et al.*, 1979). The effects of such programmes and the early initiation of treatment is still being assessed, but there is already evidence that pre-symptomatic treatment may make a significant contribution to the prevention of mental handicap (*Lancet*, Nov. 14th 1981, p. 1095). Transient cases of hypothyroidism seem to be uncommon (Hulse *et al.*, 1982).

Rett syndrome

It is now known that this syndrome (Fig. 5.5) is one of the more common causes of severe mental retardation. It only affects girls with an incidence of about 1 in 15 000 girls, although a few boys have been suspected of having the syndrome. Almost always early development appears normal, but at the age of 18 months to 2 years skills are lost and the girl becomes increasingly and, sometimes rapidly, physically and mentally retarded. The diagnosis is most often suggested by mannerisms such as hand clapping and teeth grinding movements, and by autistic-type behaviour. Hyperventilation when agitated is a common feature. Progress of the disease slows into a chronic stage, with rigidity and involuntary movements being more common than spasticity; and at this stage a wrong diagnosis of ataxic cerebral palsy may be made. Epilepsy often occurs, and typically the EEG shows diffuse abnormalities, especially during sleep. Survival into adult life is frequent, and then severe wasting may occur and a clinical picture not unlike spastic tetraplegic cerebral palsy. No definite chromosome or biochemical abnormalities have been found, but intensive research is being carried out, and there may be disorders of transmitter amines (Lekman *et al.*, 1989). Neuropathological studies have not been very helpful. There is moderate

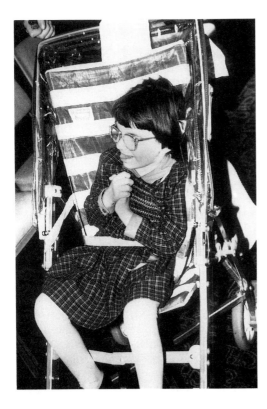

Figure 5.5   Child with Rett syndrome.

cortical atrophy and shrinkage of the brain. Microscopically there is mild gliosis and some underpigmentation in certain nigral structures. Slight degenerative changes have been found in the spinal cord. The differential diagnosis is from disorders such as epileptic encephalopathies, types of cerebral palsy, infantile autism and infantile neuronal ceroid lipofuscinosis. There is no specific treatment (Hagberg *et al.*, 1983; Hagberg, 1989), but giving drugs such as bromocriptine may be of benefit, especially in alleviating the impaired motor function (Zappella *et al.*, 1990).

There are many other postnatal causes of acquired damage to the brain, but perhaps enough has been said to emphasize their diverse nature and the increasing number that can be treated so that lifelong handicap is prevented.

Assessment and care of the mentally handicapped

A particular responsibility of the doctor is to try to establish the cause of retarded development, and, if possible, institute specific treatment. Assessment of the child's development must then begin, and may have to be continued over a period of time. Certainly, re-assessment must be considered if the child's progress is not as expected. First of all, developmental tests are given to infants and children under the age of 5 years (Egan, Illingworth and MacKeith, 1969). As the child grows older, standardized tests of intelligence will be used, depending on the age of the child and the type of disability, e.g. the Stanford-Binet Scale, the Wechsler Intelligence Scale for Children and the Merrill-Palmer test. These will be discussed again in Chapter 8.

The object of examining children with the aid of such tests is not so much to produce a figure denoting the level of intelligence as to highlight the particular needs of an individual child and indicate ways in which he can best be helped. It is also important to highlight a child's assets. Developmental and intelligence tests may have to be repeated on a number of occasions over a period of several years. The need for repeated assessment is not only to enable a more exact prognosis to be given but to identify changes that occur in the pattern of a child's development which may well alter as he or she grows older.

Controversy and changes in the care of the severely mentally handicapped will continue to occur (Bavin, 1970). The exact form these will take is likely to vary, but whatever decisions are taken they should be in the interests of both the patient and the family. Family care probably provides the best environment for the severely affected child, but it is not always appropriate. There are instances where the strain placed on the family may be more than they can bear, and alternatives have to be considered. If there were more facilities for temporary care, crises could be avoided; parents must feel that they are not being left in isolation but that there are a number of people who can help them and are only too willing to do so. Other children in the family will react to the presence of a handicapped sibling in different ways, and perhaps the family doctor is in the best position to judge if they are coming to any harm. In the future there may be an expansion of fostering and adoption facilities for handicapped children as an alternative to institutional care.

Temporary care has a number of advantages, apart from giving the parents some relief from their exacting role. It may prevent them from becoming over-protective and help them to a better adjustment to the situation. Problems tend to look different to anyone after a short holiday and to assume more realistic proportions. Also, a period away from home does give the child some degree of independence, even if this has to be very limited. If a crisis occurs, due to the parents' illness for instance, the child may then be able to return to a familiar environment, and no hasty and unplanned decision will have to be taken.

It has been shown that even severely subnormal individuals can benefit from suitable training, and there is a great need for further research in this field (Clarke, 1970). There is also controversy over the best way to educate the less severely handicapped child. Should this be in special schools, in special classes in ordinary schools, or as part of the 'streaming' that occurs in many schools; in short, segregation or integration? There is unlikely to be an answer that covers all eventualities. The aim should therefore be for flexibility and for as varied facilities as are compatible with efficient organization and economic resources. Handicapped children are almost always multiply handicapped, and this applies particularly to children of below average intelligence. Minor defects of vision and hearing, if unrecognized, may easily tip the balance, leading to an erroneous assessment of the child's potential and preventing him or her from benefiting from appropriate education. A thorough physical examination of the child is essential, with the correction of any remediable condition as early in life as possible. Also, as will be seen later, various specific disorders of learning are no respectors of the intelligence level. Identification of specific learning difficulties is therefore important so that special help can be given when it is indicated, and the child shown how to overcome the defect. Physical disabilities will often be associated with mental handicap, and it will be apparent that there are many problems common to both conditions.

Parent counselling

There are numerous agencies capable of helping the mentally handicapped child and the family, but they tend to be scattered, some working under the auspices of the hospital services, some in the local authority services, and some organized by voluntary bodies. There needs to be someone, whatever his or her title, who is responsible for coordinating the help given to an individual child and interpreting this this to the parents, for they often remain ignorant of what can be done. Many feel that there is no-one to whom they can turn for advice, or even to talk over their problems with. However, there are signs that much more will be done for the mentally handicapped child in the future, and the paediatric neurologist has a very definite part to play in this work.

Whoever does accept the role of counselling the parents of handicapped children must be prepared to give advice on a number of occasions. This is particularly true if, as is often the case, the answer to the parents questions cannot be the ones they really want to hear. If it is evident that the child is suffering from a handicap which is going to persist throughout life it will rightly take a long time for the parents to accept this. Also a balance will have to be maintained between encouraging a realistic attitude to the child's potential so that he or she is put into a situation which is meaningful to him or her, and maintaining a reasonably hopeful outlook. Growth and development are with few exceptions bound to result in some improvement (Gordon, 1972).

Freeman and Pearson (1978) have stressed that parents need information about what has happened to their child, how it can be treated and what the future holds. Parents must be involved in the management of their child whenever possible, and must know who is primarily responsible for the child's care.

There are grave dangers of making a diagnosis, unaccompanied by adequate guidance, as this may do little more than add another handicap. This will be referred to again in the next chapter in the context of speech development. The diagnosis of mental retardation can result in deprivation because of the way people treat 'backward' children, and parents in particular must be advised on how to stimulate their child to the best advantage. However irrational it may often be parents do experience guilt about their child's condition and their efforts to help may mitigate this. These efforts must be given expert guidance or otherwise they can get out of hand to the detriment of all the family.

MacKeith (1973) considers grief and shock are more common reactions than guilt among parents of handicapped children. He defines the crisis periods during the growth of the handicapped child as when the parents first learn about or suspect handicap in their child; when at about the age of five years decisions have to be taken about schooling; when the time comes to leave school; and when the parents become older and no longer able to look after their child, and may be unaware of the statutory services which can give help. In the field of paediatrics there has not been sufficient concern over the care of mentally handicapped children. Fortunately, this is now changing, and paediatricians are becoming more involved in the problems of these children, and are in a particularly advantageous position to mobilize all the various services which should be aiding and supporting the handicapped child and the family; and this involvement must continue throughout childhood at home and in hospital.

References

Anderson, J.M., Miner. R.D.G. and Stritch, S.I. (1967) Effects of neonatal hypoglycaemia on the nervous system: a pathological study. *Journal of Neurology, Neurosurgery and Psychiatry*, **30**, 295

Anderson, J.M., Bain, A.D., Brown, J.K. *et al.* (1976) Hyaline membrane disease, alkaline buffer treatment and cerebral intraventricular haemorrhage. *Lancet*, **i**, 117

Bavin, J. (1970) Subnormality in the seventies: priority in resources. *Lancet*, **i**, 285

Berry, C. (1981) X-linked mental retardation. *Archives of Disease in Childhood*, **56**, 410

Brock, D.J.H. (1984) Maternal serum alpha-fetoprotein as screening test for Down's syndrome. *Lancet*, **i**, 1292

Chisolm, J.J. and Barltrop, D. (1979) Recognition and management of children with increased lead absorption. *Archives of Disease of Childhood*, **54**, 249

Clarke, A.D.B. (1970) Stretching their learning skills. *Special Education*, **59**, 21

Clarke, C.A. (1967) Prevention of Rh-haemolytic disease. *British Medical Journal*, **iv**, 7

Davis, I. (1970) The effects of early environment on later development. *Developmental Medicine and Child Neurology*, **12**, 98

de Courten, G.M. and Robinowicz, Th. (1981) Intraventricular haemorrhage in premature infants: reappraisal and new hypothesis. *Developmental Medicine and Child Neurology*, **23**, 389

Dobbing, I. (1970) Undernutrition and the developing brain. The relevance of animal models to the human problem. *American Journal of Diseases of Children*, **120**, 411

Drillien, C.M. (1967) The long-term prospects for babies of low birth weight. *Hospital Medicine*, **2**, 937

Egan, D.F., Illingworth, R.S. and MacKeith, R. (1969) *Developmental Screening 0-5 Years*, Clinics in Developmental Medicine no. 30. SIMP, Heinemann, London.

Elek, S.D. and Stern, H. (1974) Development of vaccine against mental retardation caused by cytomegalovirus infection in utero. *Lancet*, **i**, 1

Elliott, S., Morten, R.E. and Whitelaw, R.A.J. (1988) Atlantoaxial instability and abnormalities of the odontoid in Down's syndrome. *Archives of Diseases in Childhood*, **63**, 1484

Emery, A.E.H. (1977) Folates and fetal central nervous system malformations. *Lancet*, **i**, 703

Forbes, G.B., Bryson, M.F., Manning, I., Amirhakini, G.H. and Reiha, I.C. (1972) Impaired calcium homeostasis in the infantile hypercalcaemic syndrome. *Acta Paediatrica Scandinavica*, **61**, 305

Fredrick, I. and Butler, N.R. (1970) Certain causes of neonatal death. 11. Intraventricular haemorrhage. *Biology of the Neonate*, **15**, 257

Freeman, R.D. and Pearson, P.H. (1978) Counselling with parents. *Care of the Handicapped Child* (ed. J. Apley), William Heinemann Medical Books, London

German, J., Kowal, A. and Ehlers, K.H. (1970) Trimethadione and human teratogenesis. *Teratology*, **3**, 349

Gordon, N. (1972) Parent counselling. *Developmental Medicine and Child Neurology*, **14**, 657

Gordon, N., King, E. and Mackay, R.I. (1967) Lead absorption in children. *British Medical Journal*, **i**, 480

Gordon, N. and Thursby-Pelham, D. (1969) The Sanfilippo syndrome: an unusual disorder of mucopolysaccharide metabolism. *Developmental Medicine and Child Neurology*, **11**, 485

Gutler, F. and Hanson, G. (1977) Different phenotypes for phenylalanine-hydroxylase deficiency. *Annals of Clinical Biochemistry*, **14**, 124

Hagberg, B. (1975) Pre-, peri- and postnatal prevention of major neuropaediatric handicaps. *Neuropädiatrie*, **6**, 331

Hagberg, B. (1989) Rett syndrome: clinical peculiarities, diagnostic approach, and possible cause. *Pediatric Neurology*, **5**, 75

Hagberg, B., Aicardi, J., Dias, K. and Ramos, O. (1983) A progressive syndrome of autism, dementia, ataxia and loss of purposeful hand use in girls: Rett's syndrome: report of 35 cases. *Annals of Neurology*, **14**, 471

Hambleton, G. and Appleyard, W.I. (1973) Controlled trial of fresh frozen plasma in asphyxiated low birth-weight infants. *Archives of Disease in Childhood*, **48**, 31

Hanson, J.W. and Smith, D.W. (1975) The fetal hydantoin syndrome. *Journal of Pediatrics*, **87**, 285

Hanson, J.W., Jones, K.L. and Smith, D.W. (1976) Fetal alcohol syndrome. Experience with 41 patients. *Journal of the American Medical Association*, **235**, 458

Harris, H. (1970) Genetical theory and the 'Inborn errors of metabolism'. *British Medical Journal*, **i**, 321

Hibbard, E.D. and Smithells, R.W. (1965) Folic acid metabolism and human embryopathy. *Lancet*, **i**, 1254

Holmström, G., Almond, G., Temple, K. and Baraitser, M. (1990) The iris in Williams syndrome. *Archives of Disease in Childhood*, **65**, 987–9

Hulse, J.A., Grant, D.B., Jackson, D. and Clayton, B.E. (1982) Growth, development and reassessment of hypothyroid infants diagnosed by screening. *British Medical Journal*, **i**, 1435

Illingworth, R.S. (1979) Why blame the obstetrician? A review. *British Medical Journal*, **i**, 797

Jackson, R.H. (1978) Hazards to children in traffic. *Archives of Disease in Childhood*, **53**, 807

Jones, K.L. and Smith, D.W. (1973) Recognition of the fetal alcohol syndrome in early infancy. *Lancet*, **ii**, 999

Jones, K.L., Smith, D.W., Ulleland, C.N. and Streissguth, A.P. (1973) Patterns of malformations in offspring of chronic alcoholic mothers. *Lancet*, **i**, 1267

Jordan, B.R. (1987) Human genetics: fragile sites still a mystery. *Lancet*, **i**, 492

Komrower, G.M. (1969) Metabolic abnormalities and mental retardation. *British Journal of Hospital Medicine*, **2**, 840

Komrower, G.M., Lambert, A.M., Cusworth, D.C. and Westall, R.G. (1966) Dietary treatment of homocystinuria. *Archives of Disease in Childhood*, **41**, 666

Lammer, E.J., Sever, L.E. and Oakley, G.F. (1987) Teratogen update-valproic acid. *Teratology*, **35**, 465

Larroche, I.C. (1972) Post-haemorrhagic hydrocephalus in infancy. Anatomical study. *Biology of the Neonate*, **20**, 287

Leech, R.W. and Kohnen, P. (1974) Subependymal and intraventricular haemorrhages in the newborn. *American Journal of Pathology*, **77**, 465

Lekman, A., Witt-Engerstrom, I., Hagberg, B. *et al.* (1989) Rett syndrome: biogenic amines and metabolites in postmortem brain. *Pediatric Neurology*, **5**, 357

Levene, M.I., Wigglesworth, J.S. and Dubowitz, V. (1981) Cerebral structure and intraventricular haemorrhage in the neonate: a real-time ultrasound study. *Archives of Disease in Childhood*, **56**, 416

Lou, H.C., Lassen, N.A. and Früs-Hanson, B. (1979) Is arterial hypertension crucial for the development of cerebral haemorrhage in premature infants. *Lancet*, **i**, 1215

Macfaul, R., Dorner, S., Brett, E.M. and Grant, D.B. (1978) Neurological abnormalities in patients treated for hypothyroidism from early life. *Archives of Disease in Childhood*, **53**, 611

MacKeith, R. (1973) The feelings and behaviour of parents of handicapped children. *Developmental Medicine and Child Neurology*, **15**, 524

Manley, G. and Williams, U. (1969) Urinary excretion of glycosaminoglycans in the various forms of gargoylism. *Journal of Clinical Pathology*, **22**, 67

Marshall, W.J S. (1967) Herpes simplex encephalitis treated with idoxuridine and external decompression. *Lancet*, **ii**, 579

Meadows, R. (1989) Poisoning. *British Medical Journal*, **298**, 1455

Neligan, G.A., Kolvin, I., Scott, D. and Garside, R.F. (1976) *Born Too Soon or Born Too Small*, Clinics in Developmental Medicine No. 61, William Heinemann Medical Books, London

Neufeld, E.F. and Muenzer, J. (1989) The mucopolysaccharidoses. In *The Metabolic Basis of Inherited Disease*, 6th edn. (eds. Scriver *et al.*). McGraw-Hill, New York

Oliver, I.E. (1975) Microcephaly following baby battering and shaking. *British Medical Journal*, **ii**, 262

Pape, K.E. and Wigglesworth, J.S. (1979) *Haemorrhage, Ischaemia and the Perinatal Brain*, Clinics in Developmental Medicine Nos. 69/70, William Heinemann Medical Books, London

Papile, L., Burnstein, J., Burnstein, R. and Koffler, H. (1978) Incidence and evolution of subependymal and intraventricular haemorrhage: a study of infants with birth weights less than 1500 gm. *Journal of Pediatrics*, **92**, 529

Peckham, C.S., Coleman, J.C., Hurley, R. *et al.* (1983) Cytomegalovirus infection in pregnancy: preliminary findings from a prospective study. *Lancet*, **i**, 1352

Robinson, R.O. (1979) Pathogenesis of intraventricular haemorrhage in the low-birth weight infant. *Developmental Medicine and Child Neurology*, **21**, 815

Ruta, D.A. and Leece, J.G. (1988) Screening policy for Down's syndrome. *Lancet*, **ii**, 752

Rutter, M. (1980) Raised lead levels and impaired cognitive/behavioural functioning: a review of the evidence. Supplement No. 42 *Developmental Medicine and Child Neurology*, **22**, 1

Schlesinger, B.E., Butler, N.R. and Black, J.A. (1956) Severe type of infantile hypercalcaemia. *British Medical Journal*, **i**, 127

Seip, M. (1976) Growth retardation, dysmorphic features and minor malformations following massive exposure to phenobarbitone in utero. *Acta Paediatrica Scandinavica*, **65**, 617

Simmons, M.A., Adcock, E.W., Bard, H. and Battaglia, F.C. (1974) Hypernatraemia and intracranial haemorrhage in neonates. *New England Journal of Medicine*, **291**, 6

Smith, I., Clayton, B.E. and Wolff, O.H. (1975) New variant of phenylketonuria with progressive illness unresponsive to phenylalanine restriction. *Lancet*, **i**, 1108

Stern, H., Elek, S.D., Booth, J.C. and Fleek, D.G. (1969) Microbial causes of mental retardation. *Lancet*, **ii**, 443

Thalhammer, O. (1973) Prevention of congenital toxoplasmosis. *Neuropädiatrie*, **4**, 233

Towbin, A. (1969) Mental retardation due to germinal matrix infarction. *Science*, **164**, 156

Tsiantos, A., Victorin, L., Relier, I.P. *et al.* (1974) Intracranial haemorrhage in the prematurely born infant. *Journal of Pediatrics*, **85**, 854

Turner, G. and Opitz, J.M. (1980) X-linked mental retardation. *American Journal of Medical Genetics*, **7**, 407

Turner, G., Robinson, H., Laing, S. and Purvis-Smith, S. (1986) Preventive screening for the fragile X syndrome. *New England Journal of Medicine*, **315**, 607

Udwin, O. (1990) A survey of adults with Williams syndrome and idiopathic infantile hypercalcaemia. *Developmental Medicine and Child Neurology*, **32**, 129

Walfish, P.G., Ginsberg, J., Rosenberg, R.A. and Howard, N.J. (1979) Results of a regional cord blood screening programme for detecting neonatal hypothyroidism. *Archives of Disease in Childhood*, **54**, 171

Ward, N.J., Cuckle, H.S., Densem, J.W. *et al.* (1988) Maternal serum screening for Down's syndrome in early pregnancy. *British Medical Journal*, **297**, 883

Westall, R.G. (1963) Dietary treatment of a child with maple syrup urine disease (branch chain ketoaciduria). *Archives of Disease in Childhood*, **38**, 485

Whitley, R.J., Soong, S., Dolin, R. *et al.* (1977) Adenine arabinoxide therapy of biopsy proved herpes simplex encephalitis. *New England Journal of Medicine*, **297**, 289

Wigglesworth, J.S. and Husemeyer, R.P. (1977) Intracranial birth trauma in vaginal breech delivery: the continued importance of injury to the occipital bone. *British Journal of Obstetrics and Gynaecology*, **84**, 684

Yu, I.S. and O'Halloran, M.T. (1970) Children of mothers with phenylketonuria. *Lancet*, **i**, 210

Zackai, E.H., Mellman, W.J., Neiderer, B. and Hanson, J.W. (1975) The fetal trimethadione syndrome. *Journal of Pediatrics*, **87**, 280

Zappella, M., Genazzani, A., Facchinetti, F. and Hayek, G. (1990) Bromocriptine in the Rett syndrome. *Brain and Development*, **12**, 221–225

Zellweger, H. and Simpson, J. (1977) *Chromosomes of Man*, William Heinemann Medical Books, London

6 Specific disorders of learning

Specific learning difficulties are present when a child's acquisition of a particular skill seems more difficult than would be expected from his or her overall development, and when there are no obvious social or environmental factors adequate to account for all the problems. External factors that can accentuate learning difficulties include absence from school due to illness or truancy, inappropriate teaching, emotional disturbances due to discord in the home, and disabilities such as defective vision and high-tone deafness which may well go unnoticed. Such specific disorders of learning can be genetically determined, as will be discussed later; but in many instances they seem to occur for the same acquired reasons that can result in major disorders of cerebral function. Whether the outcome is severe mental or physical handicap or a more subtle type of disability will depend on the degree of damage, its timing and the part of the brain involved. The concept of a 'continuum of reproductive casualty' cannot be accepted as it stands (Pasamanick and Knobloch, 1960), with the implication that everyone suffers a degree of damage during pregnancy and birth, for which there is no evidence. There are a number of other models: the additive model, in which socio-economic variables are added to the medical events; the threshold model, suggesting that there is a limit to human adaptability and that if a series of medical and social risk factors occur a point will come when evidence of a disability will be inevitable; the interaction model, in which a 'continuum of caretaking casualty' is added to the 'continuum of reproductive casualty'; and perhaps the most favoured model, the transactional model which recognizes the continuing interplay of influences throughout development so that the child elicits responses from his or her environment according to his or her characteristics at the time, the influence of the environment will produce a response from the child, which may in turn modify his or her environment, and so on. In particular this model emphasizes the complexity of the problem (Stratton, 1977).

In this chapter certain learning disorders will be discussed in the chronological order in which learning abilities usually develop. Perceptual motor skills are acquired first, then spoken language and, with rare exceptions, it is only after having acquired these functions that the child learns to read.

Developmental disorders of perceptual motor skills

Analysis of perceptual motor function

Wedell (1968) has listed the many components that may be involved in perceptual motor function. Adequate peripheral sensory mechanisms are of importance; even a simple squint can lead to perceptual difficulties (Abercrombie, 1960). Then the information from the various sensory inputs must be integrated. Sensory perception will be influenced by such factors as attention span, memory and concept formation. Children with physical handicaps in early life are particularly liable to have lacked the experience essential for the development of concepts. Some of them perform badly on certain tasks until they are given a few clues as to what is involved; such children fail from lack of opportunity and not from any specific learning disability. Other children can perform perceptual tests quite well, but suffer from an obvious failure of motor organization; these children are more likely to have an inadequately developed body-image. Anyone who tries an unfamiliar task is likely to be clumsy until they have practised the movements for a while. Motor organization constitutes this develop-ment of patterns and memory of movements which underlie the acquisition of skills so that they can be done automatically. This applies to such tasks as playing the piano and the use of tools, which for skilful use have to become part of the body image. This simplified framework can be applied to learning difficulties of all types.

There will be some overlap between different kinds of disorder, but it is important to analyse the child's disability before planning treatment, and just as it is incorrect to teach all late readers by the same method, so also there is a danger in categorizing children as 'clumsy' and trying to help them all in the same way. Those with mainly perceptual difficulties will need tasks to be broken down into their component parts which can be frequently demonstrated in detail. The child's verbal ability must also be used in training. If these children are just told to do something they may not know what you are talking about. When the difficulties seem to be due to defects of motor organization, practice suitably motivated and rewarded, is likely to be the solution. The higher the intelligence and the more stable the child's emotional state, the more easily will these difficulties be overcome.

Although caution must be used in applying the results of studies on adults who have lost skills, to children who are trying to acquire them, the observations of Bogan (1969) may be of some relevance. Bogan examined patients who had been operated on for intractable epilepsy, the operation consisting of a division of one half of the brain from the other. The results are compatible with the left side of the brain being concerned mainly with speech or propositional functions, while the right side is involved in perceptual motor or appositional functions. Acquired dyspraxia due to a left hemisphere lesion presents as a defect in the organization of movement, while a right hemisphere lesion is manifest as a disorganization of spatial perception. Also, as McFie (1970) pointed out, left hemisphere lesions show disorders of body image such as finger agnosia and right-left disorientation, while right hemisphere lesions confirm that this part of the brain is concerned in the integration of data from the various senses which enables us to orientate in space.

If such disorders occur in an acquired lesion among adults, one cannot help speculating whether similar distinctions between left and right hemisphere dis-turbances of function cannot be made in childhood. If genetic and environmental factors play a part in the failure of the development of higher cerebral functions in childhood, there seems to be no reason why they should not affect one cerebral hemisphere more than another. In fact, there is evidence to suggest that generalized cerebral insults cause the most severe damage in that part of the brain which is functionally less active at the time (Taylor, 1969).

The proportion of clumsy children who are left-handed is higher than average, but the importance of this finding is difficult to assess (Touwen, 1972). It may be related to both genetic and acquired factors (Gordon, 1986a). We live in a 'right-handed world', so it does not help to prefer the left hand, but more important than this is the possibility that in some children left-handedness is a symptom of cerebral dysfunction. Certain families contain a number of left-handers, but the genetic factor is of little relevance to learning disorders. Other children may take a long time to show any evidence of cerebral dominance, or may prefer to do some things with the right hand, suggesting an acquired or forced left-handedness. The importance of the findings lies in the support they give for an acquired cerebral lesion causing the disabilities, rather than in the fact that the child prefers to use one or other hand (Bishop, 1983).

The clumsy child

The very clumsy child is easy to recognize, although as he or she grows older the clinical picture may become more and more obscured by the complicating emotional and behavioural disorders. Developmental milestones may be delayed, and there may be difficulties with articulation. The child will always be dropping things and falling, tripping over his or her own feet. He or she will be late in learning tasks such as doing up buttons and tying up shoelaces. The child's movements are awkward and inco-ordinated, and he or she lacks the grace of the normal child after infancy. He or she is likely to be bad at doing puzzles and building models, and may not even attempt them. He or she tends to be poor at ball games, on which popularity at school is likely to depend, and one of the main difficulties at school may arise from the child's illegible writing (Fig. 6.1). On examination, apart from the difficulties of co-ordination, there may be fine, jerky (choreiform) movements of the unsupported limbs, persistence of associated movements, slight abnormalities of the reflexes and other 'soft' neurological signs (Touwen, 1979). There may also be obvious failures in perceptual tasks, e.g. recognizing objects and fitting shaped blocks into appropriately shaped holes. Behaviour may be unrestrained, with difficulties of concentration and rapid swings of mood, but this is by no means always so, and the child can become increasingly depressed and withdrawn as time goes on.

In a survey carried out on 810 children in Cambridge (Brenner *et al.*, 1967) the affected children had been regarded as being abnormally awkward, clumsy, untidy, difficult and irritating for a very long time. Of the 54 children identified as having this type of disability only one had been referred for help, and this child had attended a child psychiatric clinic on account of an emotional disorder, rather than a perceptual

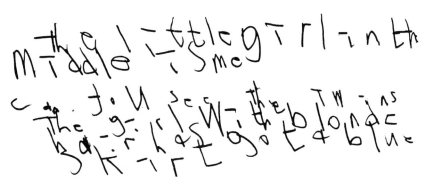

Figure 6.1   An example of illegible handwriting. It reads: 'The little girl in the middle is me. Can you see the twins? The girl with the blonde hair has got a blue skirt'.

motor disability or difficulty in learning. Information on the incidence of clumsy children is scanty, but the figure may be about 6% of children (aged 5–11 years) in normal schools. The problem is probably greater than this as the disability affects all levels of intelligence.

Aetiology

'Clumsy' children do show an increased incidence of complications before, during and after birth (Prechtl and Stemmer, 1962), although in an unpublished study carried out in Manchester it was not possible to involve any single factor in the past history of clumsy children, except possibly for anoxia during pregnancy, which occurred more frequently than in controls. Brown (1976) followed up a group of infants with symptomatic neonatal asphyxia, and compared with normal controls there was evidence of an association between the asphyxia and a variety of handicaps, including motor incoordination, epilepsy, speech retardation and school problems.

Learning depends so much on associations; between various sensory inputs, patterns of past experience, memories, and emotional content. Specific learning disorders are therefore most likely to result from a failure to establish these links, rather than from an absence of neurons, which tends to occur from cerebral insults in early pregnancy causing severe mental retardation. Cerebral connections may fail to develop, be destroyed or not used, and the concept of non-connection syndromes is referred to again when discussing specific disorders of language development.

Malnutrition, either from maternal starvation or from starvation of the fetus due to deficient food supply through the placental circulation, can have a permanent effect on brain development during the spurt of brain growth starting in mid-pregnancy and lasting at least until the end of the second year of life (Dobbing, 1970). This spurt of growth is mainly due to dendritic and axonal arborisation, and myelination, but it is of interest in relation to co-ordination that during this period microneurons are developing in the cerebellum (Shimada and Morikawa, 1978). A total of 14% of the series of 115 clumsy children studied in Manchester had a birth weight of 2.5 kg or less, compared with the overall incidence of 6–7%. In the context of learning disorders in general Francis-Williams and Davies (1974) found that 20% of 105 children weighing less than 1.5 kg at birth had learning difficulties.

In his studies on the effects of hypoxia during pregnancy as well as at birth, Towbin (1969) stresses that intra-uterine life and birth are a somewhat perilous time. It may be hard to accept his contention that if it were not for the hypoxia and mechanical damage occurring at this time there would be more geniuses among us, but it may nevertheless explain the difference between two brothers, one a dextrous athlete and one an 'awkward child'. If the hypoxia during pregnancy is not too severe the fetus will survive to be born normally at full term but of low birth-weight. Hypoxia occurring during birth at full term, or after birth from conditions such as hyaline membrane disease, may also be of significance, as any lack of oxygen to the brain can cause irreparable destruction to the interneuronal connections which are developing so rapidly at this time. Drillien (1972) also stresses that adverse factors in late pregnancy are more likely to be related to minor neurological abnormalities resulting in subtle disabilities such as learning disorders, rather than to very severe handicaps. It has been shown by CT scan that about one third of children with inco-ordination difficulties have cerebral abnormalities such as cerebral atrophy, asymmetry or anomalies, marked enough to be demonstrated by this technique (Bergström and Bille, 1978). Arrested hydrocephalus is another fairly common cause of clumsiness.

It is intriguing to ask to what extent learning can determine and maintain these dendritic connections. Animal experiments have shown that function exerts an effect on them after birth. When studying visual responses their maintenance depends on the interaction of stimuli from the two eyes: is it not possible that lack of experience also affects brain structure (Gaze, 1970)? Associations may not be developed at critical periods of learning due, for example, to lack of stimulation or emotional disturbances, and it is interesting to speculate how far the average individual falls below his or her potential because of lack of appropriate stimulation at the optimum time. It has been convincingly shown by positron emission tomography (PET) that connections do disappear during childhood, presumably if they are not used.

Although genetic factors seem to be relatively uncommon among 'clumsy' children, they cannot be ignored. They will be discussed again in relation to reading retardation, but the fact that gross disorders such as absence of the corpus callosum can sometimes be genetically determined raises interesting possibilities. Skills definitely run in certain families, so it is not unreasonable to consider that the opposite may occur.

Recognition of the disability

If the child is to be given the necessary help to cope with this disability it must be identified at an early age. Assessment is started by the mother and other members of the family. Although she may feel her child is awkward and clumsy she probably says nothing of this when the child starts school. Children attending nursery schools are also quite likely to be recognized if they are unduly clumsy. However, it does seem important to have a few simple tests which can be given soon after school entry at the age of 5 years, perhaps as part of the initial school medical examination, to identify those children who may for one reason or another be at risk (Bax and Whitmore, 1973). Such an assessment of clumsy children is best carried out at this age (rather than earlier as in the case of children with disorders of language development) because, unless very severely affected, they are unlikely to be under significant pressure, or their parents unduly worried, until they enter school. Also, as Piaget has shown, it is not until the age of 4–7 years that children can see one thing in relation to another and take account of proximity, separation, order and continuity (Beard, 1969).

Those severely affected will need to be examined in more detail to see what form their clumsiness takes and in what spheres they need special help. The 'routine' neurological examination is usually not sensitive enough to demonstrate adequately these children's disability, and the doctor may have to employ special techniques as part of his or her neurological assessment. Some will work out standardized tests of their own (Peters, Romine and Dykman, 1975), but two tests that have proved useful in this respect are Stott's test of Motor Impairment, a modification of the Gollnitz-Oseretsky test of motor ability, and the Frostig Developmental Test of Visual Perception. In the former there are five items for each year of the chronological age from 5 to 15 years. A start is made with the test items for the child's chronological age, and the testing is continued until the subject passes a complete year-level. The Frostig test, standardized for 3–9-year-olds, is subdivided into tests for eye-hand co-ordination, figure-ground perception, form constancy, perception of position in space and spatial relationships. Other tests that can be of assistance include the Imitation of Gesture, standardized for 3–8-year-olds by Bergès and Lézine. These tests can be used as an extension of the routine neurological examination. If more expert help is available the Griffiths Mental Development Scale can be used. This is now standardized for children up to 8 years old, and is now being revised. It is subdivided into locomotion, personal-social, hearing and speech, eye and hand co-ordination, performance, and practical reasoning scales. The Weschler Intelligence Scale for Children is also helpful so long as the mental age is not under seven, as the disparity between the performance scale and verbal scale IQs may be particularly striking. Under this age, the Weschler Pre-School and Primary Scale of Intelligence can be used. With information from such tests, it should be possible to identify the needs of a particular child, although it is not always easy to ensure that appropriate help is given.

Management of children with perceptual-motor disabilities

Many children have difficulties in acquiring perceptual-motor functions, but, as with other learning difficulties, only a few will be severely affected. The majority are likely to progress satisfactorily if given extra help and understanding in the early stages of their school careers. Teaching methods likely to help these children, such as the Montessori technique, are used in infant classes. Ideally, the more severely affected child should be given individually-programmed help in a remedial class where he or she can receive a fair amount of individual attention, whether this is based on such methods as the Frostig programme for the development of visual perception or on programmes devised by individual teachers. Special use will need to be made of the child's verbal skills, as these will almost certainly be better than his or her ability to carry out actions; for instance, the child may find it easier if he or she names what he or she has to discriminate. The child may not at first be able to draw a diamond, but if this concept is verbalized to the figure with the four points then he or she may be able to do so. The teacher obviously has an essential part to play, not only in helping the child to overcome or circumvent his or her learning difficulties, but in building up the child's confidence and demonstrating that he or she can succeed in tasks he or she may be reluctant to attempt. It is of the utmost importance to impress on the parent and the teacher that the child must be given the opportunity to succeed, and must be given every credit for trying. Occasionally a child will be so severely affected that he or she may be unable to manage in an ordinary school, and such alternatives as schools for physically handicapped children may have to be considered in order to obtain the help needed.

Apart from the analysis of clumsiness already considered, Paine and Oppé (1966) have stressed that the underlying inco-ordination may affect these children in various ways. These include impairment of gross movements such as walking, running or climbing; finer co-ordination, of individual finger movements or of movements of the bulbar muscles; and visuo-motor co-ordination as in drawing, writing or catching a ball. Clumsy children of average or above average intelligence have a reasonable chance of finding ways of compensating for their disability, although not all of them succeed. As has been stated, children of below average intelligence almost certainly will not do so, and are therefore in particular need of help (Dare and Gordon, 1970). As with other disabilities of this kind there is a considerable overlap between different types of handicap, and there is a high incidence of speech disorders among 'clumsy' children. When the disability is unrecognized the child is often referred to the out-patient clinic because of such complaints as headaches or abdominal pain, behavioural disorders, slow progress at school and emotional disturbances, and only later is found to have perceptual-motor disorders.

When the child's disability is unrecognized he or she will attempt tasks which seem to present no particular difficulty to his or her peers, and fail. This may happen many times, until the child quite naturally gives up the struggle. But by then he or she may have acquired such labels as 'a lazy child', 'a behaviour problem', or 'a child who could do better if he or she tried'. The trouble is that many of these children have tried many times and failed, as no-one has understood their problems. There can be few things so disheartening to a child as failure in the first few years at school, particularly if the child is unjustly treated. Many of the secondary problems that occur among these children, and which tend to be so hard to treat could surely be prevented to a great extent by early recognition of the disability and by giving appropriate help. If the child's difficulties are carefully analysed, the physiotherapist and the occupational therapist can plan various ways of helping the co-ordination of both large and fine movements, depending on the child's needs. The exercises can be supervised by the parents, as it is almost always an advantage to involve the parents in the child's treatment (Gordon and Grimley, 1974; Gordon and McKinlay, 1980).

Developmental speech and language disorders

Specific disorders of language development

It may be argued that the acquisition of one's mother tongue does not have to be learnt; that the human brain is so structured that it has propensities which enable it to extract from the linguistic input the relevant data needed to organize language into a consistent system. That may be so for the average child, but not for the child who, for one reason or another, is slow to develop language; and even for the average child it is only a half-truth. The child's environment will affect the richness and complexity of language and the ability to express feelings and ideas. The baby will convey messages to its mother by the way it vocalizes, and when babbling commences at about the age of 6 months links are formed between tactual, kinaesthetic and auditory stimuli, and so the relationship between hearing and uttering. Soon the sounds produced by babbling begin to resemble those produced in the child's environment. Some draw a sharp division between babbling and speech, but it seems more likely that language slowly arises from babbling by means of selective reinforcement, mainly by the pleasure of the parents. The child begins to associate sound combinations with particular situations, people or objects, and the use of symbolic utterances arises on this foundation, but the comprehension of symbols so they have meaning is a task of some complexity. The formation of concepts is an essential foundation of language which puts the physically handicapped child at a particular disadvantage. For example if the motor disability is severe it may not be possible for the child to pour water from a jug into a glass, and to realize just what this involves. Once this inner language is established, the acquisition of receptive language can proceed with the association of symbols with meaning; and finally expressive language. The use of symbols to communicate is a vast step even when their meaning is well understood, and will depend a great deal on memory and imagery. It is relatively easy to learn to understand a foreign language but how much more difficult to speak it, and the same must surely apply to your mother tongue.

The age when a child of average intelligence first uses words with meaning varies widely, and many who are late in speaking develop quite normally. However, if a healthy child of average intelligence is not using words by 18 months to 2 years a specific disorder of language development will have to be considered. As with any other type of disability, speech disorders, unrelated to other handicaps, can vary from mild to very severe (Ingram, 1969); but the majority are in the first category and the children are likely to develop normally if given a little help in their early years. In mild cases there will be a delay in acquiring speech sounds; the infantile stages of speech development will persist for longer than normal, with difficulties of articulation. Speech therapy is not usually required. When the condition is more severe, comprehension of speech as well as its expression will be affected; if comprehension is fairly adequate by the age of 3 years, and provided that a severe dysarthria does not exist, the prognosis for the spoken word is fairly good. The children with severe disorders, quite apart from their disorder of language development, may have difficulty in distinguishing between less specialized sounds, and then may be said to suffer from congenital auditory imperception. Children with the semantic-pragmatic deficit disorder have defects of the higher order processing of language. They speak quite fluently, but the content of their speech is confused and often without much meaning; and they have great difficulties in expressing ideas.

The most severely affected children may show evidence of central deafness or auditory agnosia in early life; sounds of all kinds will lack meaning and sometimes will fail to elicit a response of any kind, even when the peripheral pathways appear to be intact. This emphasizes that we do not hear with our ears; or see with our eyes. They are excellent microphones and cameras to generate electrical currents in response to appropriate stimuli, but if the brain is unable to attach meaning to these electrical impulses you are just as deaf as if you have no ears or as blind as if you have no eyes. However, the cause of the abnormal response to auditory stimuli can be very difficult to assess, especially as central and peripheral damage are often associated. The cerebral cortex and auditory nuclei in the brain-stem may be equally vulnerable to causal factors such as anoxia at birth, so that both central and peripheral deafness will result. It may sometimes be necessary to use a number of investigations to establish the level of the lesion, including stapedial response audiometry, electrocochleography, crossed acoustic response audiometry (Henderson, 1975), and even such sophisticated techniques as auditory-evoked potentials to ascertain if the impulse reaches a cortical level, the EEG trace being averaged by a computer. The latter has largely superseded tests like the EEG audiogram, which shows only a non-specific alerting response to sounds during sleep (Gordon and Taylor, 1964). However, evoked-response audiometry can give false-negative and false-positive results, and needs to be interpreted with the repeated application of other investigations. A few of these very disabled children will never acquire the spoken word, although they may learn to read and write if given the necessary teaching (Gordon, 1966). As they grow older they characteristically begin to react to sounds and all but the most severely affected will show increasing evidence of language function, that is as long as their disability is fairly specific and does not involve a fundamental defect of symbolization.

When a child with normal ears and normal auditory nerves does not respond to sound there is a possibility that the stimulus never reaches a cortical level, or if it does, it is not transmitted to the association areas which will give it meaning. Many acquired disorders of cerebral function among adults are ascribed to 'disconnection' of one area of the brain from another (Geschwind, 1965). Therefore, why should there not be 'non-connection syndromes' as suggested in the discussion on perceptual-motor disorders.

As with 'clumsy' children, a failure of such connections to be made, resulting in a disorder of language development, is likely to be due to acquired and to genetic factors. For example, Woods (1976) found that in a survey of children with various disabilities perinatal morbitity caused delay in language development in a significant number of children. This perinatal damage caused both receptive and expressive disorders of language and defects of articulation. One point of importance to the problem of delayed language development may be the effects of inhibition. The concept of the 'lazy eye' is accepted, the child with a squint ceasing to appreciate the stimulus from what may be a healthy eye in order to avoid the intolerable burden of double vision. The fact that it may become permanent shows the power of the brain to inhibit afferent stimuli. If auditory stimuli lack meaning for a prolonged period, may not the brain inhibit these, with the result that the child has 'lazy ears'? Obviously, the assessment of children with such a severe disability takes a long time, but having as far as possible excluded peripheral deafness, is it sufficient to sit back and await events? It may be that it is equally important to keep alive an awareness of sound in children with severe auditory agnosia as it is to fit a peripherally deaf child with a hearing aid. One way of doing this is to convert auditory stimuli into visual ones by converting the sounds a child makes into patterns on a television screen.

Management

Many children with disorders of speech development will overcome their difficulties, but often at considerable cost. The price may be their other intellectual attainments and their emotional well-being. Expansion of speech therapy services and closer co-operation between speech therapists and teachers may well help these children, but there is a need for more research into methods of treatment and for follow-up studies on those already in use. Children with disorders of language development are among the most difficult to assess, and many of the intelligence scales in use are too verbally orientated. It may be necessary to use a battery of tests and repeat them over a period of time. Some of these, such as the Reynell Developmental Language Scales, are undoubtedly helpful. The education of these children raises many problems, as language is so fundamental to thought and intelligence. Those most severely affected will need individual attention in special units, as so often applies to children with a variety of disabilities. Those less severely affected should, as far as possible, be given the help they need in a normal environment. Children may learn language from adults but they tend to practise it on other children. Admission to a nursery school may help the under fives as long as they have sufficient understanding not to become increasingly confused by the variety of sounds they hear.

The use of language in relation to objects and movements gives the child the best chance of associating the sounds we make with meaning. It is essential to talk in a loud voice, as the child with delayed language development is likely to be running around the room and not sitting on his or her mother's knee. Also important is learning to listen. It is helpful to emphasize to parents that the first word a child uses with meaning can occur only when comprehension of speech is well advanced. The first word is therefore a late stage in language development, and to reach it the parents will have to talk to the child for months on end and ask very little in return. But this does not mean that nothing is happening, although the time-lag stresses the tremendous advance that has to be made between the comprehensive and expressive stages of language development. As already stated a limited analogy is that it is obviously easier to understand a foreign language than to speak it.

A number of teaching techniques have been developed: some depend on the building up of the memory and sequence of sounds in words, and then associating the word with meaning; another uses different colours to denote nouns, prepositions, adjectives and adverbs, and bases sentence structure on this (Gordon, 1966). There is no doubt that these children have difficulties in building up the associations which give sensory stimuli their meaning, and it seems reasonable to encourage all possible means of overcoming this. Occasionally, because of a severe disorder of language development or from some other reason such as physical and mental handicap, it becomes apparent that the child is never going to make reasonable use of the spoken word. Then the use of some other means of communication must be considered using signs or symbols. Such methods include the American Sign Language, the British Sign Language, the Paget-Gorman Sign System, Bliss Symbols, the Premark System and the Rebus System (Kiernan, 1977). Whatever method of teaching is used the needs of the individual child should be paramount, and the educational programme should be kept as flexible as possible. It is also important to take into account the emotional disturbances that these children can so easily develop, and not to ask them to attempt tasks beyond their capabilities. If they fail too often they may later on refuse to attempt skills which further development has in fact placed within their grasp. Any child who has suffered from and overcome delayed language development will be at risk later on from problems with reading and writing.

Disorders of language development related to other handicaps

Apart from these specific disorders, the development of language may be delayed for various other reasons (Ingram, 1969), and these must be assessed as a matter of urgency. Speech and language disorders are common enough, as Peckham (1973) has shown. Among children starting school at the age of 5 years in the UK, the speech of 14.4% of boys, and 9.7% of girls is not fully intelligible, and among 1.8% of boys and 0.9% of girls most of their words are unintelligible.

Deafness

When a child is not talking at the expected age the first responsibility is to exclude peripheral deafness, although this is not always easy in early life, even in the most skilled hands. High-tone deafness can be particularly hard to diagnose, but the effect of this on a child attempting to acquire language can only be realized when listening to speech from which the high tones have been extracted. The omission of 'e', 'f', 'sh', 'th' and 's' sounds in the child's speech is a very suggestive finding. As has been mentioned, the diagnosis of peripheral deafness is quite often complicated by central factors; for example, if there is a combination of central and peripheral deafness the fitting of a suitable hearing aid may be particularly difficult. Certain children are especially at risk from peripheral deafness, and need to be examined with care. These include children with a family history of deafness, or a history of rubella during pregnancy, anoxia at birth or jaundice after birth, premature babies who have been nursed in noisy incubators (Douek *et al.*, 1976), or those who have suffered from meningitis or have been treated with aminoglycosides during infancy. Also, deafness can easily be acquired during early life from inadequately treated infections of the ear. Children with cleft palate and palatal disproportion are very liable to middle ear infection. Such deafness is likely to vary from time to time, and consequently the diagnosis may be missed. If it occurs at an age when language function is rapidly progressing its effect may be critical and cause delayed development (Gordon, 1986b).

Guidance for parents of deaf children is essential, as has been shown by Williams

(1969). He found that if the diagnosis of deafness was made before the age of 2 years, language development might be slower than if the diagnosis was made at a later age. It was considered that this might be due to associated brain damage, the difficulty of supplying the correct type of hearing aid, or the effect of changed parental attitudes. This study is not a criticism of early diagnosis but of our methods. If the implications of the diagnosis and management are not discussed with the parents there is no doubt that the recognition of a disability may add to the parents' anxieties, rather than reassure them. The parents' approach to the child is likely to change when they know what is wrong; for instance, they may stop talking to their partially deaf child, and his or her language development is bound to be affected as a result of this. The undeserved stigma of deafness may lead some parents to reject the deaf child to a surprising degree.

Mental retardation

Once hearing has been examined, the problem is often to assess the child's mental development as a cause for delayed speech. It may be difficult to come to any definite conclusion without a prolonged period of observation, and it is always necessary to give the patient the benefit of the doubt. Once a child has been labelled as mentally handicapped he or she will be at a disadvantage from the point of view of social contacts and stimulus to speech development. Parents always tend to talk to their mentally handicapped children in a restricted way. They may correct the child's sentence structure, but will not enrich the child's experience of language, presumably because they have been told to talk to the child in as simple a fashion as possible (Cashdan, 1969); although to a degree this may well be necessary. By such means children tend to fulfil the expectations made for them, even though the expectations are too low.

Physical handicap

Physically handicapped children are at a particular disadvantage owing to their lack of experience. Their world can consist of home and special school, and anything outside this has little meaning for them. There is no doubt that it is sometimes difficult to be sure if the child's speech retardation is due almost entirely to environmental factors or if there is any underlying defect. Speech therapy has a particular role to play in the management of mentally and physically handicapped children, by enlarging their horizons and trying to give them experiences they have lacked. This in itself may result in a rapid improvement in language function. Surely the one thing that can make the life of a handicapped child tolerable is a means of communication, even if this must be mainly by gestures, word-cards, typing or writing.

Severe emotional disorders and psychoses

Emotional disorders such as anxiety or depression in early childhood will often affect language development. There is confusion over the diagnosis of childhood psychosis and autism. To 'diagnose' a child as *autistic* is to recognize a behaviour pattern in which the child is withdrawn from the environment and lives in a world of his or her own. There may be many associated phenomena, such as acute anxiety, odd mannerisms and fixed habits. The effect on language development will depend on the time of onset and the cause of the disorder. If the behaviour pattern is present from birth, expressive speech may be absent and the understanding of speech may be very variable. If the onset is later in childhood, speech already acquired before this time will then be lost. It seems that the condition can be related to disorders of perception and language development, mental retardation and other evidence of brain damage, and sometimes blindness and deafness are complicating factors. Often there is no apparent cause that can be established for certain, but there is no reason to consider the condition is synonymous with schizophrenia among adults. Perhaps the common factor, whatever the related disability, is the inability of the child to make any sense of his or her environment because of a basic cognitive defect resulting in severe perceptual difficulties combined with delayed language development (Rutter, 1970). Current concepts on the cause of autism recognize the cognitive deficits, combined with deviant development and that they are most probably the result of some kind of developmental disorder of organic origin. So treatment can be based on the fostering of normal development, a reduction of rigidity and stereotypy that effects so much of these children's functioning, the elimination of non-specific maladaptive behaviour, and alleviation of family distress (Rutter, 1984).

Admittedly, these children are among the most difficult to assess, and a prolonged period of observation and 'education' is almost always necessary before it can be said if the child will respond or not. There is therefore a great need for special units, even if these are very demanding in terms of staffing ratios; and they should be closely linked to all the diagnostic services available.

When a girl presents with autistic behaviour and gives a history of rapid dementia in the first few years of life, followed by slow progression with symptoms such as ataxia, hyperventilation and stereotyped washing and clapping movements of the hands, the possible diagnosis of Rett syndrome must be considered (Hagberg *et al.*, 1983). Asperger's syndrome shows lesser degrees of withdrawal, and although affected children are often very clumsy, language function can be relatively well preserved. This syndrome will be discussed in Chapter 13.

Loss of speech

Loss of already acquired speech is always a worry. If this occurs only in certain situations it may be due to elective mutism, a condition which is difficult to treat, probably because it is a symptom of a profound emotional disorder. A radical change in the child's environment may have some effect, for example admission to a hospital or a residential school, but the prognosis tends to be bad, as the emotional disorder is so severe. Cerebral degenerative diseases have to be considered, as well as focal space-occupying lesions. There is a rare syndrome of acquired dysphasia of unknown cause, although some type of 'encephalitis' has been suggested (Landau and Kleffner, 1957), in which there is a loss of language function, often for long periods, in association with an EEG showing spike-wave activity with temporal lobe predominance. The child may or may not have clinical seizures (*acquired auditory agnosia* or the *Landau Kleffner syndrome*). The prognosis is very variable and treatment has to be symptomatic (Shoumaker *et al.*, 1974; Gordon, 1990).

In these days trauma is a common cause of brain damage. Such injuries in children affecting the dominant hemisphere will retard subsequent speech development and cause a loss of speech already acquired, although the younger the child the more readily will the contralateral hemisphere be able to adapt. Such acquired dysphasia is characterized by reduced expressive activity of the spoken and written word and gesture. There is often a complete lack of spontaneous speech, and disorders of articulation are common. These children have particular difficulties in finding words and in the construction of grammatical sequences (Alajouanine and Lhermitte, 1965). Those interested in the effects of brain damage on language ability will be fascinated by Charles Dickens' account of Laura Bridgeman (Gordon, 1969).

Reading retardation

Much that has already been discussed also applies to children with reading retardation, and it must again be emphasized that there is a considerable overlap between various disabilities of this kind. Although it is obviously important to recognize a child's particular problems there are dangers in too rigid a categorization when it comes to trying to help them. Reading backwardness may result from defective vision, inappropriate teaching, absenteeism from school, emotional disturbances, adverse social conditions, or mental retardation. Reading retardation can occur in apparent isolation while other aspects of the child's development proceed reasonably satisfactorily. However, although such alternative terms as 'dyslexia' or 'word blindness' are of use in drawing attention to a group of children who need special educational provision, they are apt to cause some confusion. Almost inevitably they will be applied to children who do not have specific learning difficulties but who are generally retarded or severely emotionally disturbed. Rutter (1969) has shown that there is nothing to suggest that dyslexia is a single condition distinguished by its purity and gravity. He suggests that there may be several dyslexias all due to different factors, linked because they are each due to some developmental neurological anomaly; in other words there are no clear-cut syndromes, and reading retardation is the end-product of the interaction of a number of only weakly related features. He also stresses that whatever is the basic cause of the different types of reading retardation, the final state is often the result of a combination of biological, social and psychological factors. Rutter, Tizard and Whitmore (1970) have defined reading backwardness as an attainment in reading accuracy or comprehension which, on the Neale test, is 28 months or more below the chronological age, and reading retardation when this attainment is 28 months or more below the level predicted on the basis of the child's age and IQ on a modified WISC (Weschler Intelligence Scale for Children).

Aetiology

The causes of reading retardation are likely to be as varied as for the other learning disorders already discussed. Genetic factors have always been emphasized, but in terms of a disorder with a dominant mode of inheritance there seems little evidence for this (Childs, 1972). There seems to be no single mode of genetic transmission which suggests genetic heterogenicity (Finucci, 1976). Also it cannot be assumed that a reported familial incidence is necessarily evidence of a genetic origin when there can be so many causes for a particular disability (Naidoo, 1972). There may, for example, be social reasons such as the size of the family. Complete concordance has been reported in uniovular twins but only in a third of binovular twins, which is certainly suggestive evidence for genetic influences; and as so often in conditions of this type there is likely to be an interaction of genetic and environmental factors. However, one finding which has to be explained is the predominance of boys with learning disorders, especially in the case of dyslexia. There could be polygenic expression which has a lower threshold for males than females, or the expression of a mutant at a single locus may be modified by sex. Also a possible explanation is the message of the Y chromosome (Ounsted and Taylor, 1972). It is suggested that this is effected through a regulation of the pace of development. If the development of boys is slower it will allow more time for learning, and will affect its pattern. The linguistic function of girls, at least in terms of fluency, will be more advanced than in boys of the same age, but often not in verbal comprehension and reasoning. Apart from this, the delayed maturation of boys will expose them over a longer period to increased risks derived from information resulting from imperfections in their genome; and, if it is accepted that immaturity of the brain is directly related to vulnerability to noxious agents, this will also mean that males will be more exposed to adverse environmental events for a longer time. This slower rate of development among boys in early childhood may result in some boys, compared with girls, being at a disadvantage in mixed classes when starting school.

Classification

Ingram (1960) classifies reading and writing difficulties in three separate groups, with considerable overlap between them; and the more complex the disorder, the worse the prognosis is likely to be.

Children with visuo-spatial disorders often run into difficulties when they start to learn to read. They have difficulties in recognizing the shapes of letters, and in orientating them correctly, so that they are perceived in their appropriate order. Mirror writing often persists, and the sequence of letters in short words or syllables may be reversed. It is therefore no wonder that reading and writing can be difficult for these children. Because of the problems of sequencing, the child has particular troubles with spelling. Also the visuo-spatial difficulties often result in clumsiness and inco-ordination, and as a result, illegible writing may be added to almost incomprehensible content.

In the second group, any child who is slow in acquiring the spoken word is at risk of having difficulties with reading and writing. Just as the child found it hard to give meaning to the symbolic sounds he or she heard, he or she then finds the symbolic signs that are read have no significance. He or she may be able to write mechanically to dictation, but cannot convert the meaning that needs to be conveyed into the written word.

The third group consists of children with correlating and synthesizing difficulties. The ability to relate visual symbols to the spoken sound is impaired and the child finds it difficult to identify what a group of letters represents and to build up the components of a word into the word itself. Equally, when writing, there is a difficulty in breaking words down into syllables and finding their written equivalents. In a study of children with reading disabilities Ingram, Mason and Blackburn (1970) found evidence of both visual-perceptual and audio-phonic inadequacy; the latter was particularly marked when there was under-achievement in reading and spelling only. This emphasizes that audio-phonic skills are the most important for reading.

Boder (1973) has suggested a somewhat similar classification. Her dysphonetic group have a defect in symbol/sound integration so that the child cannot develop phonetic word analysis/synthesis skills. The child recognizes words globally, and reading is easier in context as he or she can then make intelligent guesses. Spelling is by sight and not by ear, and tends to remain poor in later life. The dyseidectic group cannot perceive letters and whole words as configurations. They have a good auditory memory and, although poor spellers, their errors are not bizarre. These children are the only ones who can truly be said to be word-blind, although they form only 10% of the total numbers studied. They are especially slow and laborious readers. The third group who have both types of disorders are obviously in most serious trouble. Boder and Jarrico (1982) have constructed a useful test which helps to assign dyslectic children to these three groups.

Other children do not fit neatly into any of these groups. For example some seem to have a very specific defect of visual recognition. They have no difficulties with spoken language development and are not clumsy. They can spell words verbally without difficulty but not when they write it down as they cannot seem to recognize certain visual symbols correctly. This type of analysis showing the exact nature of the disability is essential in order to plan the methods for helping these children.

Management

Boder (1973) emphasized that in teaching these children it is logical to use the good channel; a 'look-and-say' approach, such as 'Breakthrough to Literacy' for those with a predominantly audio-phonic defect, and a phonetic approach when there is mainly a visual-perceptual disability. Other teaching methods include use of the Initial Training Alphabet. More books are needed which are of interest to older children and are written in simple language.

There is a great need for more detailed research of such complex functions as reading, writing and spelling. Kinsbourne (1973) has analysed some of these: discriminating forms, discriminating their orientation, and the sequence in which they are presented, breaking up a word into its phonemes, putting it together again, associating groups of shapes with a word, associating individual shapes with phonemes, and so on.

Those children with severe reading retardation, although their condition will certainly improve, may continue to have difficulties when they reach adult life. There are many bad spellers among us. It seems that there are a number of reasons for reading retardation, and one of the dangers of using such terms as 'dyslexia' is the implication that there is one cause and therefore one method of helping children with such a disability; quite apart from the frequent overlap of different types of learning disabilities. Once the child's difficulties have been recognized it is far more important to analyse these than to attach a label. As with many disabilities of this type there is a high association with emotional and behavioural complications, and these must receive due consideration (Critchley, 1968). They may be another indication of cerebral dysfunction or may be due to maladjustment to educational failure. Society is so orientated to an ability to read and write that it is easy enough to see how a child's failure to acquire this skill may cause him or her to rebel. Social factors such as large families, the attitude of the parents, and poor living conditions can also aggravate the difficulties of the child.

The hyperkinetic child

It has been emphasized that learning difficulties are liable to be associated with emotional and behavioural disorders, and it is easy to understand how the child's difficulties may lead to these complications. Sometimes the disorder is of a primary rather than a secondary nature, and this applies particularly to overactivity or hyperkinetic behaviour, although the *attention deficit disorder* or hyperkinetic syndrome is rare (Sandberg, Rutter and Taylor, 1978). Overactivity, and related symptoms, are most likely to be due to emotional disorders, possibly due to disturbances of the family background; boredom in school due to inappropriate teaching; and oversedation with drugs such as phenobarbitone, for example given in the treatment of epilepsy. The true syndrome like many other manifestations of 'minimal cerebral dysfunction', may follow complications before, during, or after birth, or may occur for no obvious reason. No doubt genetic and acquired factors both play their part. Certainly this behaviour pattern overlaps other disabilities such as epilepsy (Ounsted, 1955), specific learning disorders, and mental retardation. Although more common among children of below average intelligence, it can occur at all intelligence levels. The child is not able to settle to anything for long, has no powers of concentration, and is seemingly distracted by the slightest stimulus. This must have a profound effect on the child's ability to learn, quite apart from the strain it imposes on those caring for the child, particularly the parents. One of the most interesting features of the condition is the paradoxical response to certain drugs. There is no doubt that sedatives such as barbiturates may aggravate the overactivity of these children, and occasionally certain stimulants result in a dramatic improvement.

There may be a number of reasons for this pattern of behaviour, but one possibility seems to be the effects of over-stimulation. Much of the sensory input to the brain is inhibited and never reaches a conscious level. Factors such as concentration, attention and interest are of obvious importance, and the selection of sensory input appears to be one of the most active and complex functions that we ask of our brains. If this system is defective, due to injury or dysfunction of the diencephalon and brain-stem in early life, too many stimuli may reach a conscious level and the child responds first to one and then another in a seemingly endless series of disassociated actions. One hypothesis which may account for such a disorder is a disturbance of catecholamine metabolism at a diencephalic level. Then the giving of a sedative would further depress a system already working inefficiently, and, conversely, stimulants may improve its function by altering synaptic transmission. The child often seems to respond to a teaching situation in which stimulation is reduced to a minimum. The furniture and decorations in the room are few and simple, and only objects necessary for the task in hand are permitted. If the child can be on his or her own for a period, and be given individual attention the results may be particularly rewarding. The general paediatric ward is one of the most unsuitable situations for such a child.

Also, it is suggested that the behaviour of these children is characterized by short sampling. They cannot retain short-term memory traces so do not become familiar with their environment, and therefore explore it constantly. They respond on the basis of the immediately preceding event, and react very quickly, but inaccurately. In addition, they show inconsistency of response, and are little affected by past experiences. If sampling time can be increased this will improve the capacity to learn (Hutt and Hutt, 1964). It has been suggested that hyperkinetic children are under-aroused, which at least could explain the occasional beneficial action of stimulant drugs. However, in experiments with hyperkinetic children and controls, those of the former group who demonstrated a diminished response of the autonomic nervous system also showed that their abnormal behaviour was particularly related to anxiety (Conners, 1976).

When the condition is severe and a correct diagnosis has been made there is some justification for trying to modify it with medical treatment; as this may prevent such overactivity from interfering with learning and will obviously help in the management of the child. However, before doing this it is essential to exclude other causes, as already suggested. Dexamphetamine sulphate, pemoline or methylphenidate in increasing doses may be the most effective drugs, but in view of possible side-effects, such as lack of appetite, loss of weight and insomnia, it is probably justifiable to try others first. Phenothiazine derivatives can be helpful in this, as in other types of behaviour disorder. Haloperidol and diazepam are alternatives worthy of a trial. If anxiety is evident this will have to be treated and psychiatric advice may well be needed. Special help must be given in school if this is indicated.

If some degree of improvement can be obtained, relationships within the family will alter. When a child's behaviour causes considerable stress to others this is bound to affect their attitude to the child, and can easily result in a vicious circle, as all such relationships are a two-way process. When representing the interests of the hyperkinetic child, which is certainly the duty of the doctor involved in the care and management of such an individual, these interests must be related to the family situation. As has been discussed in relation to mentally handicapped children, many families appear to be able to adapt very well to the inevitable strains that will develop, but it is dangerous to generalize, and there must be provision for members of the more unstable families in the community. There is no doubt that more could be done in terms of support and help, such as more facilities for temporary care, better parent counselling services, and more and better assessment units within the community.

The role of the doctor

When so many of the problems of children with learning difficulties are educational it is reasonable to ask what role the doctor should play, and how he or she can be most effective. First of all, he or she must be a member of a team, his or her colleagues being physiotherapists, occupational therapists, speech therapists, psychologists, social workers and, last but not least, teachers (Gordon and McKinlay, 1980). From the medical point of view, the contribution of the first three will be most relevant to the child up to about the age of 7 years. The physiotherapists, for example, can play an important part in helping the child overcome inco-ordination of larger movements, and can advise on enjoyable activities such as swimming or riding at which the child may succeed; the occupational therapist may be more concerned with improving the child's finer movements and devising ways of bettering the activities of daily living; and the speech therapist must be involved in the assessment and treatment of disorders of language development as soon as these have been recognized. All three must involve the parents in helping their child as far as this is possible. Most parents are eager to do so, and, if they do not also become members of the team, the effectiveness of everyone else's efforts is likely to suffer.

Handicapped children rarely suffer from a single disability; the very presence of a disability is likely to result in emotional disturbances. Quite trivial handicaps, if they occur in conjunction with others, can have a significant effect on a child's progress. Therefore, all such children must have their vision and hearing carefully checked. To give another example, it is often stated that about 10% of children at schools for the deaf do not progress as expected, and this may well be due to such factors as difficulties with abstract thought, disorders of language development, marked perceptuo-motor disabilities, and emotional disturbances.

Also, children may be referred not because of learning difficulties but with a history of headache, abdominal pain, bed-wetting and behaviour problems, and it is only after taking a careful history that it is realized that stresses at school are the cause of the symptoms.

Ways in which the doctor can help with the analysis of the child's difficulties have already been indicated. In giving advice to the older child he or she can point out that the child does have certain handicaps which have interfered with learning, and stress that the child can be helped by methods other than those he or she has endured. It is also important to indicate that difficulties can be circumvented as well as overcome.

When talking to the parents it must be emphasized that the child has a real handicap which is no-one's fault. It is of the utmost importance to ensure that the child succeeds in some activities, and that everyone's efforts are not solely directed toward the child's disabilities. The doctor can offer to contact the Education Authorities over particular problems that arise, and he or she can certainly act as a questioner, for example checking if remedial teaching really has been of benefit to the child.

Discussions with teachers are likely to be of mutual benefit. They may react to the poor results of a child's work by blaming either themselves or the child, and it may help if they see themselves as diagnosticians of learning disorders, and as members of the therapeutic team. If the child has been under undue pressure at home and at school, removal of this pressure and ensured success in some field or other may be very effective in many instances. It should be realized that these children often have to try much harder than the average, and they must be given due credit for this. As a result, they are likely to tire towards the end of the school day, and the school term. They usually respond best to a structured classroom situation, with distractions reduced to a minimum. Considerable thought will have to be given to ways in which the child can be helped, for example if poor writing is one of the main problems, using a thick pencil, and writing on alternate lines may be of benefit. In view of fatigue, homework may need to be limited and carefully planned. At a later age it may be necessary to negotiate concessions for the child, such as extra time during examinations or the use of a typewriter. As the child grows older, it seems increasingly important to concentrate on the child's assets and to exploit his or her expressed interests rather than give too much time and effort to his or her weaknesses.

If the child with specific learning difficulties is of below average intelligence a realistic view must be taken of the child's potential. It may help to point out to parents that the greatest disservice you can do to a child is to place him or her in a situation which is not meaningful to the child, and where repeated failure may discourage him or her.

A major contribution of the doctor is surely to try to resolve some of the emotional problems so often related to learning disorders. It is so easy for the situation to get out of hand and involve the whole family, especially if learning is high on their list of priorities. The doctor can be willing to discuss the problems and, with the help of social workers, health visitors and teachers, may well be able to modify adverse home and school conditions.

Apart from emotional disturbances, behaviour disorders are common enough among children with learning difficulties, and the doctor must try to contribute to the treatment of these. Overactivity, truancy from school, destructive behaviour and aggression may well be the result of abnormal stresses at home and at school, just as depression and anxiety are, but may also result from failures of cerebral integration. Drugs are likely to have a limited role to play except in emergency situations. Stimulant drugs in the treatment of the hyperkinetic syndrome have been mentioned, and while other solutions are being sought anxiety and depression may have to be treated.

The doctor can also play his or her part in pressing for more efficient services, but sometimes he or she has to point out to parents that in this life there is rarely an ideal solution and that the school may be doing all it can to help. Occasionally it may be justifiable to ask for a second opinion on a child's assessment, but care must be taken not to play one expert off against another.

In the case of disabilities of a subtle kind such as learning disorders, children coming to hospital clinics are likely to be mainly from the higher social classes, which is an argument for a specialized role for the hospital-based assessment units, and for as much of this work as possible being done in the community.

Finally, the doctor has a particular role to play as a coordinator of all the services available, and as an adviser to the parents of the availability of these services and the contribution they can make to the welfare of the child, and as an interpreter of the results of assessments. Enough has been said to indicate that the doctor cannot opt out of this situation; in fact, in the future he or she must be increasingly involved in attempts to try to solve these problems.

References

Abercrombie, M.L.J. (1960) Perception and eye movements. Some speculation on disorders in cerebral palsy. *Cerebral Palsy Bulletin*, **2**, 142

Alajouanine, T. and Lhermitte, F. (1965) Acquired aphasia in children. *Brain*, **88**, 653

Bax, M. and Whitmore, K. (1973) Neurodevelopmental screening in the school entrant medical examination. *Lancet*, **ii**, 368

Beard, R.M. (1969) *An Outline of Piaget's Developmental Psychology*. Routledge Kegan Paul, London

Bergström, K. and Bille, B. (1978) Commuted tomography of the brain in children with minimal brain damage: a preliminary study of 46 children. *Neuropädiatrie*, **9**, 378

Bishop, D.V.M. (1983) How sinister is sinistrality? *Journal of the Royal College of Physicians of London*, **17**, 161

Boder, E. (1973) Developmental dyslexia: a diagnostic approach based on three atypical reading-spelling patterns. *Developmental Medicine and Child Neurology*, **15**, 663

Boder, E. and Jarrico, S. (1982) *The Boder Test of Reading-Spelling Patterns*. Grune and Stratton, New York

Bogan, J.E. (1969) The other side of the brain. *Bulletin of the Los Angeles Neurological Society*, **34**, 73, 135, 191

Brenner, M.W., Gillman, S., Zangwill, O.L. and Farrell, M. (1967) Visuo-motor disability in school-children. *British Medical Journal*, **iv**, 259

Brown, J.K. (1976) Infants damaged during birth. Perinatal asphyxia. In *Recent Advances in Paediatrics*. (ed. D. Hull), Churchill Livingstone, London

Cashdan, A. (1969) The role of movement in language learning. In *Planning for Better Learning* (eds. P. Wolff and R. MacKeith), Clinics in Developmental Medicine No. 33. SIMP, Heinemann, London

Childs, B. (1972) Genetic analysis of human behaviour. *Annual Review of Medicine*, **23**, 373

Conners, C.K. (1976) Learning disabilities and stimulant drugs in children: theoretical implications. In *The Neuropsychology of Learning Disorders* (eds. R.M. Knights and D.J. Bakker), University Park Press, London

Critchley, E.M.R. (1968) Reading retardation, dyslexia and delinquency. *British Journal of Psychiatry*, **114**, 1537

Dare, M.T. and Gordon, N. (1970) Clumsy children: a disorder of perception and motor organisation. *Developmental Medicine and Child Neurology*, **12**, 178

Dobbing, J. (1970) Undernutrition and the developing brain. The relevance of animal models to the human problem. *American Journal of Diseases of Children*, **120**, 411

Douek, E., Bannister, L.H., Dodson, H.C. *et al.* (1976) Effects of incubator noise on the cochlea of the newborn. *Lancet*, **ii**, 1110

Drillien, C.M. (1972) Aetiology and outcome in low-birthweight infants. *Developmental Medicine and Child Neurology*, **14**, 563

Finucci, J.M., Guthrie, J.T., Childs, A.L. *et al.* (1976) The genetics of specific reading disability. *Annals of Human Genetics*, **40**, 1

Francis-Williams, J. and Davies, P.A. (1974) Very low birth weight and later intelligence. *Developmental Medicine and Child Neurology*, **16**, 709

Gaze, R.M. (1970) *The Formation of Nerve Connections: a Consideration of Neural Specificity Modulation and Comparable Phenomena*, Academic Press, London

Geschwind, N. (1965) Disconnection syndromes in animals and man. *Brain*, **88**, 237, 585

Gordon, N. (1966) The child who does not talk. Problems of diagnosis with special reference to children with severe auditory agnosia. *British Journal of Disorders of Communication*, **1**, 78

Gordon, N. (1969) A history of Laura Bridgeman—from American Notes by Charles Dickens. *British Journal of Disorders of Communication*, **4**, 107

Gordon, N. (1986a) Left-handedness and learning. *Developmental Medicine and Child Neurology*, **28**, 656

Gordon, N. (1986b) Intermittent deafness and learning. *Developmental Medicine and Child Neurology*, **28**, 364

Gordon, N. (1990) Acquired aphasia in childhood: the Landau-Kleffner syndrome. *Developmental Medicine and Child Neurology*, **32**, 270

Gordon, N. and Grimley, A. (1974) Clumsiness and perceptuo-motor disorders in children. *Physiotherapy*, **60**, 311

Gordon, N. and McKinlay, I. (1980) *Helping Clumsy Children*, Churchill Livingstone, Edinburgh

Gordon, N. and Taylor, I.G. (1964) The assessment of children with difficulties of communication. *Brain*, **87**, 121

Hagberg, B., Aicardi, J., Dias, K. and Ramos, O. (1983) A progressive syndrome of autism, dementia, ataxia and loss of purposeful hand use in girls: Rett syndrome: a report of 35 cases. *Annals of Neurology*, **14**, 471

Henderson, A.G. (1975) Electrophysiological tests of hearing. *Developmental Medicine and Child Neurology*, **17**, 96

Hutt S.J. and Hutt C. (1964) Hyperactivity in a group of epileptic (and some non-epileptic) brain-damaged children. *Epilepsia*, **5**, 334

Ingram, T.T.S. (1960) Paediatric aspects of specific developmental dysphasia, dyslexia, and dysgraphia. *Cerebral Palsy Bulletin*, **2**, 254

Ingram, T.T.S. (1969) Disorders of speech in childhood. *British Journal of Hospital Medicine*, **4**, 1608

Ingram, T.T.S., Mason, A.W. and Blackburn, I. (1970) A retrospective study of 82 children with reading disability. *Developmental Medicine and Child Neurology*, **12**, 271

Kiernan, C. (1977) Alternatives to speech: a review of research on manual and other forms of communication with the mentally handicapped and other non-communicating populations. *British Journal of Mental Subnormality*, **23**, 6

Kinsbourne, M. (1973) School problems. *Pediatrics*, **52**, 697

Landau, W.M. and Kleffner, F.R. (1957) Syndrome of acquired aphasia with convulsive disorder in children. *Neurology*, **7**, 523

McFie, J. (1970) The other side of the brain. *Developmental Medicine and Child Neurology*, **12**, 514

Naidoo, S. (1972) *Specific Dyslexia*, Pitman, London

Ounsted, C. (1955) The hyperkinetic syndrome in epileptic children. *Lancet*, **ii**, 303

Ounsted, C. and Taylor, D.C. (1972) *Gender Differences: Their Ontogeny and Significance*, Churchill Livingstone, Edinburgh

Paine, R.S. and Oppé, T.F. (1966) *Neurological Examination of Children*, Clinics in Developmental Medicine. Nos. 20/21. SIMP, William Heinemann, London

Pasamanick, B. and Knobloch, H. (1960) Brain damage and reproductive casualty. *American Journal of Orthopsychiatry*, **30**, 298

Peckham, C.S. (1973) Speech defects in a national sample of children aged seven years. *British Journal of Disorders of Communication*, **8**, 2

Peters, J.E., Romine, J.S. and Dykman, R.A. (1975) A special neurological examination of children with learning disabilities. *Developmental Medicine and Child Neurology*, **17**, 63

Prechtl, H.F.R. and Stemmer, C.J. (1962) The choreiform syndrome in children. *Developmental Medicine and Child Neurology*, **4**, 119

Rutter, M. (1969) The concept of dyslexia. In *Planning for Better Learning* (eds. P.H. Wolff and R. MacKeith), Clinics in Developmental Medicine, No. 33. SIMP, William Heinemann, London

Rutter, M. (1970) Psycho-social disorders in childhood and the outcome in adult life. *Journal of the Royal College of Physicians*, **4**, 211

Rutter, M. (1984) Autism-aetiology, therapy and the family. *Communication*, **18**, 3

Rutter, M., Tizard, J. and Whitmore, K. (1970) *Education, Health and Behaviour*, Longman, London

Sandberg, S.T., Rutter, M. and Taylor, E. (1978) Hyperkinetic disorders in psychiatric clinic attenders. *Developmental Medicine and Child Neurology*, **20**, 279

Shimada, M. and Morikawa, Y. (1978) Effects of early experimental undernutrition on brain development. *Asian Medical Journal*, **21**, 476

Shoumaker, R.D., Bennett, D.R., Bray, P.F. and Curless, R.G. (1974) Clinical and EEG manifestations of unusual aphasic syndrome in children. *Neurology*, **24**, 10

Stratton, P.M. (1977) Criteria for assessing the influence of obstetric circumstances on later development. In *Benefits and Hazards of the New Obstetrics* (eds. T. Chard and M. Richards), Clinics in Developmental Medicine No. 64., William Heinemann Medical Books, London

Taylor, D.C. (1969) Differential rates of cerebral maturation between sexes and between hemispheres. *Lancet*, **ii**, 140

Touwen, B.C.L. (1972) Laterality and dominance. *Developmental Medicine and Child Neurology*, **14**, 747

Touwen, B.C.L. (1979) *Examination of the Child with Minor Neurological Dysfunction*, 2nd Edn, Clinics in Developmental Medicine No. 71, William Heinemann Medical Books, London

Towbin, A. (1969) Mental retardation due to germinal matrix infarction. *Science*, **164**, 156

Wedell, K. (1968) Perceptual-motor difficulties. *Special Education*, **57**, 25

Williams, C.E. (1969) Early diagnosis of deafness and its relation to speech in deaf, maladjusted children. *Developmental Medicine and Child Neurology*, **11**, 777

Woods, C.E. (1976) The incidence of handicapping conditions in childhood resulting from perinatal morbitity. *Developmental Medicine and Child Neurology*, **18**, 394

7   Disorders and diseases of the motor system

Hypotonia in the newborn period

The assessment of muscle tone is always very subjective and varies from one observer to the next. Much depends on the state of arousal of the child and whether he or she is placid or irritable. It must be emphasized that there are also wide variations from one normal infant to another, and at different gestational ages.

Assessment of tone can be made by a number of tests, for example by pulling the supine infant into the sitting position, assessing rebound after extension of the limbs, by passive movements of the limbs, by holding the forearm and flapping the wrists, or in ventral suspension when the head may be flexed and the limbs hang down loosely. Movements will be poor, with a weak suck and cry and difficulties with breathing.

In the immediate newborn period the most common causes of hypotonia are cerebral depression due to hypoxia, birth trauma, infections and drugs. There is often an associated difficulty in establishing adequate respiration, and this can result in the death of the infant. Some neuromuscular disorders can present with hypotonia in the same way, for example infantile spinal muscular atrophy, the congenital type of dystrophia myotonica and neonatal myasthenia gravis.

Hypoxia and birth trauma are usually obvious, but the diagnosis of infections may need a careful screening of all body systems. Drugs include not only sedatives given to the mother during labour but analgesics, especially those used for epidural anaesthesia, and sedatives given later to mothers who are breast-feeding.

If such disorders are not found to be the cause of the baby's floppiness, diseases of the motor system are the most likely diagnosis. However, there are a few rare metabolic disorders worth considering, such as the most severe form of glycogenesis, i.e. type II glycogenesis or Pompe's disease, which will be described later. The various types of hyperglycinaemia can cause profound hypotonia in infancy, but there should be a few days of normal development before the effects of protein feeding become apparent.

Diseases of the motor system in the newborn period

Spinal cord injury due to birth trauma

Spinal cord injury due to birth trauma was more frequently referred to in the early literature than it has been in recent years. In a survey of previous reports, and on the basis of his own studies, Towbin (1969) found that more than 10% of autopsies in the neonatal period showed evidence of spinal cord or brain-stem injury. He considered that this was caused by excessive longitudinal traction, especially when combined with flexion and torsion of the spinal axis. This may occur with breech delivery when applying traction to the trunk and manipulating the head. Injudicious traction with forceps during vertex delivery can have the same effect. Contributing factors include prematurity, primiparity, disproportion and precipitous delivery. Transection of the cervical cord has been reported in about a fifth of infants born with hyperextension of the head associated with breech and transverse presentations; and it is recommended that all such babies should be delivered by Caesarean section (Abrams *et al.*, 1973). The baby may be limp, with impaired movements of the limbs, and chest deformities can occur. Respiratory complications are common. The spinal cord may show almost complete disruption (De Souza and Davis, 1974). Spinal cord transection can also occur *in utero*, possibly due to attempts at version during pregnancy (Chapman *et al.*, 1978). In contradistinction to progressive spinal muscular atrophy there is no muscle fasciculation, and although there may be a flaccid paralysis of the arms with absent reflexes, there will be spasticity of the legs with brisk reflexes and a strong withdrawal response on plantar stimulation. It is particularly important to consider these possibilities before confirming the diagnosis of infantile spinal muscular atrophy and giving the parents genetic advice.

Brachial plexus injuries

Injury to the brachial plexus can result from traction at birth, particularly in breech presentations. The degree of improvement depends on whether the nerves are stretched or torn. If the lesion is mild, weakness may not be noted for a while after birth.

The most common type is involvement of the upper roots of the brachial plexus (Erb's palsy). This will lead to wasting and paresis of the deltoid, superspinatus, infraspinatus, biceps, brachioradialis and sometimes of the extensors of the wrist and fingers. The arm will be held in the 'tip position' due to weakness of abduction at the shoulder and of external rotation of the arm. The biceps and radial reflexes will be absent. If the lower roots of the plexus are injured (Klumpke's paralysis) there will be weakness and wasting of the hand muscles, and often a Horner's syndrome on the affected side with ptosis, enophthalmos, a small pupil, and absence of sweating on the side of the face. In both types the growth of the limb will be impaired. Treatment consists of rest for a few days after birth, the sleeve of the affected arm being pinned to the sheet in 30 degrees abduction. After one week, passive movements are begun and spontaneous recovery to some degree takes place in more than half of the cases. Later on, if recovery is unsatisfactory, reconstructive surgery can be considered, especially if there is dislocation of the shoulder, rotation deformity or dislocation of the head of the radius. Tendon transplants may be possible, especially in Klumpkle's paralysis. If the arm remains useless, the adolescent may choose amputation (Matson, 1969).

Infantile spinal muscular atrophy (Werdnig-Hoffmann's disease)

This is one of the more common causes of very severe muscular hypotonia in the young infant. It is a condition with much variation in clinical presentation as well as age of onset, and there has been disagreement whether early and late onset in childhood represent genetically separate entities or are variants of the same disease. Now the gene for all types of spinal muscular atrophy has been located to chromosome 5q, which settles that argument (Gordon, 1991). The disease shows autosomal

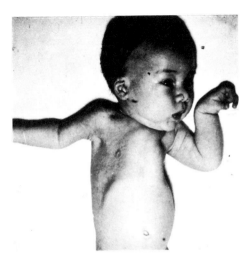

Figure 7.1   Werdnig Hoffmann's disease with chest deformity.

recessive inheritance, but rare cases have been described in successive generations. The discovery of the gene for spinal muscular atrophy raises exciting possibilities for diagnosis, more accurate classification and, it is hoped, for treatment (Brzustowicz *et al.*, 1990). Although no specific treatment is available it is important to make an exact diagnosis so that genetic advice can be given.

Werdnig-Hoffmann's disease (Fig. 7.1) is the most severe form of infantile spinal muscular atrophy, with an incidence of 1 in 20 000; and can have its earliest clinical manifestations *in utero* when the mother notes markedly reduced fetal movement. The child can be very hypotonic at birth, resembling a rag doll, or can initially show a normal pattern of muscle tone and movement, only to develop acute paralysis some weeks after birth. Head control is often virtually absent, and the legs assume a position of complete abduction, known as the frog position. Movement in the fingers, toes, face and diaphragm is mostly spared. The intercostal musculature is nearly always involved, causing impaired respiratory excursion. Pulmonary infection and collapse is common, and causes death within a few years. Muscle fasciculation can be observed in many muscles but is best seen in the tongue. Tendon reflexes are absent. Contractures develop rapidly, especially at knee, ankle and elbow level. The chest often shows a 'bell-shaped' deformity due to diaphragmatic action on a chest with paralysed intercostal muscles. Paradoxical respiration is occasionally seen. The feet frequently develop an equinus deformity due to constant pressure of the bed on the lateral border of the foot.

Hypotonia in infants

In addition to those entities which are often detectable in the newborn period, a wide range of conditions can cause muscular hypotonia in young children. Before discussing the more well-defined neuropathies and myopathies, there are other conditions, some not usually thought to have neurological side effects, which need to be considered.

Mental retardation

Conditions in which mental retardation is an important feature will very frequently be associated with muscular hypotonia. Some will have a clearly demonstrable cause, for example Down's syndrome. The mucopolysaccharidoses are also commonly associated with hypotonia, as are some of the aminoacidurias. In many cases no specific causation can be found and muscle tone improves with advancing maturation.

Cerebral palsy

Children with cerebral palsy will at times show marked hypotonia in their first year, particularly in the dyskinetic and ataxic forms. Ataxic cerebral palsy presents with early hypotonia and, as the child grows older, motor development is delayed and incoordinate movements become apparent.

Hagberg, Sanner and Steen (1972) have emphasized that some children are disabled by a disturbance of posture. They define the dysequilibrium syndrome (Chapter 8) as a non-progressive neurological condition dominated throughout childhood by an inability or difficulty in maintaining an upright body position and of experiencing the position of the body in space. Affected children lack equilibrium. Cerebellar signs are present but may be obscured by the main disability. Motor development is markedly retarded, with hypotonia lasting several years. Standing may be delayed until the age of 6 or 9 years, and walking occurs even later. These children often fall full length without showing protective responses. As in other forms of cerebral palsy, the aetiology varies from environmental factors, such as cerebral hypoxia at birth, to genetic influences.

Benign congenital hypotonia

Many children presenting with muscular hypotonia as an isolated feature, and in whom no other pathological condition can be demonstrated, have been grouped under this heading (Walton, 1961). The prognosis is often good, and, after a variable period, improvement is the rule, with a proportion of cases recovering completely. With recent diagnostic advances, especially in muscle biopsy examination by histochemical staining and with the electron microscope, some cases formerly included under this heading are identified as having a muscular abnormality and should be excluded from this group.

Hagberg and Lundberg (1969) have followed up a group of children whose disability was of a limited type. Head control and motor development of the arms and hands was normal. The legs had always been less active than the arms, and the ability to sit up, crawl, kneel and stand was markedly retarded. Although muscle power was normal the children could not use their legs for walking or staying in an upright position as expected for their age. Muscle tone of the legs was usually decreased, and the feet were poorly developed. When supporting their weight the children showed recurved valgus knees and planovalgus feet. Tendon reflexes were usually normal. These typical clinical findings suggest a syndrome of *dissociated motor development*, only the development of gross and not fine motor skills being delayed. Many of the children progress normally in the end. A negative prenatal, perinatal and postnatal history, combined with an hereditary tendency to shuffle and a development pattern of late learning to sit, favours a good prognosis (Lunberg, 1979).

It is possible that some of the children diagnosed as suffering from benign congenital hypotonia are in fact suffering from the effects of delayed development of certain parts of the motor system. A disturbance of cerebellar function may prevent facilitating effects on the gamma motor system, reducing its activity and causing hypotonia. There are other developmental disorders in childhood which are dependent on delay in the integration of one part of the central nervous system, for example children who are of normal intelligence but are late in learning to talk or read. In most cases improvement eventually occurs by processes of compensation for any cerebral deficiencies. There seems no reason, therefore, why defects in motor function resulting in hypotonia should not do likewise.

Parents may have to be told that it is not possible to make an exact diagnosis at present, that the nature of the child's disability will in time become more apparent, that a pattern of development will become clearer after a period of observation, and that plans for future management can then be made.

Nutritional and metabolic disorders

A number of metabolic diseases have to be considered in the differential diagnosis of the floppy infant, especially the organic acidaemias which can often be treated successfully (Keeton and Moosa, 1976). Children with renal tubular acidosis may also have muscular hypotonia as an associated feature. Classically, *idiopathic infantile hypercalcaemia (William's syndrome)* presents in a child whose regular weight gain and developmental advance ceases. The affected child has reduced subcutaneous fat and a generalized hypotonia. The serum calcium level is raised and the urinary calcium excretion is excessive. The calcium loading test shows a lag curve, and skeletal X-rays show excessive calcium deposition at the metaphyses as well as in the orbits and iliac crests. Vitamin D administration must be restricted and the dietary calcium intake temporarily reduced. The facial characteristics and the mild mental retardation persist, and these children are found to have infundibular aortic stenosis or other large blood vessel stenosis. This condition is also referred to in Chapter 5. Hypothyroidism can be another cause of hypotonia, and amongst nutritional disorders it is seen in infants with gluten enteropathy, as well as in those with rickets.

Connective tissue disorders

Generalized disorders of connective tissue are not infrequently associated with reduced muscle tone. Children with arachnodactyly (Marfan's syndrome) often show this clearly. They are usually tall and thin, and have characteristic long fingers, hands, feet and toes. The joints are excessively mobile and there are associated cardiac lesions, particularly auricular septal defects.

The Ehlers-Danlos syndrome is notable because of the excessive skin and joint laxity, a liability to trauma, and healing with tissue-paper scars. Young infants with this disorder show an associated muscular hypotonia.

In osteogenesis imperfecta (fragilitas osseum) both the congenita and tarda forms can be associated with hypotonia, and in the latter the muscular features with motor retardation can precede the occurrence of fractures.

Prader-Willi syndrome

Prader-Willi syndrome (Fig. 7.2) consists of obesity, dwarfism, mental retardation and cryptorchism. Muscular hypotonia and feeding difficulties are outstanding

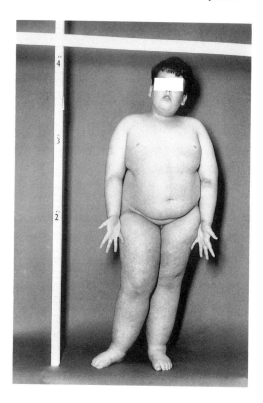

Figure 7.2   Prader-Willi syndrome.

features in the newborn period. The hands are narrow, with long slim fingers, and the feet and head are relatively small. Puberty is delayed, and the secondary sex characteristics are poorly developed. Later in life diabetes mellitus may complicate the picture (Prader and Willi, 1963). There is sometimes a striking similarity between the children's facial appearance, with almond-shaped eye sockets and slightly over-hanging eyelids, high cranial vault, prominent forehead, retroussé nose and slightly open, fish-like mouth (Laurence, 1967). It has been suggested that the syndrome may be related to the presence of insulin antagonists (Evans, 1964). Another possibility seems to be a defect at hypothalamic and brain-stem level occurring in early life. This might result in various endocrine disorders, mental retardation and hypotonia. Certainly it seems likely that the lack of tone is of central and not peripheral origin, and children with this condition contribute to the larger group of benign congenital hypotonia. In infancy the condition may be confused with infantile spinal muscular atrophy, but the diagnosis can usually be made on clinical grounds. Whatever the exact causal mechanisms of the syndrome are, it is now known that its genetic origins are related to a deletion in the long arm of chromosome 15 inherited from the father, in the same region as deletions found in Williams' syndrome and Angelman's or happy puppet syndrome (Fig 7.3) (Punnett and Zakai, 1990). In the latter syndrome, inheritance is from the mother; and the inheritance of the Prader-Willi and Angelman's syndromes is a good example of genomic imprinting or uniparental disomy. There can be exceptions to the parent involved due to complex disorders of the genes. For instance when there are no cytogenetically visable deletions, two chromosomes 15 may be inherited from one parent, the mother in the Prader-Willi

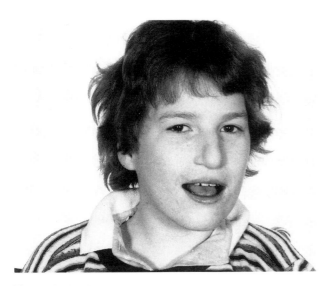

Figure 7.3   Angleman's or happy puppet syndrome.

syndrome and the father in Angelman's syndrome; showing that it is the lack of the particular part of chromosome 15 from the relevant parent which is significant (Malcolm *et al.*, 1991). The risk of recurrence is about 1 in a 1000.

Diseases of the motor system in infancy and childhood

Infantile spinal muscular atrophy (Kugelberg-Welander syndrome)

Having already described the most severe form of this disorder, Werdnig-Hoffman's disease, with its onset in the neonatal period, it is necessary to emphasize that infantile spinal muscular atrophy can start at a later age and run a much more prolonged course, although it is most probable that all forms of spinal muscular atrophy are due to mutation at the same gene locus (Melki *et al.*, 1990).

Kugelberg and Welander (1956) described a milder type, in which the onset is usually later and the children characteristically show proximal muscle weakness. Affected children do learn to walk, though they may develop skeletal deformities, particularly scoliosis and kyphosis. The condition often seems static, and there may even be improvement with age and maturation. An intercurrent illness can precipitate a sudden deterioration, when muscle fasciculation is particularly easily detected. It may mimic muscular dystrophy, with a tendency for the child to 'climb up his or her legs'. The child falls easily and has difficulty in getting up from the floor and in climbing stairs. Involvement of the arms may follow that of the legs, and there is often a tremor of the hands (Moosa and Dubowitz, 1973). The tendon reflexes are sluggish or absent, and occasionally the plantar responses are extensor. Progressive disability is often due to contractures and not to increased weakness. Measures must be taken to try to prevent these. Respiratory failure can occur even in the mild forms of spinal muscular atrophy. Weakness of the axial musculature may warn of this complication (Benardy, 1978).

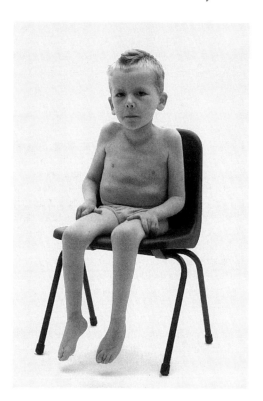

Figure 7.4 Infantile spinal muscular atrophy: intermediate type.

In cases with a relatively late onset, the condition has been described under the title of 'juvenile amyotrophic lateral sclerosis', and in some instances there may be involvement of the bulbar muscles (Gordon, 1968). The possibility of an intermediate form between Werdnig-Hoffmann's disease and the Kugelberg-Welander syndrome, with an onset in the first year of life, has been suggested by Fried and Emery (1971) (Fig. 7.4). Another variant of this syndrome has been described by Pearn and Hudgson (1978), with onset in adolescence and a slowly progressive course. Gross calf hypertrophy is a particular feature and the inheritance appears to be sex-linked recessive, rather than autosomal recessive, as usually found in spinal muscular atrophy. There are, in fact, a variety of conditions which can be classified under the term spinal muscular atrophy, which come on at various ages up to adult life and with dominant, recessive and sex-linked modes of inheritance (Pearn, 1980).

Serum creatine phosphokinase estimations are normal or only slightly raised, though electromyography will show a denervation pattern with high amplitude polyphasic potentials of long duration, reduced interference pattern on voluntary movement, and fibrillation potentials at rest. Histological appearance on muscle biopsy shows groups of atrophic fibres interspersed with fascicles containing hypertrophied fibres.

Management should centre on keeping the child mobile for as long as possible, with light calipers where practicable, as well as support to the spine with well-fitting spinal braces to prevent deformities; and meticulous care of the respiratory tract with physiotherapy and postural drainage. The child should have a wheelchair of appropriate size, with a horizontal seat, and platforms that give good support to the feet.

Peripheral neuropathies

Peripheral nerves can be involved in a number of acute and chronic disease processes which may involve some or all of the neuronal elements carried in the nerve. Motor, sensory and autonomic fibres are affected singly or in combination. Muscle weakness is the predominant clinical feature and is more obvious distally than proximally, though proximal weakness occurs in some cases and can imitate a myopathy. Patients are at times noted to tire easily, requiring differentiation from myasthenia gravis. Diminished or absent tendon reflexes are the most common sign, and loss of muscle bulk develops fairly rapidly. Sensory changes occur: older children will complain of pain and tingling or even numbness, whilst infants and young children present mainly with irritability, and may rub hands, feet and occiput, as in Pink disease following mercury poisoning. Autonomic involvement is clinically reflected by unusual erythema or pallor, peripheral cyanosis and excessive sweating.

Neuropathies can be associated with infections, bacterial and chemical toxins, metabolic disturbances and inborn errors of metabolism. They occur as acute conditions or can be subacute and chronic relapsing.

Infectious polyneuritis (Guillain-Barré syndrome)

While the precise aetiology is not known, there is often a preceding respiratory or gastrointestinal illness. Viruses have been isolated in a few cases of polyneuritis with rising antibody titres. They include mumps, chicken-pox, herpes simplex, herpes zoster, coxsackie B, Echo 6, and the Epstein-Barr virus. A variety of mechanisms of action are postulated: the virus may act by acute and direct invasion, by release of a latent infection, or by setting up an auto-immune phenomenon, though the condition has been known to occur even during adequate immunosuppression for renal transplantation (Drachman et al., 1970). Circulating demyelinating factors have been demonstrated during the acute phase of the disease (Cook et al., 1971).

There is usually a rapid onset of generalized weakness of all limbs which may start in the legs and spreads upwards. Muscles may be tender, and paraesthesia, pain, and sensory loss occur quite often, though they are usually transitory. Unilateral or bilateral facial paralysis is often present, and is a finding which particularly suggests the diagnosis; ophthalmoplegia is very uncommon. Tendon reflexes are diminished or absent. Urinary retention is sometimes a problem, and very occasionally respiration becomes seriously embarrassed and endangers the patient's life. Frequent assessment of respiratory function is therefore mandatory. Rarely, intracranial hypertension occurs, with headache, vomiting and papilloedema. This may be due to impaired absorption of the cerebrospinal fluid due to blocking of the arachnoid villi, or to cerebral oedema. The nephrotic syndrome is also an unusual complication.

A marked increase in the cerebrospinal fluid protein with few, if any, cells is a characteristic and helpful finding, but it may take 7–14 days to develop from the onset of the disease. In around 15% of cases the gamma-globulin fraction of the serum and of the spinal fluid protein are raised (Dyck et al., 1975). It is suggested that the very raised level of protein in the cerebrospinal fluid is the result of vascular congestion, but it seems possible that swelling of the nerve trunks in the intervertebral foramina can interfere with the absorption of spinal fluid. The pathology is one of segmental demyelination. Motor and sensory nerve conduction studies are useful, both in diagnosis and to assess recovery.

The prognosis tends to be worse among children than adults. It is claimed that the most significant predictor of incomplete recovery is the interval between the greatest weakness that occurs and the beginning of improvement. A period of longer than 18 days is indicative of incomplete recovery (Eberle *et al.*, 1975).

On the theory that oedema of the nerves may be of allergic origin, treatment with steroids has been given. It is difficult to estimate the effect of this form of treatment in a condition which usually improves without therapy of any kind, but it may be justifiable to give steroids if the paralysis is severe and spreading. Doubts have certainly been raised about the efficacy of steroids in the treatment of acute polyneuropathies (Hughes *et al.*, 1978), but it is possible that treatment may have to be continued for long periods before failure is certain. It is equally difficult to assess the effects of giving a polyunsaturated fatty acid (PUFA) diet. This has been suggested in long-standing cases because of the possibility of auto-immunity in this condition and the fact that these acids do cause immunosuppression (Bower and Newsholme, 1978). If the patient continues to deteriorate, or fails to improve over a long period, plasma exchange, intravenous immunoglobulin, and immunosuppressive drugs can be tried (Fowler *et al.*, 1979). There is suggestive evidence that plasma exchange can be of benefit in the treatment of infectious encephalomyelitis and transverse myelitis (Newton, 1981), but this still has to be proven. Respiratory failure may necessitate tracheostomy as well as the use of a respirator.

If this condition is due to an allergic type of reaction to infection, it seems that this may occur at various levels of the nervous system; an acute disseminated encephalomyelitis in which the brain and spinal cord are affected, a myelo-radiculitis when there is evidence of damage to the spinal cord and nerve roots, and infectious polyneuritis with involvement of the nerve roots and peripheral nerves. Occasionally, nerve roots and peripheral nerves can be individually affected.

One variety of this extended group of diseases is the Miller-Fisher syndrome with external ophthalmoplegia, ataxia and areflexia. Computerized axial tomography scans may show evidence of lesions in the brain-stem and cerebellum (Littlewood and Bajada, 1981).

Diagnostic difficulties can occur with Lyme disease, and a good review of this condition is given by Cryan and Wright (1991).

Neuralgic amyotrophy

In neuralgic amyotrophy, the nerves to the arm (especially at C5 and C6 level) are involved, sometimes after vaccination or various infections. The onset is acute, with pain spreading from the neck to the shoulder and down the arm. This is soon followed by muscle weakness and wasting. Sensory loss is rare, but may sometimes be found over the outer side of the upper arm. The cerebrospinal fluid can show a slightly raised cell count. The course of the condition may be prolonged, but recovery is usually complete in the end. Treatment with steroids may at least relieve the pain, but it is doubtful if it affects the muscle weakness.

A hereditary form can occur (heredofamilial brachial plexus neuropathy). It has a greater tendency to start in childhood and is more liable to relapse. Sufferers often have peculiar facies with close-set eyes, and syndactyly of the second and third toes, cleft palate and small stature. Even if the symptoms are confined to the arms, EMG and nerve conduction studies may reveal a more widespread involvement. Treatment with steroids is also controversial in this condition (Dunn, Daube and Gomez,1978).

Toxic neuropathies

Biological toxins include diphtheria, which causes palatal palsy followed by cranial nerve involvement and, occasionally, a sensorimotor neuropathy. Antitoxin and penicillin should be given promptly and in large doses. Ingestion of the toxin from *Bacillus botulinus* produces symptoms in 18–36 hours, with diplopia, photophobia, dysphagia and generalized weakness. Death from respiratory failure or cardiac arrest can occur. Antitoxin should be given.

Chemical toxins include lead poisoning (Chapter 12), which usually presents with acute symptoms of vomiting, convulsions and coma, but occasionally wrist and foot drop may occur, with associated abdominal pain and anaemia (Boothby, De Jesus and Rowland, 1974). Calcium disodium versenate and penicillamine are usually the treatments of choice, and the child must be protected from further exposure to lead. Drinking water can be contaminated by flowing through lead pipes, paint containing lead is still found in old properties, and toys can be made in moulds with a high lead content.

Ingestion of thallium can result in a polyneuropathy, and acute ingestion is complicated by ataxia, coma and death. Alopecia results in less severe cases.

Pink disease (acrodynia) is caused by mercury poisoning. Mercury was once incorporated in teething powders. Affected children are irritable and photophobic, are generally weak and floppy and have vasomotor disturbances, with red but cold hands and feet and increased sweating and salivation. Mercury excretion is measured in the urine, and treatment with dimercaprol (British anti-lewisite) is useful. It can be given in four doses of 2.5 mg/kg body weight daily for 4–5 days, and then in gradually diminishing doses.

Insecticides such as DDT, aldrin, parathion and malathion have caused polyneuropathies, as have such drugs as isoniazid and nitrofurantoin. Vincristine used as an anti-neoplastic agent often results in loss of tendon reflexes and may also produce a sensory and motor neuropathy. Autonomic disorders and a painful proximal myopathy can also occur. There are an increasing number of drugs known to cause axonal degeneration, and occasionally segmental demyelination (Argov and Mastaglia, 1979).

Metabolic neuropathies

Diabetic neuropathy, typical of the affected adult, with paraesthesiae, sensory changes, weakness and diminished reflexes is not common in childhood, but it does occur and abnormal signs with prolonged nerve conduction times have been reported (Lawrence and Locke, 1963). Strict control of the diabetes can help to alleviate the condition, but may not result in complete recovery.

Acute intermittent porphyria may present with a predominantly motor neuropathy, and this subject has been well reviewed by Ridley (1969). The proximal muscles are often affected to a greater extent than the distal groups, and the arms are affected more than the legs. Diagnostic features are the paradoxical preservation of the ankle jerks and a 'bathing trunks' distribution of sensory loss. The particular danger in this neuropathy is its aggravation by barbiturates which may be given for associated mental disturbances and epileptic seizures. Respiratory paralysis or cardiac arrest can cause death. There can be a remarkable recovery even from severe generalized paralysis. Excess porphyrins in the urine are suggestive of the diagnosis, but these also occur in lead poisoning. The urine may darken on standing due to the formation of various porphyrins, but porphyrin precursors are not always found in the urine even during an acute attack. Supportive measures and various forms of treatment including large doses of pyridoxine (vitamin B6), carbohydrate loading with fructose (400 g/day) and haematin (4 mg/kg body weight/12h) (McColl *et al.*, 1979), if given early enough in the illness, may be worth a trial. The onset may occasionally be pre-pubertal. The condition is also discussed in Chapter 3.

Metachromatic leucodystrophy usually presents with intellectual regression, spasticity and convulsions, but it can start with a peripheral neuropathy. Nerve conduction is slow, and nerve biopsy shows the accumulation of metachromatically staining sulphatide, particularly in the Schwann cells. Low arylsulphatase-A levels are found in peripheral leucocytes and cultured fibroblasts (Beratis, Aron and Hirschhorn, 1973).

Chronic Neuropathies

Refsum's syndrome (heredopathia atactica polyneuritiformis) is a rare condition showing autosomal recessive inheritance, but one of particular interest to the author for several reasons, not least that it originally described a variety of apparently unassociated system disorders and was then found to manifest a very significant metabolic disturbance. The main clinical features are hemeralopia (better night than day vision), concentric limitation of visual fields associated with an atypical retinitis pigmentosa, a hypertrophic polyneuritis with paresis of a peripheral distribution, and ataxia of cerebellar origin with nystagmus. The pupils are small and react sluggishly to light; there is a perceptive deafness, cardiac enlargement with ECG changes (Gordon and Hudson, 1959), and a marked rise in cerebrospinal fluid protein. In children the condition may be associated with ichthyosis (Refsum, Solomonson and Skatvedt, 1949), and the infantile form is characterized by facial dysmorphia, retinitis pigmentosa, neurosensory hearing loss, hepatomegaly, osteopenia (reduced bone mass), delayed growth and psychomotor development. In this form there is elevation of the plasma long chain fatty acids (Poll-Thé *et al.*, 1986), as in Zellweger's syndrome and adrenoleukodystrophy, compatible with peroxisomal dysfunction. Excessive amounts of phytanic acid (tetramethyl hexadecanoic acid) have been demonstrated in the tissues, related to a complete or partial absence of phytanic acid-a-hydroxylase (Steinberg *et al.*, 1967). As phytanic acid is not synthesized in the body, limitation of intake should prevent storage. In adults, a diet low in phytanic acid, and high in calories, to prevent mobilization of phytanic acid from fat stores, reduces serum levels of phytanic acid with improvement in muscle strength, sensation and nerve conduction (Refsum, 1981). Large-volume plasma exchange has also been used to advantage (Gibberd *et al.*, 1979). Vision and hearing have shown little recovery.

Peroneal muscular atrophy (Charcot-Marie-Tooth) is usually dominantly inherited, though some cases occur as autosomal or sex-linked recessive traits (Dyck and Lambert, 1968). Pes cavus, clawing of the toes and scoliosis are early features in children, as are decreased or absent reflexes. The symptoms usually start with the involvement of the peroneal muscles becoming obvious and spreading to other muscles below the knee. The preservation of the upper thigh muscles gives the legs the characteristic inverted 'champagne bottle' appearance. Eventually foot-drop develops, with a high-stepping gait. The distal muscles in the arms usually become weak and wasted after those in the legs, but there is sometimes a surprising preservation of power, especially in the hands, even in the presence of severe wasting. Fasciculation may occur, and there may be sensory changes; these are often slight, but vibration sense is usually impaired. Sensory loss is more marked if there is a segmental demyelination, and then there may be severe ataxia. Four groups are recognized by some according to the pathological presentation; the hypertrophic neuropathy group with nerve hypertrophy and marked segmental demyelination with onion bulb formation; the intermediate group with the latter two findings but with no nerve hypertrophy and with axonal degeneration and regeneration; the neuronal sensori-motor group which shows some onion bulbs, paranodal demyelination and evidence of axonal degeneration and regeneration; and the neuronal motor group with no major abnormalities apart from some cluster formation, indicating axonal regeneration (Madrid, Bradley and Davis, 1977). In the first group the onset is often within the first decade. Nerve conduction velocity will be markedly reduced. When there is axonal degeneration, the onset is usually in the teens and nerve conduction velocities will be normal or moderately reduced. Neuropathies showing both segmental demyelination and axonal degeneration can have a prenatal origin. If the symptoms and signs are very slight, the eponym Roussy-Lévy has been used. The lifespan is not necessarily shortened and, the cause being unknown, there is no specific treatment.

Hypertrophic interstitial polyneuritis, first described by Dejerine and Sottas, has a similar clinical picture to peroneal muscular atrophy and is inherited as a dominant or autosomal recessive trait (Dyck and Lambert, 1968). As the symptoms and signs are comparable, it may be best to regard peroneal muscular atrophy and hypertrophic interstitial polyneuritis as 'heredity motor and sensory neuropathy' of different inheritance and possibly aetiology, but a more satisfactory classification will have to wait for increased knowledge of underlying causes.

Although the clinical classification is still confused, the most widely accepted and simple is undoubtedly *heredity motor and sensory neuropathy* of three types, as follows:

Type 1: peroneal muscular atrophy to include the hypertrophic form of Charcot-Marie-Tooth disease and Dejerine-Sottas disease, with onset in the first decade, reduced conduction velocity below $38 \, \text{mS}^{-1}$ and segmental demyelination.

Type 2: neuronal peroneal muscular atrophy to include the neuronal form of Charcot-Marie-Tooth disease, progressive spinal muscular atrophy of the Charcot-Marie-Tooth type, heredity spastic paraplegia and spinocerebellar degeneration with peroneal atrophy, with onset in the second decade or later, relatively preserved nerve conduction and little evidence of segmental demyelination.

Type 3: confined to cases of severe infantile neuropathy, with hypomyelination and markedly reduced nerve conduction velocity (Harding and Thomas, 1980). Recent studies have suggested that this group is an artificial entity made up of a number of different disorders, and that it should be abandoned (Hagberg and Westerberg, 1983).

Hypertrophic interstitial polyneuritis often has its onset in childhood. Weakness of the legs is apparent some time before the arms are affected and is maximal distally. Atrophy may be marked and may be accompanied by paraesthesiae and shooting pains, though sensory impairment can be minimal. The tendon reflexes are diminished or absent. Striking deformities of the feet can occur, and there may be severe kyphoscoliosis. The peripheral nerves can be palpated subcutaneously as thickened bands, and histological examination shows proliferation of the perineural and endoneural connective tissue. Proliferation of the Schwann cells causes a concentric, laminated appearance, referred to as 'onion bulbs'.

A-β-lipoproteinaemia (Bassen-Kornzweig syndrome). This rare disease is also discussed in the chapter on genetically-determined conditions. It can result in an ataxic neuropathy which may appear in association with a progressive retinopathy from the age of 18 months onwards. A malabsorption or coeliac-like syndrome with steatorrhoea is present from birth, and is sometimes associated with secondary mineral and vitamin deficiencies. Acanthocytes (crenated red cells with spines), although not pathognomonic, are a useful finding on a blood smear, and a jejunal biopsy shows massive accumulations of fat droplets in the epithelial cells. Arrythmias and cardiac enlargement occur.

Neuropathies due to lack of vitamin E can also occur in malabsorption syndromes, such as congenital biliary atresia and cystic fibrosis (Bieri *et al.*, 1983). Treatment with vitamin E should be considered in any condition associated with lipid malabsorption, and also in spinocerebellar syndromes of unknown cause. Lack of α-lipoprotein (Tangier disease) can also be associated with a neuropathy (Haas, Austad and Bergin, 1974).

Deficiency neuropathies are well known in nutritional vitamin B deficiency but can also occur with intestinal malabsorption and anorexia nervosa.

Collagen diseases, sarcoidosis and amyloidosis and leukaemia may rarely be complicated by a peripheral neuropathy and the diagnostic net has to be cast widely.

Congenital sensory neuropathy has been reported in infancy (Barry, Hopkins and Neal, 1974). Among older children a similar condition is referred to as 'hereditary sensory radicular neuropathy' and has occurred in several generations of a family. There may be shooting pains in various parts of the body, and dissociated sensory loss is occasionally found in association with impairment of the autonomic nervous system. Trophic ulcers may occur on the feet. Degeneration of the nerve cells in the dorsal root ganglia has been described, and also abnormalities of the sensory nerves. It has to be diagnosed from conditions such as congenital indifference to pain which is of cortical origin.

Familial dysautonomia (Riley-Day syndrome) is a difficult condition to identify, and one which is limited to Ashkenazi Jews. There is evidence of motor inco-ordination, with sluggish or absent tendon reflexes and there may be sensory impairment. The child is sometimes mentally retarded and feeding difficulties are common. The most typical findings are defective lacrimation, and hypertension, skin blotching, and sweating in response to anxiety. The most likely cause is a disturbance of autonomic function, probably at a diencephalic level (Riley *et al.*, 1949), although reduction of cells has been demonstrated in autonomic and sensory ganglia. The diagnosis is helped by an absence of fungiform papillae on the tongue, a very diminished reaction to 1 in 1000 intradermal histamine, and miosis on installation of methacholine into the conjunctival sac. Management has recently been well reviewed by Axelrod, Nachtigal and Dancis (1974).

Myasthenia gravis

Myasthenia gravis is an interesting, if uncommon, condition at any age, but is particularly rare among children (Mackay, 1951). It was thought there was a defect in the synthesis and storage of acetylcholine at the neuromuscular junction in this condition, in distinction to the impaired release of acetylcholine in the myasthenic syndrome associated with malignant disease (Eaton and Lambert, 1957), and this may still play a part in its aetiology. It has also been suggested that it is related to the possible secretion by the thymus of a substance (thymin) which inhibits acetylcholine synthesis (Newsom Davies, 1974). Now there is little doubt that the disorder in myasthenia gravis is due to a reduced number of functioning acetylcholine receptors and that this results from immunological damage caused by circulating antibodies to the receptors (Harvard, 1977). Between 80 and 90% of patients with this disease have these antibodies in their serum. The titres fall after thymectomy and after remissions induced by steroids. The exact reason why the body sometimes treats the acetylcholine receptor as an autoantigen is not known, but may be related to the presence of these receptors within the thymus and the ability of certain thymic cells to produce neoantigens. Another possible cause of myasthenia gravis is that antibodies to acetycholine receptors may damage the thymus and cause a release of thymopoietin, the hormone responsible for the differentiation of thymocytes,which is known to have a neuromuscular blocking action (Goldstein and Schlesinger, 1975).

Myasthenia in infancy

Very rarely true myasthenia may be seen in infancy. The clinical presentation differs little from that seen in older age groups and there is no family history.

More commonly, however, babies born to mothers with myasthenia gravis present in the newborn period with considerable muscular hypotonia, poverty of movement, feeding difficulties and respiratory problems. The condition is self-limiting, and the babies show a dramatic improvement after a few weeks and subsequently develop normally. This supports the suggestion that antibodies to acetylcholine receptors cross the placenta and take about three weeks to disappear following separation from the mother.

Congenital myasthenia syndromes: various types are seen, and there may be evidence of some form of Mendelian inheritance. Although responsive to anticholinesterase drugs, in some instances no benefit is obtained from immunosuppressive therapy. There may be an enzymatic defect of acetylcholine re-synthesis; and a form associated with small nerve terminals, reduced acetylcholine release and end-plate acetyl-cholinesterase deficiency; and one form that may relate to a defect of the ion channels of membranes that are normally induced by acetylcholine release (Barlow, 1981). A congenital deficiency of acetylcholine receptors, and a congenital paucity of secondary synaptic clefts, have been described (Smit et al., 1986).

Myasthenia gravis in children

Myasthenia gravis very occasionally starts in childhood and, as in older age groups, the most common mode of onset is with weakness of the external ocular muscles. Occasionally only one muscle, for example the external rectus show this weakness and then the diagnosis is not likely to be apparent until other muscles are affected. Ptosis is relatively common, and bilateral facial palsy should always suggest this disease (Fig. 7.5). When the jaw and limb muscles start to be involved pathological fatigueability, the main characteristic of the condition, really becomes evident. Chewing, talking and any use of the arms and legs results in a more rapid loss of power than can be passed as normal, though recovery will occur quite quickly when the relevant muscles are rested.

The diagnosis is established by the rapid recovery of muscle power after intravenous injection of edrophonium chloride. In children weighing less than 30 kg,

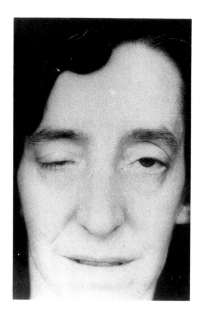

Figure 7.5   Myathenia gravis: face.

1 mg of edrophonium chloride ('Tensilon') is injected in 15 seconds. If there has been no change after 30 seconds, a further 4 mg is slowly injected. Very rarely, patients with myasthenia gravis may be unresponsive to edrophonium chloride, and if the clinical picture is suggestive an injection of neostigmine (0.04 mg/kg body weight) combined with atropine (0.01 mg/kg body weight) should be tried. Many patients with myasthenia gravis, unassociated with thymoma, have an HLA association (Scadding and Havard, 1981). Excessively rare as it may be, it is worthwhile recording that botulism can occur in infancy (Turner *et al.*, 1978), and is part of the differential diagnosis of myasthenia gravis at this age.

Treatment consists of the administration of neostigmine bromide in the first instance, starting in a young child with 7.5 mg two or three times a day and gradually increasing the dose until an optimal effect has been achieved. There is a danger of overdosage and of increasing the muscle weakness by precipitating a cholinergic crisis. This may have serious consequences if the respiratory muscles are particularly sensitive to anti-cholinergic drugs. An edrophonium chloride test can resolve this dilemma, as an increase of muscle power after an injection will suggest a myasthenic crisis, while in a cholinergic crisis the condition will tend to worsen. Side-effects, such as nausea, vomiting, diarrhoea, and cramp, may be treated with atropine or belladonna. Sometimes pyridostigmine bromide may be used as an alternative or an addition to treatment with neostigmine bromide, a 60 mg tablet of the former corresponding to a 15 mg tablet of the latter. Ephedrine, 30 mg three times a day, may also be helpful.

Treatment with prednisolone (an alternative day regime, or slowly incrementing dosage), or thymectomy, will seldom have to be considered during childhood. However, when the acute form of the disease, with widespread weakness, occurs and does not respond to medical treatment, then a decision on operation should not be delayed. The possibility of treating myasthenia gravis with other immunosuppressive agents, has been discussed (Mertens, Balzereit and Leipert, 1969). Azathioprine (1–2 mg/kg body weight) and cyclophosphamide (1–2 mg/kg body weight) have been given with benefit, in addition to cholinesterase inhibitors, and seem to help to stabilize the condition, especially in the presence of a thymoma. Also in view of the inverse relationship between the clinical state and the titre of antibodies specific for acetylcholine receptors plasmapheresis has been tried when all else has failed to control severe symptoms (Dau *et al.*, 1977).

The myopathies

Muscular dystrophies

Aetiology

Muscles form the final link in the neuromuscular chain producing movement. Although the term 'muscular dystrophy' implies disease of the muscle cell the disorder need not necessarily be limited to it. The initial assumption, that the disorder was limited to muscle, was based on the absence of demonstrable pathological findings in the nervous system, but some recent evidence indicates that both muscular dystrophy and myasthenia gravis may also be related to a disorder of motor neurons which are thought to have difficulty in maintaining satisfactory synaptic connections with muscle fibres (McComas, Sica and Campbell, 1971). This is manifested by impaired transmission on maximum volitional effort and on repetitive nerve stimulation, or by an inability of the neuron to make contact with previously denervated muscle fibres because axonal sprouting is ineffective.

Electrophysiological studies have shown a loss of motor units in both myasthenia gravis and muscular dystrophy, and further support for the importance of a neuronal disorder in muscular disease has come from the finding of abnormalities of motor end plates in muscles from dystrophic Bar Harbor 192 mice on electron microscopy (Ragab, 1971). Also, murine dystrophic muscle has been found to regenerate normally when cultured with spinal cord from normal mice, but regeneration of both normal and dystrophic muscle is severely affected when coupled with spinal cord from dystrophic mice. The neurons and neuritic growth of these spinal cords was normal but functional neuromuscular junctions did not develop, so that a chemical or physiological fault may be responsible (Gallup and Dubowitz, 1973). The concept has been criticized by others who have found the number of motor units to be within normal limits (Scatpalezos and Panayiotopoulos, 1973). Another theory, which seems less likely, seeks to relate the muscle degeneration to ischaemia from abnormal skeletal muscle blood flow (Hathaway, Engel and Zellweger, 1970). In view of the abnormalities in erythrocytes and lymphocytes there is suggestive evidence that the basic defect in muscular diseases may possibly lie in widespread defects in the cell membrane (Pickard *et al.*, 1978).

Classification

A number of myopathies can be recognized with reasonable certainty on clinical grounds.

1. Sex-linked muscular dystrophy
   (a) Severe form (Duchenne type)
   (b) Mild form (Becker type)
2. Autosomal-recessive muscular dystrophy
   (a) Autosomal recessive Duchenne type
   (b) Limb girdle form (Erb)
3. Dominant muscular dystrophy
   (a) Facio-scapulo-humeral muscular dystrophy
   (b) The congenital myopathies
   (c) Familial periodic paralysis
4. Muscular diseases with myotonia
   (a) Myotonia congenita
   (b) Dystrophia myotonica
   (c) Paramyotonia congenita
5. The metabolic myopathies
6. Endocrine myopathies

Such a classification must be regarded as only a rough framework and there will be many exceptions; for example, some instances of the Duchenne type and of the facio-scapulo-humeral dystrophy have an autosomal recessive form of inheritance, and some of the limb girdle forms have a dominant one. Moreover, many congenital myopathies are sporadic (Moosa, 1974).

Sex-linked muscular dystrophy

Severe form (Duchenne type)
This is the most common and one of the most severe forms of muscular dystrophy, with a prevalence rate of 2.48/100 000, and few affected individuals survive beyond the mid-teens. The condition shows sex-linked recessive transmission due to mutation at Xp21, a specific locus on the short arm of the X chromosome (Rowand, 1988), and carrier mothers will pass it to 50% of their sons. About one third of all cases arise as spontaneous new mutations, in which case the mother does not herself carry the gene and will not pass it on to subsequent offspring. Carrier status in females can be detected with an 80% accuracy by serum creatine phosphokinase estimations, although the estimation may have to be repeated several times before abnormalities are found. The younger the carrier, the higher the detection rate is likely to be (Nicholson *et al.*, 1979). More rarely, carrier females have been found in the past by electromyography, electrocardiography, or even muscle biopsy (Emery 1969a,b). It has also been suggested that examination for myoglobinaemia may be a useful adjunct to other methods of carrier detection (Adornato, Kagan and Engel, 1978). The recent work on abnormalities of the cell membrane, which in the case of B lymphocytes can result in an interference with the aggregation of fluorescent antigen-antibody complexes on their surface (capping phenomenon), can possibly be used (Pickard *et al.*, 1978). Research into other methods of carrier detection has helped, for example carrier detection can be improved by ultrasound (Steinbicker *et al.*, 1984). However, the use of cDNA probes is now the major advance in diagnosis. This involves carrier determination with cloning of the Duchenne gene and in-corporation of DNA (which codes for dystrophin) from affected boys into micro-organisms to allow full sequencing of the dystrophin gene and its abnormalities; and the testing for the presence or absence of the abnormalities in other affected people

(Speer *et al.*, 1989). Recent studies have confirmed that the gene linked to the Duchenne type of muscular dystrophy and to the Becker type is the same. The difference in their clinical presentation may be due to changes in the structure of the gene. Once a child with this type of muscular dystrophy is diagnosed in a family and, if possible, the mother has been identified as a carrier, sexing in early pregnancy by amniocentesis can be offered; and abortion in the case of the male fetus. Unfortunately, diagnosis is often only made after another sibling has been born, and it has therefore, been suggested that a more effective approach may be to screen all boys who are not able to walk at 18 months of age for an increase of serum creatine kinase (Gardner-Medwin, Bunday and Green, 1978). This would involve about 3% of boys. It will not be so effective as screening all newborns for affected boys and carrier girls, but may be more feasible, and in some instances be more desirable. Telling parents that their baby will develop an incurable disease must carry considerable risks to the well-being of the family involved (Gardner-Medwin, 1979). Prenatal studies with DNA restriction fragment length polymorphisms of pregnancies at risk seems to be an effective means of preventing the birth of boys affected with Duchenne muscular dystrophy (Cole *et al.*, 1988). The discovery of a missing protein 'dystrophin' in muscle from affected boys opens up all kinds of possibilities for the future (Hoffman, Brown and Kunkell, 1987). The function of dystrophin is not yet known, but may be involved with factors such as stabilization of plasma membranes. Hopes for effective treatment may soon be fulfilled, for example by myoblast transfer.

Most affected boys learn to walk quite normally before the gait becomes stumbling and unsteady, though in a few the weakness may show itself early enough to present as delay in attaining independent walking. Most present in the third year of life, though they are occasionally seen as late as 6 or 7 years. There is a characteristic lordosis and they walk with a waddle. Pseudohypertrophy is seen in the calves in about 80% of patients, and less commonly in the temporal and deltoid muscles. The affected muscles feel firm and waxy. Contractures in the calves lead to toe-walking with the feet widely splayed. Weakness in the hip extensors and spinal muscles results in difficulty in

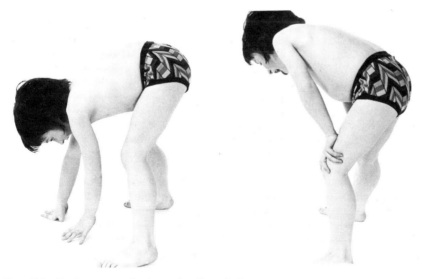

Figure 7.6   Duchenne muscular dystrophy. Gower's sign.

raising the body to the erect position without help. A characteristic manoeuvre described by Gower is seen, during which the boy pushes himself up by the arms against his own legs and body until he reaches the standing position (Fig. 7.6). Weakness in the upper limbs is first noticed in the shoulder girdle and spreads down the arm. Some finger function is usually preserved until very late. The tendon jerks are diminished or absent, but the ankle jerks can remain brisk for a long time. Intercurrent illness will often hasten the weakening. Whilst these children should be encouraged to remain ambulant for as long as possible, which helps to prevent scoliosis, the boys eventually have to resort to a wheelchair. Muscle contractures occur quite early, especially in the calves and hip flexors, and develop with frightening rapidity when the patient is immobile. Finally, the patient becomes bedridden and is able to move only the fingers and toes. Death usually occurs in the second or third decade from chest infection or cardiac failure. Cardiac involvement is common and ECG findings are characteristic with deep Q-waves in the standard leads and tall R-waves in the right precordial leads (Manning and Cropp, 1958). Tachycardia and other disturbances of rhythm are seen. Serum levels of phosphocreatine kinase and aldolase are very high in this type of myopathy, particularly in the early stages, and sometimes before abnormalities are found on clinical examination.

Many of the affected boys are dull, and discussions have centred on the causation of the mental handicap. Deprivation of opportunity to learn has been blamed and undoubtedly occurs, but as the delay in development of speech and social skills often precedes the muscular weakness, and can be of a severe degree, it is likely that it is in part the genetic expression of the disease; possibly due to a mutation in a separate gene near that for Duchenne muscular dystrophy (Rowland, 1988). Severe mental retardation and epilepsy is associated with the myopathy in the Fukuyama type of congenital muscular dystrophy (Fukuyama, Kawazura and Haruna, 1960). Children with other types of congenital muscular dystrophy, confirmed by muscle biopsy, have been reported to have normal intelligence (Dubowitz, 1980).

It is possible that treatment with predisone, continuous or intermittent, can increase muscle power in this condition, but further research is needed (Dubowitz, 1991).

Mild form (Becker type)

Becker (1962) described the milder form of sex-linked recessive muscular dystrophy with a prevalence rate of 2.38/100 000 (Bushby, Thambyayah and Gardner-Medwin, 1991). Dystrophin levels are abnormal in both Duchenne muscular dystrophy and in Becker's muscular dystrophy, but the two conditions can be differentiated because the amount of dystrophin is higher in the latter disease. The condition tends to manifest itself later (from 5–20 years) and runs a milder course, with serious interference with ambulation occurring only in the third decade after symptoms are first noted. The heart is rarely involved and contractures are also uncommon. If affected individuals marry, the condition is seen to pass through carrier daughters to grandsons. About half of the carriers of this type of muscular dystrophy have a raised serum level of creatine phosphokinase (Emery et al., 1967). It has been shown that there is no clear way of differentiating clinically between Duchenne muscular dystrophy and the early onset of the Becker form, except the later age of becoming chair-bound. From the point of view of genetic counselling, the diagnosis from limb-girdle muscular dystrophy is important because of the risk of sisters of sufferers of the Becker type being carriers. The finding of a raised serum level of creatine kinase in the mother, sister or daughter of such a male would be evidence in favour of X-linkage (Emery and Skinner, 1976).

Autosomal recessive muscular dystrophy

Autosomal recessive Duchenne type

Gardner-Medwin and Sharples (1989) have shown that this type of muscular dystrophy can cause diagnostic difficulties. Among the criteria that can differentiate this dystrophy from the sex-linked type are prominent toe walking before walking is difficult, a normal ECG and a normal intelligence. When the pseudohypertrophic type of muscular dystrophy has a recessive mode of inheritance the progress of the disease may be slower, and the clinical picture milder, than in the sex-linked form. The muscle biopsy may show differences, with less fibrosis, more fibre splitting and central nucleation, less active necrosis or regeneration, and often ring fibres (Gardner-Medwin, 1977). It must also be remembered that women who are carriers of the Duchenne gene may show slight muscle weakness, probably related to the number of affected X chromosome which are preserved (Lyon hypothesis).

Limb girdle muscular dystrophy (Erb)

Whilst most cases of this type of muscular dystrophy have their onset in the second decade of life, it can occur earlier. Both sexes are affected and initial symptoms depend on whether the pelvic or shoulder girdle are involved first. Pelvic girdle weakness presents as difficulty with rising from sitting to standing or with climbing stairs, and weakness is found in the gluteus maximus, quadriceps, and hip adductors. The anterior tibial and peroneal muscles are affected later, whilst the calf muscles are often spared. Shoulder girdle weakness may occur early and can remain the only feature for many years (scapulo-humeral type). Involvement of the trapezius and pectoralis major will result in sloping shoulders, and serratus anterior and rhomboid weakness causes winging of the scapulae. The biceps, triceps and brachioradialis are affected subsequently, as is the forearm and hand musculature. One side of the body is often more severely affected than the other. Pseudohypertrophy of calves and lateral vasti can occur in 30% of cases. Contractures develop late and are dependent on the degree of immobility. The intellect is unaffected.

Diagnostic confusion may also occur between limb-girdle muscular dystrophy and the Becker type of sex-linked muscular dystrophy. This can now often be resolved by the use of dystrophin cDNA probes so that correct genetic advice can be given (Norman *et al.*, 1989).

Dominant muscular dystrophy

Facio-scapulo-humeral muscular dystrophy (Landouzy-Dejerine)

There is considerable clinical variation in this condition, and care must be taken to differentiate it from some of the congenital disorders of muscle, such as nemaline myopathy, mitochondrial myopathy, central core disease, and (especially) myo-tubular myopathy, as these can show a clinical picture not unlike that of facio-scapulo-humeral muscular dystrophy.

As is common in dominantly inherited conditions, the severity varies quite markedly in different members of the same family; whilst some patients can be incapacitated quite early in life, many show symptoms only in the second or third decade. They are often only mildly affected and may be unaware that they have the condition. Children can present with a speech disturbance caused by nasal escape (hyperrhinophonia) and poor facial movements which result in a lack of emotional expression. There is often no frowning or smiling, which can be disconcerting to the casual observer. Closing the eyelids and whistling may be difficult. The shoulder girdle will be affected at some time and winging of the scapulae will occur. Pelvic girdle weakness is usually manifest later and results in a waddling gait which is accentuated by weakness of the anterior tibial group of muscles when the feet tend to be slapped down. The intellect is unaffected. Mild elevation of serum enzymes is usually found and the EMG shows myopathic potentials. Muscle histology often shows an increase in mean fibre diameter. Also, the histological findings can resemble those of polymyositis, supporting the possibility that this is a 'syndrome' of varying aetiology and sometimes justifying a trial of treatment with steroids (Munsat et al., 1972). However, the gene for this type of myopathy may well be on chromosome 4, which argues against genetic heterogenicity (Wijmenga et al., 1990).

The congenital myopathies

Recent years have seen a veritable explosion in the delineation of disorders of muscle in young children which, because of their clinical presentation, have at times been called 'non-progressive congenital myopathies'. Whilst they usually present with hypotonia from birth, and clinical signs and symptoms improve with age and developmental advance, a few do show clinical deterioration (Fenichel and Bazelon, 1966). The majority have a myopathic basis, but this is occasionally open to doubt; so far, characteristic histological findings have been identified in only some of them. Typical clinical features include deformities of the feet at birth and proximal muscle weakness, and constitute some of the myopathic forms of arthrogryposis multiplex congenita. The creatine phosphokinase level may be slightly raised in the serum, and the electromyogram suggests the diagnosis of myopathy. Muscle biopsy may only be abnormal if special staining techniques are used (Dubowitz, 1980). If there are no structural charactcristics on biopsy it may not be possible to classify the myopathy. There are various types of congenital muscular dystrophy which can be established as genetic and clinical entities: the Fukuyama type with contractures, weakness of limbs, trunk and facial muscles, mental retardation, speech disturbances, epilepsy and, occasionally, ocular lesions (Tsutsumi et al., 1989); and the Ullich atonic-sclerotic type with proximal joint contractures, hyperextensibility of distal joints, hyperidrosis and normal mental development (Lenard and Goebel, 1980). In instances of the Fukuyama type of congenital progressive muscular dystrophy, and even more rarely among other types of congenital muscular dystrophy, CT scanning may show a marked increase of radio-translucency of the white matter due to hypomyelination (Egger et al., 1983). This is not always associated with retarded development (Fukuyama, Makiko and Sazuki, 1981). There is some evidence that on repeating the CT scan, low density areas and other evidence of cerebral atrophy may decrease, suggesting that this may not be a degenerative disorder but perhaps an infection during interuterine life (Yoshioka et al., 1981). Apart from the Fukuyama type which shows evidence of brain and muscle disorders, there is the Santavuori type with involvement of the muscles eyes and brain, and the Walker-Warberg syndrome. In the latter there is hydrocephalus and other cerebral malformations as well as ocular abnormalities, and in some patients evidence of changes in the muscles. It is possible all three syndromes are variants of the same disease (Pavone et al., 1986).

Central core disease is a dominantly inherited condition, first described by Shy and Magee (1956) in five members of a family in three generations. Many cases have since come to light. The clinical presentation is usually that of hypotonic musculature in early infancy with occasional delay in motor milestones. Affected individuals may show a positive Gower's sign or just an inability to run as fast as their peers. Proximal muscles are more prominently affected than distal groups. Climbing steps may be difficult. The musculature is usually thin and lordosis is common. Some affected individuals may show a ptosis with weakness of facial muscles. Contractures around the hips, knees and ankles are rarely described.

Electromyography and serum enzymes are usually normal. Findings on muscle biopsy are of interest. Sections stained with haematoxylin and eosin show few abnormalities except for some small fibres. Oxydative enzyme stains, the periodic acid-Schiff (PAS) and phosphorylase reaction, show central cores which lack oxidative enzymes, and phosphorylase, and ATPase stains reveal that these findings are often limited to Type I fibres. It is suggested that the disease depends on some neural influence during development, as similar histological findings have been demonstrated in muscles from patients with long-standing neurogenic atrophy (Engel, 1961). Age makes the condition less obvious or more acceptable. No treatment is known.

Nemaline myopathy (rod-body myopathy)—this term was first used because of the rod or threadlike structures seen in histological sections of muscle from a girl aged 4 years with hypotonic musculature (Shy *et al.*, 1963). Most cases subsequently described have been mildly affected, with reduced muscle bulk, though occasionally the handicap has been quite profound (Shafiq *et al.*, 1967). Patients often have a long face and a high, arched palate; skeletal development is poor with a kyphoscoliosis; pigeon chest and pes cavus also occur. Although wasting with weakness is most marked in the trunk and proximal limb muscles it can also affect the temporalis and facial muscles and the sternocleidomastoids (Hopkins, Lindsey and Ford, 1966).

Serum enzymes are usually normal, though the EMG may show myopathic features. On muscle biopsy the rod-bodies are best demonstrated with Gomori trichrome stain. They have been found in all muscle fibre types and are variably distributed within the muscle (Fig. 7.7). Electron microscopy shows the rods to be dense and rectangular in shape and forming a fairly regular lattice pattern. They are most probably composed of tryptomyosin, and the condition is an abnormality of muscle protein (Dubowitz, 1969). The condition is probably inherited as a dominant

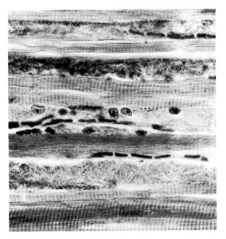

Figure 7.7   Nemaline (rod-body) myopathy. Rods and granules of different size occur in parts of muscle fibres when myofibrils have disintegrated (PTAH × 670).

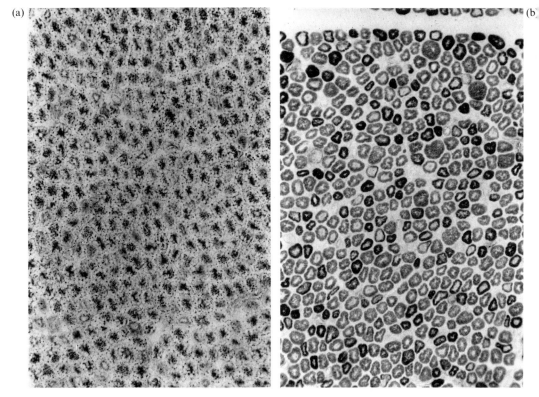

Figure 7.8   Centronuclear or myotubular myopathy. Histology of muscle biopsy. (a) ATPase pH 10.4 × 40. (b) NADH-TR × 40.

trait, and, as the clinical expression is extremely variable, many affected individuals may show few if any symptoms.

Centronuclear myopathy (myotubular myopathy)—a number of reports have appeared in the literature of a condition which presents with delayed motor development, generalized and slowly progressive muscular weakness, ptosis, external ophthalmoplegia and facial diplegia. Some of the children have a facial appearance similar to those with nemaline myopathy (Spiro, Shy and Gonatas, 1966). Not all of the cases described have been of early onset, nor do they need to have prominent facial or extra-ocular muscle weakness. Muscle enzymes may be slightly raised and the EMG may be normal. The muscle biopsy usually shows muscle fibres of normal size and a normal proportion of fibre types. More than three quarters of the fibres have centrally placed nuclei and are surrounded by an area devoid of myofibrils (Fig. 7.8). Oxydative enzyme activity is either absent or increased in these areas. The findings may indicate an arrest of muscle development, but it is not yet certain that this condition is a nosologic entity.

Mitochondrial myopathy—children with a similar type of clinical picture have been reported to show abnormalities of the mitochondria on electron microscopy (Fig. 7.9). In one, the mitochondria were abnormally large and contained inclusions, and the term 'megaconial myopathy' was suggested. Another showed increased numbers

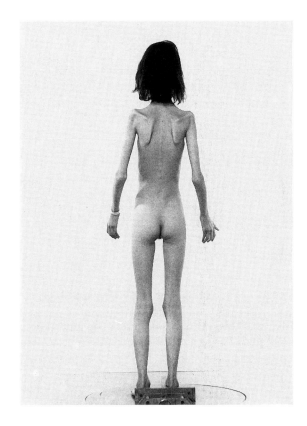

Figure 7.9   Child with mitochondrial myopathy.

of mitochondria in many fibres and was designated 'pleoconial myopathy' (Shy, Gonatas and Perez, 1966). Mitochondrial-laden fibres react excessively to stains for oxidative enzymes, and have been termed 'ragged-red fibres'.

Among myopathies with abnormal mitochondria is the Kearns Sayre syndrome (KSS). This includes external ophthalmoplegia of myopathic type, ptosis, pigmentary retinal degeneration, sensorineural deafness, cerebellar ataxia, spasticity, growth failure, heart block and dementia, as well as a mitochondrial myopathy. The cerebrospinal fluid protein is raised. The disease starts after the age of 3 years and progresses to death from heart failure or spongiform encephalopathy. Partial forms of the condition are common and the form of inheritance is uncertain (Kearns and Sayre, 1958). However, a syndrome with so many variations is likely to be of multiple aetiology, especially as mitochondria can only react in a few ways to a large number of influences (Egger *et al.*, 1981). A number of other syndromes are now included in the rubric of mitochondrial encephalopathies and myopathies, especially myoclonus epilepsy with ragged-red fibres (MERRF), and mitochondrial myophathy, encephalopathy, lactic acidosis and stroke-like episodes (MELAS) (Di Mario *et al.*, 1985). The expression of MELAS can be varied, and inheritance is uncertain. Mitochondrial inheritance has been proposed, but autosomal and X-linked dominant are also possible (Driscoll, Larsen and Gruber, 1987). Other mitochondrial encephalopathies include Leigh's and Alper's syndromes. Classification will have to await identification of the underlying metabolic defect. A temporary classification of

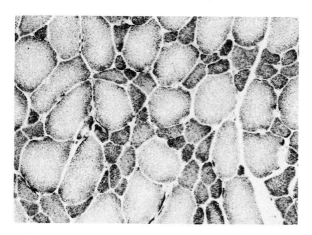

Figure 7.10   Congenital fibre-type disproportion. Cryostat section stained for NADH. The dark Type I fibres are all much smaller than the lightly stained Type II fibres (× 2770).

these *myopathies* has been devised by Walton and Mastaglia (1981): A hypermetabolic state with myopathy; the Kearns-Sayre syndrome; a myopathy with paralytic attacks provoked by exercise, alcohol or cold; and a facio-scapulohumeral or limb girdle syndrome with or without cardiomyopathy, diabetes mellitus, lactic acidaemia and cerebral degeneration.

In the diagnosis of mitochondrial disorders, apart from muscle biopsy, a pyruvate loading test may be useful (Trijbels *et al.*, 1988), but this test can be dangerous if cardiac function is impaired (Matthys, Van Coster and Verhaaren, 1991).

Congenital fibre type disproportion (Type I fibre hypotrophy) — children who have been described under this heading present as floppy babies in the immediate postnatal period and may show contractures of the hands or feet. Dislocated hips are quite common and, although all muscle groups appear to be affected, the legs are often weaker than the arms. Weakness is occasionally severe enough to result in almost complete immobility for the first two years of life, though a mild delay in milestones is more common. Many of these children are small and underweight, and some show high arched palates, kyphoscolioses and either flat or highly arched feet. Respiratory infections can be troublesome, particularly in the first year of life.

Serum enzymes are normal. The electromyogram can be normal or show a reduced interference pattern, complex motor unit potentials of high amplitude and prolonged duration, and occasional fibrillations; findings suggestive of a neurogenic lesion (Lenard and Goebel, 1975). Histochemical staining techniques demonstrated the two basic types of muscle fibres (Fig. 7.10). Type I fibres have a high mitochondrial oxidative enzyme activity and a low content of glycogen, phosphorylase and myofibrillar ATPase. Type II fibres have the opposite staining characteristics. In this condition there is a selective involvement of Type I fibres which appear smaller in diameter than normal and the nuclei are central. Type II fibres are normal or enlarged (Engel, 1970).

There are still doubts about the entity of this condition, but it is thought that the histological findings may represent a failure of development, a dysgenesis of Type I muscle fibres. Differential diagnosis is from spinal muscular atrophy, arthrogryposis multiplex congenita, neonatal myotonic dystrophy, and in particular nemaline myopathy as there is an overlap of the pathological findings (Cavanagh, Lake and McMeniman, 1979). Spontaneous improvement with age is possible. The pattern of inheritance has not been finally settled, but if nemaline myopathy is carefully excluded, the evidence is more in favour of a recessive than a dominant mode of transmission. Other combinations of predominance or variation in size of type I or type II fibres are reported, but their specificity is doubtful.

Familial periodic paralysis

Hyperkalaemic periodic paralysis (adynamia episcodica hereditaria) shows a dominant inheritance with the gene mapped to chromosome 17; and is associated with a rise in serum potassium during an attack (Gamstorp, 1963). The onset is in the first decade, and the attacks tend to be mild and of short duration. Muscle weakness is often seen after periods of rest and can be induced by the administration of potassium. Sitting still in a classroom is followed by an inability to stand up. Myotonia has been described, and it is possible that this condition and paramyotonia congenita are identical, though the precise status of these entities is still confused. Occasionally permanent weakness and wasting may occur. The administration of acetazolamide or chlorthiazide to produce potassium depletion has been recommended for prophylaxis, and 1–2 g of calcium gluconate, given intravenously, will bring relief if the paralysis is prolonged. Inhalation of salbutamol can also be effective (Wang and Clausen, 1976). Prophylactic treatment may help to prevent muscle degeneration, and is particularly indicated if frequent attacks are occurring, and the serum level of creatine phosphokinase is elevated, suggesting the presence of muscle damage.

Hypokalaemic periodic paralysis is the most common type of periodic paralysis, and is also of dominant inheritance, but clinical presentation is usually delayed until early adulthood. Paralytic attacks are associated with a fall in potassium level and are most prominent in the early morning after a night's rest. They also occur with rest after vigorous exercise, a meal containing carbohydrates, anxiety or cold. Death during an attack has been reported, and permanent weakness and loss of reflexes can occur. Administration of glucose and insulin as a test procedure will provoke hypokalaemia and an attack. The patients are unduly sensitive to the fall in potassium level, but the exact mechanism of the disorder is not known. It may be related to increased aldosterone activity (Conn and Streeten, 1960). The administration of 12 g oral potassium is helpful in stopping attacks, and prophylaxis includes a high potassium, low sodium and low carbohydrate diet, giving potassium salts at night, and trying the effect of diuretics and aldosterone antagonists.

Normokalaemic periodic paralysis has been reported (Poskanzer and Kerr, 1961). Attacks of weakness occur from an early age and may last several days. They are also precipitated by rest after exercise and by large doses of oral potassium, though the serum potassium remained normal. The administration of intravenous sodium chloride may be beneficial, and prevention can be tried with a combination of 9-α-fluorohydrocortisone and acetazolamide (McArdle, 1963).

Muscular diseases with myotonia

Myotonia congenita (Thomsen's disease)

This dominantly inherited condition characteristically presents with an inability to relax the handgrip. All muscle groups are affected, and this can result in a generalized stiffness which can lead to loss of balance. When detectable in infancy the cry may be weak and feeding difficult. Extra-ocular and facial muscles are affected, and it may take the child a considerable time to open the eyes. Lid-lag can occur on looking down after elevation of the eyes. The myotonia is worst in the morning after periods of rest and is aggravated by cold. Most affected muscle groups show a hypertrophy which usually persists throughout life, and although this also occurs in Duchenne muscular dystrophy the generalized hypertophy in this condition is such that it is referred to as the *Infant Hercules Syndrome*. Percussion of the muscle belly will cause prolonged contractions and slow relaxation, and the EMG shows a typical 'dive-bomber' pattern when it is heard on the loudspeaker of the electromyograph. Muscle biopsy reveals relatively few changes, though there is a total absence of type 2B fibres. In this condition, and in allied ones, troublesome myotonia justifies the trial of phenytoin up to 400 mg a day or procaine amide 1 g daily (Munsat, 1967), but neither drug may relieve the symptoms. An alternative may be nifedapine 10–20 mg three times a day (Grant, Sutton and Ballantyne, 1987).

Dystrophia myotonica (Steinert's disease)
This disease of dominant inheritance affects many systems, though the effect on muscles is particularly striking. It usually starts in early adult life and men are more severely affected than women. It tends to show anticipation, with children affected at an earlier age than their parents, and with an increase in severity in succeeding generations (Vanier, 1960). The fully developed picture includes slowly progressive muscle weakness, wasting and myotonia. This is very obvious in the face, where it involves the temporalis, the masseters and sternomastoid muscles. Ptosis is often noted. Cataracts are common as age increases, and slit lamp examination reveals lens lesions in 90% of cases. The testes are small and atrophic, and females may show menstrual irregularities. Cardiac involvement is usually demonstrated as a conduction defect on electrocardiography, and routine testing is justified so that pacing can be used if necessary. Contrast radiography may show inco-ordinate oesophageal contractions. Dementia may develop in individuals who have initially shown normal intellectual development.

Presentation in the paediatric age group
Many affected infants show severe muscular hypotonia in the first years of life (Gordon and Hilson, 1967). At birth there may be failure to establish adequate respiration, with resulting risk to life. They have immobile, fish-like facies, resembling Moebius' syndrome, and often have feeding difficulties. In pre-term babies with neonatal dystrophia myotonica oedema and unexplained haematoma have been described (Pearse and Höweler, 1979). Talipes equinovarus is also common. The facial appearance remains characteristic, and affected children are easily recognized by their small mandible with maloccluded teeth, and there is usually a marked dysarthria. The mouth hangs open and they dribble saliva. The expressionless face usually gives the mouth a pouted appearance (Fig. 7.11). The hypotonia persists, and these children are often clumsy and mentally backward. Occasionally ptosis is a prominent feature. Myotonia has been described in the first year of life, but is rare in infancy. To begin with, it is difficult to elicit, even by percussion of thenar and limb muscles. Then the grip may be slow to relax, and the eyes slow to open if tightly shut. It is demonstrated more readily by the electromyograph in some cases. The myotonia can cause the child to fall when balance is upset and corrective action cannot be taken quickly enough. The level of IgG may be decreased and there may be evidence of a hypersecretion of insulin. There is an increased anaesthetic risk. It is always worth

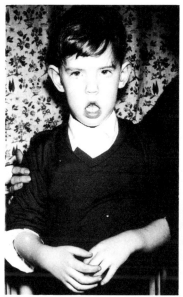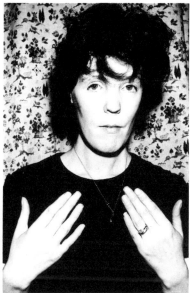

Figure 7.11 Dystrophia myotonica (congenital type).

Figure 7.12 Dystrophia myotonica. Affected mother of child in Figure 7.11.

examining the mother when the condition is suspected, for she may show only mild muscle wasting, weakness and myotonia, and often has not consulted a doctor (Fig. 7.12). The fact that the infantile form is almost invariably inherited through the mother suggests a maternal factor acting *in utero* on a fetus with the abnormal gene (Harper, 1975). No such factor has been identified, and mitochondrial inheritance may be an explanation with variation of DNA content (Flannery, 1978), or the influence of a substance such as deoxycholic acid which is markedly raised in affected mothers (Tanaka, Takishita and Takita, 1981). An attractive alternative hypothosis is a genomic imprinting effect making the disease more severe in the affected offspring of a proportion of affected mothers (Hodgson, 1991). It may be that DNA studies will, in the future, help in diagnosis.

Muscle biopsy shows fairly characteristic myopathic changes in the fully developed case. Type I fibre atrophy is often, though not invariably, present. Type II fibre hypertrophy is an important feature. The nuclei are situated centrally and fibrosis is prominent. In childhood the myotonia is generally not severe enough to require modification with procaine amide or phenytoin.

Paramyotonia congenita

The difficulty in distinguishing this condition from hyperkalaemic periodic paralysis and the possibility that it may not be a separate entity have already been mentioned. As with other types of myotonia, there is slowness and stiffness of movement, and the symptoms are precipitated by cold. If mild, the symptoms may be restricted to the hands, eyelids and tongue. If myotonia is improved, for example by giving acetozolamide or inducing hypokalaemia, muscle weakness may develop; while potassium loading increases myotonia but improves muscle strength. These findings suggest that the symptoms have different mechanisms (Wiles and Edwards, 1977).

The metabolic myopathies

The Glycogenoses with muscle involvement

Table 7.1   Disorders due to errors in glycogen metabolism

Deficiency	Type	Name	Enzyme deficiency
Acid maltase	Type II	Pompe's disease	Alpha glucosidase
Debrancher enzyme	Type III	Forbes' disease	Amylo-1,6 transglucosidase
Brancher enzyme	Type IV	Anderson's disease	Amylo-transglucosidase
Myophosphorylase	Type V	McArdle's disease	Myophosphorylase
Phosphofructokinase	Type VII	Tarui's disease	Phosphofructokinase

Greater understanding of the pathways of glycogen synthesis and breakdown have resulted in the isolation of a number of errors of glycogen metabolism which produce symptoms in the organs in which glycogen is stored, or in those for which glucose release is vital (Table 7.1). Liver and muscle are most prominently affected, and nine types have been defined to date, though international agreement is still awaited for the most recently described variants. Whilst most result in a degree of stunting, five of the types have fairly characteristic muscle involvement.

Acid maltase deficiency-Type II glycogenosis (Pompe's disease). Acid maltase (alpha glucosidase) is a lysosomal enzyme which hydrolyses maltase, linear oligo-saccharides and the outer chains of glycogen to glucose (Dubowitz, 1966). Its absence results in deposition of glycogen in many organs, including skeletal and cardiac muscle, the central nervous system, and liver (Hers, 1963). There may be widespread storage in neurons and glial cells, and gliosis of cerebral white and grey matter. Four principal forms have been identified on clinical presentation: (1) the cardiomegalic; (2) the generalized; (3) the muscular; and (4) the late infantile acid-maltase deficiency.

As the same enzyme is absent in all tissues tested, it is likely that the types do not represent different disease entities, but that the clinical symptoms depend on which tissue is predominantly affected by the glycogen deposition. Most cases have been described in young infants who present with severe muscle weakness and hypotonia, which can be due either to the primary muscle involvement or to glycogen deposition in the anterior horn cells of the cord. Affected children show clinical similarity to those with infantile spinal muscular atrophy. Progressive mental deterioration and respiratory failure can occur. In some the cases cardiac muscle is mainly affected, leading to enlargement of the heart and presentation with cardiac failure. In recent years a number of cases have been recorded in which acid maltase deficiency was associated with a less severe muscular weakness and with a later age of onset; even adult cases being described. The presentation was often similar to that seen in limb-girdle muscular dystrophy. It is obvious that the signs show wide variation, the disease sometimes being confined to the muscles (Hudgson *et al.*, 1968). Points of differentiation from muscular dystrophy are the involvement of the tongue and sparing of the arms. The creatine phosphokinase levels are usually raised. The EMG shows polyphasic potentials of low amplitude and there may be myotonic discharges (Lenard *et al.*, 1974). In the juvenile form the diagnosis may first be suggested by the EMG showing prominent high-frequency discharges in addition to myopathic potentials (Gardner-Medwin, 1977). Histological examination of a muscle biopsy shows large amounts of glycogen in the muscle fibres. The enzyme deficiency can be demonstrated in the muscle and in the peripheral leucocytes. Inheritance is of an autosomal recessive type.

Debranching enzyme deficiency-Type III glycogenosis (Forbes' disease)—whilst hepatic features usually predominate, some cases of debranching enzyme deficiency (amylo-1, 6 transglucosidase) have presented with definite muscle weakness which is usually mild and of proximal distribution. The enzyme defect can be detected readily in both tissues and leucocytes (Illingworth, Cori and Cori, 1956).

Branching enzyme deficiency-Type IV glycogenosis, or Anderson's disease, is a rare form of glycogen storage disease in which a glycogen of abnormal structure characteristically causes cirrhosis of the liver and ascites. Skeletal muscle is not invariably affected, although some children show quite marked muscle weakness and wasting. The substance deposited in the liver is thought to be amylopectin.

Myophosphorylase deficiency-Type V glycogenosis was first noted in 1951, when McArdle described a man who complained of muscle cramps on exertion; there was no rise in blood lactic acid after ischaemic exercise, and subsequent investigators have demonstrated an absence of muscle phosphorylase. Young children and adolescents may only tire easily, whilst cramps, transient myoglobinuria, weakness and wasting are seen only after the age of 20 years (Schmid and Mahler, 1959). Occlusion of the circulation with a sphygomanometer cuff will induce the cramp. Glycogen deposition in muscle is not so marked as in other glycogenoses, but the absence of phosphorylase can be demonstrated histochemically. The diagnosis is made by the lack of any demonstrable rise in the blood lactate level after ischaemic exercise. When the blood supply to the forearm has been obstructed the patient is asked to exercise with a spring grip for up to three minutes. Blood lactate levels are estimated at the start of the test and for up to 20 minutes afterwards. If possible a normal control is tested at the same time. The EMG shows typical electrical silence during the cramp. A muscle biopsy shows an excessive accumulation of glycogen, and muscle phosphorylase activity is found to be reduced to 0.5% of normal control levels (Sinclair, 1979). Inheritance is autosomal recessive. Treatment with oral fructose and ephedrine and intramuscular glucagon has been suggested but has not proved successful (Rowand *et al.*, 1966). A fat-rich diet may have beneficial effects (Viskoper *et al.*, 1975), or any means of supplying muscle energy in the form of medium chain triglycerides rather than glucose.

The presentation of *phosphofructokinase deficiency—Type VII glycogenosis*, also known as Tarui's disease, is similar to McArdle's disease, with excessive fatiguability, cramps and muscle weakness, and an absence of any rise in lactate after ischaemic exercise. It is also probably of autosomal recessive inheritance. Raised muscle glycogen and phosphofructokinase deficiency are found on biopsy (Layzer, Rowand and Ranney, 1967). A possible inhibition of phosphohexoisomerase may also produce this clinical picture (Satoyoshi and Kowa, 1967). The levels of serum aldolase and creatine phosphokinase are considerably raised in these two conditions.

Lipid myopathies

A number of different types of lipid myopathy have been described, mainly in association with carnitine deficiency. Carnitine is an essential co-factor in the transfer of fatty acids into mitochondria, a carrier molecule for those with chains of C12 or more, so that they can be oxidized within the mitochondria by a process of beta-oxidation. If there is a deficiency of carnitine palmityl transferase this cannot take place (Di Mario and Di Mario, 1973). This type of carnitine myopathy shows a clinical picture like that of McArdle's disease with muscle cramps and myoglobinuria after exertion or fasting which may last for hours or days, but ischaemic work produces a normal rise in lactic acid. The enzyme deficiency can be relieved by giving medium chain triglycerides or adequate carbohydrates before exercise as an alternative energy source. The serum creatine-phospho-kinase (CPK) can be very high during an attack and a muscle biopsy may show a few lipid-containing vacuoles in type I fibres (Gardner-Medwin, 1977).

In other types of carnitine myopathy there are no cramps or myoglobinuria and the term type I lipid storage myopathy has been proposed for the triad of muscle weakness, triglyceride excess and creatine deficiency. The CPK may be only slightly abnormal (Engel and Angelini, 1973). In another type there are episodes of vomiting and acidosis and the level of carnitine has been found to be deficient, not only in the muscles, but also in the serum and liver. There have been encouraging reports of improvement in the condition of patients with these types of carnitine myopathy after the oral administration of carnitine (Angelini *et al.*, 1976). Prednisolone and propanolol have been used. It is possible that muscle and systemic carnitine deficiency may be stages in the same mitochondrial disorder. The younger the patient the more rapidly the disease becomes generalized. It is suggested that a diagnosis simply of carnitine deficiency is no longer acceptable, as the disorder may well be secondary to other metabolic changes such as glutaric aciduria type II (Turnbull *et al.*, 1988).

Endocrine myopathies

A number of endocrine diseases have muscle involvement as part of the clinical picture. Most prominent amongst these are the thyroid disorders.

Thyrotoxicosis may be associated with a chronic myopathy—which can at times precede other clinical evidence of the disease; and also with hypokalaemic periodic paralysis. The acute myopathy in this condition involving the external eye muscles is probably myasthenic in nature.

Hypothyroidism with lack of thyroid hormone may at times be associated with muscle atrophy. Enlargement of the muscles is occasionally seen in cretinism, and involves the tongue, trapezius and pectoral muscles and muscles of the arms and legs. The bulky appearance disappears with treatment.

Acromegaly is also associated with muscle hypertrophy in the early stages of the disease.

Cushing's syndrome is at times associated with proximal muscle weakness which can increase in severity following adrenolectomy.

Primary aldosteronism presents commonly with periodic bouts of muscle weakness which are probably precipitated by the loss of potassium.

Arthrogryposis multiplex congenita

There are probably many different causes of this condition, apart from the myopathic form complicating congenital myopathies and congenital muscular dystrophies. The baby is born with extreme stiffness and contractures of joints with an absence of muscle development. Fixed deformities are common, including scoliosis, dislocation of the hip, and clubfoot. In some instances there is evidence of a neuropathy, with lack of anterior horn cells on *post mortem* examination. There is usually no suggestion of genetic factors, and it may be that most cases result from defective intrauterine environment, whether hormonal, vascular, mechanical or infective (Wynne-Davies and Lloyd-Roberts, 1976).

Paroxysmal myoglobinuria (Meyer-Betz syndrome)

Myoglobinuria is associated with a number of conditions, e.g. crush injuries, ischaemic necrosis and diabetic acidosis. However, it sometimes occurs with no apparent precipitating cause. The symptoms include cramp, tenderness and weakness of the limb muscles lasting several days. There may be a family history, but the metabolic defect is unknown. The danger to life is from anuria and respiratory paralysis (Borman, Davidson and Blondheim, 1963). The guaiac test on the urine will be positive in this disease in the absence of erythrocytes, and the myoglobin can be identified by the spectroscope.

Polymyositis

This is an inflammatory myopathy with a wide variability in clinical presentation. The aetiology is poorly understood and, whilst a number of cases are associated with a variety of malignancies, this association is not seen in early childhood. It can occur acutely following symptoms of upper respiratory tract infections, or may show up insidiously with muscle weakness and wasting, when it can closely simulate muscular dystrophy. It can be localized or generalized, and is quite frequently associated with lesions in the skin (dermatomyositis). A total of 17% of all cases present before the age of 15 years, some being as young as 2 or 3 years of age. The condition may be symmetrical or uneven in distribution. Children present with a history of being unable to get about as well as previously, with abnormalities of gait, difficulties in negotiating stairs, and noticeable muscle wasting (particularly around the shoulder girdle). Prominent involvement of the neck muscles is much commoner than in the muscular dystrophies. Generalized muscle tenderness is found in a proportion of cases and a few also have joint pains. The association of misery with weakness suggests polymyositis. Dysphagia and dysphonia imply involvement of the posterior pharyngeal musculature. Contractures can develop and calcification of muscle and subcutaneous tissues sometimes occurs. The skin manifestations may be slight, such as irregular patches of depigmentation or atrophy. Occasionally there are slightly raised red areas which are shiny or covered in scales, and sometimes the skin lesions are florid over the face, trunk, knees, elbows and knuckles; and are often itchy. The colour is often lilac, especially over the eyelids. The clinical course may be associated with a low-grade fever and be punctuated by remissions and relapses.

When the presentation is one of muscle weakness the most suggestive clinical features are a rapid onset, remissions, involvement of the neck muscles, dysphagia, slight muscle atrophy, preservation of the tendon reflexes, an associated arthralgia, and Raynaud's phenomenon. The serum enzymes may be elevated and the EMG may show a myopathic pattern, though evidence of denervation with fibrillation potentials and positive sharp waves also occurs. The erythrocyte sedimentation rate (ESR) is often normal (De Vere and Bradley, 1975). Muscle biopsy may or may not show changes of degeneration and regeneration, with necrosis and an atrophy of all fibre types. Inflammatory changes and fibrosis are seen but are not invariable.

Survival in children is much better than in adults. Those with a lesser disability at onset have a better prognosis for morbidity, but not for mortality, and the presence of rheumatoid arthritis or progressive sclerosis is a bad sign (De Vere and Bradley, 1975). Early treatment with steroids, commencing with doses of up to 60 mg of prednisolone a day, is important, as it is one of the few muscle disorders that responds to therapy. Reviewing the treatment of dermatomyositis in childhood, Miller,

Heckmatt and Dubowitz (1983) suggest that there are advantages in moderate dosage starting with prednisolone 1–1.5 mg/kg body weight/day, short-term treatment schedules, with gradual tapering of the dosage as soon as there is clinical improvement, and in trying to stop therapy within six months. Over-treatment may be a factor in prolonging the disease and in the failure of adequate long-term response. Cytotoxic agents have been effective, especially in cases refractory to corticosteroids (Sokoloff, Goldberg and Pearson, 1971), and so has azathiaprine (1 mg/kg body weight/day). A combination of cyclophosphamide and prednisone may be particularly effective (Niakan et al., 1980). Cyclosporin is invaluable in patients who are unresponsive to steroids or dependent on a high dose. Physiotherapy can help a great deal.

Diagnosis of muscle weakness

The complaint of weakness in a child may be due to a wide variety of conditions, some of which have no primary relationship with the central or peripheral nervous systems or the muscles, e.g. certain metabolic disorders, deficiency diseases and malabsorption syndromes. Investigations may have to be extensive, but when the differential diagnosis lies between a neurogenic and myopathic lesion, three tests have to be considered.

Estimation of the serum enzymes, particularly aldolase and creatine phosphokinase, is helpful in suggesting rapid breakdown of muscle, as in pseudohypertrophic muscular dystrophy, polymyositis and McArdle's disease. Very slight elevations of the creatine phosphokinase level do not differentiate between some types of myopathy and neuropathy. Giving 1 mg per kg body weight of hydrocortisone intravenously causes a significant rise of creatine phosphokinase 4 hours later in patients with muscular dystrophy and in many carriers, but not in other neuromuscular disorders, which may be helpful in the differential diagnosis (Sen and Das, 1978). A raised level of this enzyme can also identify patients at risk from *malignant hyperpyrexia* as a complication of a variety of anaesthetic agents (Lane and Mastaglia, 1978), but pharmacological and histological examination of muscle biopsies from all family members is much more reliable (Ellis et al., 1975). The *in vivo* contracture test for susceptibility to malignant hyperthermia requires a substantial amount of muscle tissue, but now that the gene for this condition has been located on chromosome 19 a more accurate test is available for known pedigrees using molecular genetic linkage studies (Healy et al., 1991). This condition is related to myopathies of various types, especially myotonic, although they are not always clinically detectable (King, Denborough and Zapf, 1972). The condition may be relieved by vigorous cooling, correction of acidosis, dexamethazone, and the use of drugs, such as procaine amide and dantrolene sodium, which lower sarcoplasmic calcium levels (Mastaglia, 1980). Dantrolene sodium can be used to prepare patients who are suspected of having this condition, by giving it orally for two to three days before operation. Also it can be given parenterally before emergency surgery (Hamer, 1981). A high calcium ion concentration in the myoplasm may be the fundamental disorder. It seems to have a dominant mode of inheritance.

Electrodiagnosis is the next investigation in making the diagnosis between neuropathies and myopathies (Lenman and Ritchie, 1970). The exclusion of myopathic and neurogenic lesions will favour a cerebral cause for hypotonia and weakness.

In neurogenic lesions, including both spinal muscular atrophy and peripheral nerve lesions, there may be evidence of denervation in the form of excessive insertion activity with positive sharp waves, fibrillations with positive sharp waves from denervated muscle fibres and fasciculation especially in anterior horn cell disorders. Widespread spontaneous fasciculations in all four limbs almost always indicates motor neurone disease, which is uncommon in the young. During voluntary muscular contraction, loss of motor units may be associated with a reduction in motor unit recruitment (reduced interference pattern). Even in severe lesions, retention of some motor unit activity indicates that the lesion is incomplete. Because of reinnervation, individual motor units may be of high amplitude and of polyphasic contour.

Reduction of motor and sensory conduction velocity is seen in many peripheral nerve lesions, though in purely axonal (neuronal 'dying back') neuropathies motor conduction may be either normal or absent. A marked slowing of conduction in individual nerve fibres will be found with segmental demyelination (demyelinating neuropathy) when the Schwann cells are attacked, as rapid conduction is dependent on the integrity of the myelin sheath. There will be reductions in the amplitude and a lengthened duration of the evoked muscle and sensory action potentials, and this can be the only evidence that the child suffers from a peripheral neuropathy. The findings are not always clear-cut, as both the Schwann cells and the nerve cells in the anterior horns of the spinal cord and in the posterior root ganglia can be affected by the noxious agent. However, these studies may differentiate between the two main types of neuropathy so that a nerve biopsy is unnecessary. Examples of segmental demyelination are: infectious polyneuritis, diabetic neuropathy and peroneal muscular atrophy. Axonal neuropathies occur in thiamine deficiency, toxic neuropathies and porphyria.

Conduction in both motor and sensory fibres may be studied together by the use of the mixed nerve action potential (Caine and Pallis, 1972). The amplitude of the nerve action potential, so evoked, depends on both antidromic motor and orthodromic sensory conduction in the nerve under study, and may be abnormal even when conduction velocity is unaffected.

In infantile spinal muscular atrophy a unique feature is regular discharge activity, 5–15 per second, in muscles relaxed voluntarily and during sleep. One or more of the electromyographic features characteristic of disease of the anterior horn cells are almost always found. An increased mean amplitude of motor unit potentials is the most constant finding, but depending on the severity of the disease, the other abnormalities include increased amplitude of the pattern during voluntary effort, prolonged duration of individual motor unit potentials and increased maximum amplitude in the territory of motor units. The territories of the motor units are often increased (Buchthal and Olsen, 1970). Sometimes there is a small reduction in motor conduction velocity due to a fall out of the fastest conducting fibres. A further consequence of this is that the height of action potentials may then be reduced. However, sensory conduction, if this can be carried out, will be normal (Schwartz and Moosa, 1977). High frequency discharges with a gradual decrement occur in the myotonias, and on the loudspeaker give rise to a characteristic noise which is often referred to as the 'dive-bomber' effect.

In muscle disease, as opposed to neurogenic disorders, increased insertional or spontaneous activity is usually absent. The characteristic finding, even when maximal voluntary force is weak, is a full interference pattern, except in the late stages of the disease. The motor units are of short duration, highly polyphasic, and are not increased in amplitude. A scratchy-sounding noise on the loudspeaker may be useful in interpretation.

In polymyositis there is a myopathic pattern but, in contrast to muscular dystrophy, spontaneous activity in the form of fibrillation and positive sharp waves is common. An abnormally early full recruitment pattern on moderate contraction may occur.

Progressive diminution of the amplitude of the evoked muscle-action potential in response to repetitive stimulation of the appropriate motor nerve at a rate of three shocks per second is sometimes helpful in the diagnosis of myasthenia gravis. This is especially so if the finding is reversed by an injection of edrophonium chloride (Richardson and Barwick, 1969).

Muscle or nerve biopsy may have to be considered when the preliminary tests are inconclusive. The former should be done on a moderately affected muscle, and one which has not been used for EMG studies, which can produce artefacts. Additional information can be obtained by intravital staining for end-plates (Woolf, 1962). The motor point can be identified by stimulating with surface electrodes before the biopsy is taken, and by direct stimulation of the muscle at operation. The findings are likely to be particularly striking in neuropathies and spinal muscular atrophies. In the former the terminal parts of the motor axons show fusiform or spherical swellings, and in the latter the characteristic findings are a break up of the terminal motor axons into a fine tangle of nerve bundles, and the presence of poorly formed end-plates (Woolf, 1969).

In denervation atrophy the histological picture will be one of groups of uniformly small fibres with dark clustered nuclei (Fig. 7.13). There is relatively little change in the connective tissue. On special staining there will be grouping of muscle fibres of the same histological type, indicating reinnervation, instead of the usual random distribution. Primary muscle disease, as in the genetic dystrophies, will be suggested by the diminution in the total complement of muscle fibres, necrosis of some fibres with signs of phagocytosis, enlargement of fibres, atrophy of others, central nucleation, nuclear chains, infiltration of fat cells, and increase of connective tissue (Fig. 7.14) (Adams, 1969). In polymyositis the necrosis and inflammatory reaction can be accentuated.

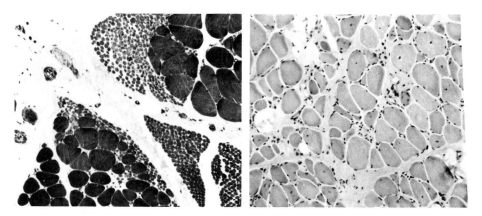

Figure 7.13 (left) Neurogenic atrophy. Denervated muscle fibres are atrophied and contrast with the normal and hypertrophied fibres. Spinal muscular atrophy (HE × 270).

Figure 7.14 (right) Myopathy. Shows variation in fibre calibre, internal nuclei, fibre splitting and fibrosis. Some of the darker fibres are regenerating (HE × 270).

To identify some muscle diseases, for example the congenital myopathies, special stains will be needed. In central core disease the central core stains blue and the periphery red with Gomori's trichrome stain. In nemaline myopathy the rods will be identified by Gomori's trichrome or phosphotungstic acid haematoxylin stains. Stains for oxidative enzymes will reveal abnormalities of the mitochondria in megaconial and pleoconial myopathies, even if this finding may be a non-specific one; and such special stains will also identify congenital fibre type disproportion.

Biopsy of a peripheral nerve will help to establish the diagnosis of certain neuropathies, such as hypertrophic interstitial polyneuritis and amyloid polyneuritis, and may be needed to differentiate an axonal neuropathy from segmental demyelination.

There can be no doubt that knowledge of neuropathies and myopathies will be advanced by intensive investigation. Tests include a search for metabolic disorders, muscle enzyme estimations, the use of electron microscopy, and tissue culture; and they may all have to be considered if a correct diagnosis is to be made in the maximum number of patients.

Treatment

Many of the conditions discussed in this chapter are not amenable to specific treatment, but this is not to suggest that there is nothing to be done for the child and the family.

If there is a known mode of inheritance, genetic advice to the parents is essential. Parents are entitled to the known facts, and if the disease is a serious one the risks of other children being affected may well be too high to be acceptable. If, as in the sex-linked form of pseudohypertrophic muscular dystrophy, it is possible to identify carriers, this service must also be offered to the family.

When a child is severely disabled, and particularly by a progressive condition, the family may need help in a number of different ways. Social problems arise and include unsuitable housing and the need to provide opportunities for holidays. Special education is often required, as is the assistance of an experienced careers advisory service. The patient and other members of the family are at considerable risk from emotional disturbances, and the doctor and the social worker can do much to anticipate situations which may lead to additional stresses and strains, and try to give practical advice and help.

Medical treatment can take a number of forms. It will obviously include treatment of such generalized diseases as malabsorption and deficiency syndromes, if these have been identified. Physiotherapy can do much to influence the course of the illness, and the advice of the orthopaedic specialist will often be needed. Not enough attention has been paid in the past to the prevention of deformities, particularly of scoliosis. The child with muscular dystrophy can remain ambulant for a longer time if provided with calipers, and when he or she is confined to a chair, scrupulous attention must be paid to its design, type and suitability, with a sloping back to help to prevent scoliosis, and adequate support for the feet to counteract the tendency for talipes equinovarus to develop. If scoliosis is progressing above 20 degrees at the start of the wheelchair stage surgical stabilization of the spine should be considered and mechanical ventilation may be necessary. Immobilization must be avoided if at all possible, and among boys with Duchenne muscular dystrophy steps must be taken to try to prevent the commonly occurring obesity, although this is easier said than done. The occupational therapist has an important part to play in the management and training of the physically handicapped child. This may include helping to solve difficulties that arise in the child's day to day living, as well as developing skills which can be surprisingly effective even in the presence of severe disability.

A small number of specific therapies have been mentioned, including neostigmine bromide for myasthenia gravis, potassium for hypokalaemic periodic paralysis, steroids for polymyositis, and the possibility of modifying metabolic disturbances affecting the function of the central and peripheral nervous systems, for example diabetes mellitus and hypothyroidism. The rarity of specific treatment means there is a special need for accurate diagnosis of children presenting with weakness, wasting and hypotonia. Only by continued study of causes will the prognosis for these children be improved.

References

Abrams, I.F., Bresnan, M.J., Zuckerman, J.E. *et al.* (1973) Cervical cord injuries secondary to hyperextension of the head in breech presentations. *Obstetrics-Gynaecology*, **41**, 369

Adams, R.D. (1969) Pathological reactions of the skeletal muscle fibre in man. In *Disorders of Voluntary Muscles* (ed. J.N. Walton), Churchill Livingstone, London

Adornato, B.T., Kagan, L.J. and Engel, W.K. (1978) Myoglobinaemia in Duchenne muscular dystrophy patients and carriers: a new adjunct to carrier detection. *Lancet*, **ii**, 499

Angelini, C., Lücke, S., Canteratti, M.S. and Canteratti, F. (1976) Carnitine deficiency of skeletal muscle: report of a treated case. *Neurology*, **26**, 633

Argov, Z. and Mastaglia, F.L. (1979) Drug-induced peripheral neuropathies. *British Medical Journal*, **i**, 663

Axelrod, F.B., Nachtigal, R. and Dancis, I. (1974) Familial dysautonomia: diagnosis, pathogenesis and management. In *Advances in Pediatrics Vol. 20* (ed. I. Schulman), Lloyd-Luke, London

Barlow, C.F. (1981) Neonatal myasthenia gravis. *American Journal of Diseases of Children*, **135**, 209

Barry, I.E., Hopkins, I.I. and Neal, B.W. (1974) Congenital sensory neuropathy. *Archives of Disease in Childhood*, **49**, 128

Bazelon, M., Paine, R.S., Cowie, V.S. *et al.* (1967) Reversal of hypotonia in infants with Down's syndrome by administration of 5-hydroxytryptophan. *Lancet*, **i**, 1130

Becker, P.E. (1962) Two new families of benign sex-linked recessive muscular dystrophy. *Revue Canadienne de Biologie*, **21**, 551

Benardy, S.G. (1978) Spinal muscular atrophy in childhood: review of 50 cases. *Developmental Medicine and Child Neurology*, **20**, 746

Beratis, N.G., Aron, A.M. and Hirschhorn, K. (1973) Metachromatic leukodystrophy: detection in serum. *Journal of Pediatrics*, **83**, 824

Bieri, J.G. Corash, L.C. Hubbart, Van, S. (1983) Medical uses of vitamin E. *New England Journal of Medicine*, **308**, 1063

Boothby, J.A., De Jesus, P.V. and Rowland, L.P. (1974) Reversible forms of motor neuron disease. *Archives of Neurology*, **31**, 18

Borman, J.B., Davidson, I.T. and Blondheim, S.H. (1963) Idiopathic rhabdomyolysis (myoglobinuria) as an acute respiratory problem. *British Medical Journal*, **ii**, 726

Bower, B.D. and Newsolme, E.A. (1978) Treatment of idiopathic polyneuritis by a polyunsaturated fatty acid diet. *Lancet*, **i**, 583

Brzustowicz, L.M., Lehner, T., Castilla, L.H. *et al.* (1990) Genetic mapping of chronic childhood-onset spinal muscular atrophy to chromosome 5q11.2-13.3. *Nature*, **344**, 540

Buchthal, F. and Olsen, P.Z. (1970) Electromyography and muscle biopsy in infantile muscular atrophy. *Brain*, **93**, 15

Bushby, K.M.D., Thambyayah, M. and Gardner-Medwin, D. (1991) Prevalence and incidence of Becker muscular dystrophy. *Lancet*, **337**, 1022–4

Caine, D.B. and Pallis, C.A. (1972) Electromyography and nerve conduction studies. *British Journal of Hospital Medicine*, **5**, 775

Cavanagh, N.P.C., Lake, B.D. and McMeniman, P. (1979) Congenital fibre disproportion myopathy: a histological diagnosis with an uncertain clinical outlook. *Archives of Disease in Childhood*, **54**, 735

Chapman, G.P., Weller, R.O., Normand, I.C.S. and Gibbens, D. (1978) Spinal Cord Transection in utero. *British Medical Journal*, **ii**, 398

Cole, C.G., Walker, A., Coyne, A. *et al.* (1988) Prenatal testing for Duchenne and Becker muscular dystrophy. *Lancet*, **i**, 262

Conn, I.W. and Streeten, D.H.P. (1960) In *The Metabolic Basis of Inherited Disease* (eds. I.B. Stanbury, I.B. Wyngaarden, and D.S. Fredricksen), McGraw-Hill, New York

Cook, S.D., Dowling, P.C., Murray, M.R. and Whitaker, I.N. (1971) Circulating demyelinating factors in acute idiopathic polyneuropathy. *Archives of Neurology*, **24**, 136

Cryan, B. and Wright, D.J.M. (1991) Lyme disease in paediatrics. *Archives of Disease in Childhood*, **66**, 1359–63

Dau, P.C., Lindstrom, J.M., Cassel, C.K. *et al.* (1977) Plasmopheresis and immunosuppressive drug therapy in myasthenia gravis. *New England Journal of Medicine*, **297**, 1134

De Souza, S.W. and Davis, I.A. (1974) Spinal cord damage. *Archives of Disease in Childhood*, **49**, 70

De Vere, R. and Bradley, W.G. (1975) Polymyositis: its presentation, morbidity and mortality. *Brain*, **98**, 637

Di Mario, S. and Di Mario, P.S. (1973) Muscle carnitine palmityltransferase deficiency and myoglobinuria. *Science*, **182**, 929

Di Mario, S., Bonilla, E., Zeviani, M. *et al.* (1985) Mitochondrial myopathies. *Annals of Neurology*, **17**, 621

Drachman, D.A., Paterson, P.Y., Berlin, B.S. and Roguska, I. (1970) Immunosuppression and the Guillain-Barré syndrome. *Archives of Neurology*, **23**, 385

Drillien, C.M. (1972) Aetiology and outcome in low-birthweight infants. *Developmental Medicine and Child Neurology*, **14**, 563

Driscoll, P.F., Larsen, P.D. and Gruber, A.B. (1987) MELAS syndrome involving a mother and two children. *Archives of Neurology*, **44**, 971

Dubowitz, V. (1966) Muscle glycogenesis. *Developmental Medicine and Child Neurology*, **8**, 432

Dubowitz, V. (1969) The 'new' myopathies. *Neuropädiatrie*, **1**, 137

Dubowitz, V. (1980) *The Floppy Infant*, 2nd edn. Clinics in Developmental Medicine, SIMP, Heinemann, London

Dubowitz, V. (1991) Prednisone in Duchenne dystrophy. *Neuromuscular Disorders*, **1**, 161

Dunn, H.G., Daube, J.R. and Gomez, M.R. (1978) Heredofamilial brachial plexus neuropathy (hereditary neuralgic amotrophy with brachial predeliction) in childhood. *Developmental Medicine and Child Neurology*, **20**, 28

Dyck, P.I. and Lambert, E.H. (1968) Lower motor and primary sensory neuron diseases with peroneal muscular atrophy. *Archives of Neurology*, **18**, 603

Dyck, P.J., Lais, A.C., Ohta, M. *et al.* (1975) Chronic inflammatory polyradiculoneuropathy. *Mayo Clinic Proc.*, **50**, 621

Eaton, L.M. and Lambert, E.H. (1957) Electromyography and electric stimulation of nerves in diseases of motor unit. *Journal of the American Medical Association*, **163**, 1117

Eberle, E., Brink, I., Azen, S. and White, D. (1975) Early predictors of incomplete recovery in children with Guillain-Barré polyneuritis. *Journal of Pediatrics*, **86**, 356

Egger, J., Lake, B.D. and Wilson, J. (1981) Mitochondrial cytopathy. A multisystem disorder with ragged red fibres on muscle biopsy. *Archives of Disease in Childhood*, **56**, 741

Egger, J., Kendall, B.E., Erdohazi, M. *et al.* (1983) Involvement of the central nervous system in congenital muscular dystrophy. *Developmental Medicine and Child Neurology*, **25**, 35

Eldjarn, L., Try, K., Stokke, O. *et al.* (1966) Dietary effects on serum phytanic-acid levels and on clinical manifestations in heredopathia atactica polyneuritiformis. *Lancet*, **i**, 691

Ellis, F.R., Clarke, I.M.C., Modgill, M. *et al.* (1975) Evaluation of creatine phosphokinase in screening patients for malignant hyperpyrexia. *British Medical Journal*, **iii**, 511

Emery, A.E.H. (1969a) Genetic counselling in x-linked muscular dystrophy. *Journal of the Neurological Sciences*, **8**, 579

Emery, A.E.H. (1969b) Abnormalities of the electrocardiogram in female carriers of Duchenne muscular dystrophy. *British Medical Journal*, **ii**, 418

Emery, A.E.H., Clack, E.R., Simon, S. and Taylor, I.L. (1967) Detection of carriers of benign x-linked muscular dystrophy. *British Medical Journal*, **iv**, 522

Emery, A.E.H. and Skinner, R. (1976) Clinical studies in benign (Becker type) X-linked muscular dystrophy. *Clinical Genetics*, **10**, 189

Engel, W.K. (1961) Muscle target fibres—a newly recognised sign of denervation. *Nature*, **191**, 389

Engel, W.K. (1970) Selective and non-selective susceptibility of muscle fiber types. A new approach to human neuromuscular diseases. *Archives of Neurology*, **22**, 97

Engel, A.G. and Angelini, C. (1973) Carnitine deficiency of human skeletal muscle with associated lipid storage myopathy: a new syndrome. *Science*, **1173**, 899

Evans, P.R. (1964) Hypogenital dystrophy with diabetic tendency. *Guy's Hospital Reports*, **113**, 207

Fenichel, G.M. and Bazelon, M. (1966) Myopathies in search of a name: Benign congenital forms. *Developmental Medicine and Child Neurology*, **8**, 532

Flannery, D.B. (1978) Mitochondrial inheritance. *Lancet*, **ii**, 1050

Fowler, H., Volpe, M., Marks, G. *et al.* (1979) Recovery from chronic progressive polyneuropathy after treatment with plasma exchange and cyclophosphamide. *Lancet*, **ii**, 1193

Fried, K. and Emery, A.E.H. (1971) Spinal muscular atrophy type II. A separate genetic and clinical entity from type I (Werdnig-Hoffman disease) and type III (Kugelberg-Welander disease). *Clinical Genetics*, **2**, 203

Fukuyama, Y., Kawazura, M. and Haruna, H. (1960) A peculiar form of muscular dystrophy. *Pediat. Univ. Tokyo*, **4**, 5

Fukuyama, Y., Makiko, O. and Sazuki, H. (1981) Congenital progressive muscular dystrophy of the Fukuyama type—congenital, genetic and pathological considerations. *Brain and Development*, **3**, 1

Gallup, B. and Dubowitz, V. (1973) Failure of 'dystrophic' neurons to support functional regeneration of normal or dystrophic muscle in culture. *Nature*, **243**, 287

Gamstorp, I. (1963) Adynamia episodica hereditaria and myotonia. *Acta Neurologica Scandinavica*, **39**, 41

Gardner-Medwin, D. (1977) Children with genetic muscular dystrophy. *British Journal of Hospital Medicine*, **10**, 314

Gardner-Medwin, D. (1979) Controversies about Duchenne muscular dystrophy. (i) Neonatal screening. *Developmental Medicine and Child Neurology*, **21**, 390

Gardner-Medwin, D., Bunday, S. and Green, S. (1978) Early diagnosis of Duchenne muscular dystrophy. *Lancet*, **i**, 1102

Gardner-Medwin, D. and Sharples, P. (1989) Some studies of the Duchenne and autosomal recessive types of muscular dystrophy. *Brain and Development*, **11**, 91

Gibberd, F.B., Billimoria, J.D., Page, N.G.R. and Retsas, S. (1979) Heredopathia atactica poly-neuritoformis (Refsum's disease) treated by diet and plasma exchange. *Lancet*, **i**, 575

Goldstein, G. and Schlesinger, D.H. (1975) Thymopoietin and myasthenia gravis. Neostigmine-responsive neuromuscular block produced in mice by a synthetic peptide fragment of thymopoietin. *Lancet*, **ii**, 256

Gordon, N. (1968) Juvenile spinal muscular atrophy. *Developmental Medicine and Child Neurology*, **10**, 617

Gordon, N. (1991) The spinal muscular atrophies. *Developmental Medicine and Child Neurology*, **33**, 934

Gordon, N. and Hilson, D. (1967) Myotonic dystrophy: its occurrence in childhood. *British Journal of Clinical Practice*, **21**, 537

Gordon, N. and Hudson, R.E.B. (1959) Refsum's syndrome. Heredopathia atactica polyneuritiformis. *Brain*, **82**, 41

Grant, R., Sutton, D.L. and Ballantyne, J.P. (1987) Nifedipine in the treatment of myotonia in myotonic dystrophy. *Journal of Neurology, Neurosurgery and Psychiatry*, **50**, 199

Greenfield, I.G., Blackwood, W., McMenemey, W.H. *et al.* (1958) *Neuropathology*, Arnold, London

Haas, L.F., Austad, W.I. and Bergin, I.D. (1974) Tangier disease. *Brain*, **97**, 351

Hagberg, B. and Lundberg, A. (1969) Dissociated motor development simulating cerebral palsy. *Neuropädiatrie*, **1**, 187

Hagberg, B., Sanner, G. and Steen, M. (1972) The dysequilibrium syndrome in cerebral palsy. *Acta Paediatrica Scandinavica*, Suppl. 226

Hagberg, B. and Westerberg, B. (1983) The nosology of genetic peripheral neuropathies in Swedish children. *Developmental Medicine and Child Neurology*, **25**, 3

Hamer, D.L. (1981) Repeat anaesthesia for emergency surgery in a patient suspected of having malignant hyperpyrexia. *Anesthesiology Review*, **8**, 37

Harding, A.E. and Thomas, P.K. (1980) The clinical features of hereditary motor and sensory neuropathy types I and II. *Brain*, **103**, 259

Harper, P.S. (1975) Congenital myotonic dystrophy in Britain. II. Genetic basis. *Archives of Disease in Childhood*, **50**, 514

Hathaway, P.W., Engel, W.K. and Zellweger, H. (1970) Experimental myopathy after microarterial embolization. Comparison with childhood x-linked pseudohypertrophic muscular dystrophy. *Archives of Neurology*, **22**, 365

Havard, (1977) Progress in myasthenia gravis. *British Medical Journal*, **ii**, 1008

Healy, J.M.S., Heffron, J.J.A., Lehane, M. *et al.* (1991) Diagnosis of susceptibility to malignant hypertension with flanking DNA markers. *British Medical Journal*, **303**, 1225

Hers, H.G. (1963) 2-Glucosidase deficiency in generalised glycogen-storage disease (Pompe's disease). *Biochemical Journal*, **86**, 11

Hodgson, S. (1991) Genomic imprinting. *Developmental Medicine and Child Neurology*, **33**, 552

Hoffman, E.P., Brown, R.H. and Kunkell, L.M. (1987) Dystrophin: the protein product of Duchenne muscular dystrophy locus. *Cell*, **51**, 919

Hopkins, I.I., Lindsey, I.R. and Ford, F.R. (1966) Nemaline myopathy. A long-term clinicopathologic study of affected mother and daughter. *Brain*, **89**, 299

Hudgson, P., Gardner-Medwin, D., Wotsfold, M. *et al.* (1968) Adult myopathy from glycogen storage disease due to acid maltase deficiency. *Brain*, **91**, 435

Hughes, R.A.C., Newsom-Davis, J.M., Perkins, G.D. and Pierce, J.M. (1978) Controlled trial of prednisolone in acute polyneuropathy. *Lancet*, **ii**, 750

Illingworth, B., Cori, G.T. and Cori, C.F. (1956) Amylo-1,6-glucosidase in muscle tissue in generalised glycogen storage disease. *Journal of Biological Chemistry*, **218**, 123

Kearns, T.P. and Sayre, J.P. (1958) Retinitis pigmentosa, external ophthalmoplegia, and complete heart block. *Archives of Ophthalmology*, **60**, 280

Keeton, B.R. and Moosa, A. (1976) Organic aciduria. Treatable cause of floppy infant syndrome. *Archives of Disease in childhood*, **51**, 636

King, I.O., Denborough, M.A. and Zapf, P.W. (1972) Inheritance of malignant hyperpyrexia. *Lancet*, **i**, 365

Kugelberg, E. and Welander, L. (1956) Heredofamilial juvenile muscular atrophy simulating muscular dystrophy. *Archives of Neurology and Psychiatry*, **75**, 500

Lane, R.J.M. and Mastaglia, F.L. (1978) Drug-induced myopathies in man. *Lancet*, **2**, 562

Laurence, B.M. (1967) Hypotonia, mental retardation, obesity and cryptorchism associated with dwarfism and diabetes in children. *Archives of Disease in Childhood*, **42**, 126

Lawrence, D.G. and Locke, S. (1963) Neuropathy in children with diabetes mellitus. *British Medical Journal*, **i**, 784

Layzer, R.B., Rowand, L.P. and Ranney, H.M. (1967) Muscle phosphofructokinase deficiency. *Archives of Neurology*, **17**, 512

Lenard, H.C. and Goebel, H.H. (1975) Congenital fibre type disproportion. *Neuropädiatrie*, **6**, 220

Lenard, H.C., Schaub, I., Keutel, I. and Osang, M. (1974) Electromyography in type II glycogenosis. *Neuropädiatrie*, **5**, 410

Lenard, H.C. and Goebal, H-H. (1980) Congenital muscular dystrophies and ultrastructural congenital myopathies. *Brain and Development*, **2**, 119

Lenman, I.A.R. and Ritchie, A.E. (1970) *Clinical Electromyography*, Pitman Medical, London

Littlewood, R. and Bajada, S. (1981) Successful plasmaphoresis in the Miller-Fisher syndrome. *British Medical Journal*, **i**, 778

Lundberg, A. (1979) Dissociated motor development. *Neuropädiatrie*, **10**, 161

Mackay, R.I. (1951) Congenital myasthenia gravis. *Archives of Disease in Childhood*, **26**, 289

Madrid, R., Bradley, W.G. and Davis, C.J.F. (1977) The peroneal muscular atrophy syndrome. *Journal of Neurological Sciences*, **32**, 91

Malcolm, S., Clayton-Smith, J., Nichols, M. *et al.* (1991) Uniparental paternal disomy in Angelman's syndrome. *Lancet*, **337**, 694

Mastaglia, F.L. (1980) Drug induced disorders of muscle. *British Journal of Hospital Medicine*, **24**, 8

Matson, D.D. (1969) *Neurosurgery of Infancy and Childhood*. Charles C. Thomas, Springfield, Illinois

Matthys, D., Van Coster, R. and Verhaaren, H. (1991) Fatal outcome of pyruvae loading test in child with restrictive cardiomyopathy. **338**, 1020–21

McArdle, B. (1951) Myopathy due to a defect in muscle glycogen breakdown. *Clinical Science*, **10**, 13

McArdle, B. (1963) Metabolic myopathies. *American Journal of Medicine*, **35**, 661

McColl, K.E.L., Thompson, G.T., Moore, M.R. and Goldberg, A. (1979) Haematin therapy and leucocyte-aminolaevulinic acid-synthesase activity in prolonged attacks of acute porphyria. *Lancet*, **i**, 133

McComas, A.I., Sica, R.E.P. and Campbell, M.I. (1971) 'Sick' motor neurones. A unifying concept of muscle disease. *Lancet*, **i**, 321

Manning, G.W. and Cropp, G.I. (1958) The electrocardiogram in progressive muscular dystrophy. *British Heart Journal*, **20**, 416

Mertens, H.G., Balzereit, F. and Leipert, M. (1969) The treatment of severe myasthenia gravis with immunosuppressive agents. *European Neurology*, **2**, 321

Melki, J., Sheth, P., Abdehak, S. *et al.* (1990) Mapping of acute (type1) spinal muscular atrophy to chromosome 5q12-q14. *Lancet*, **336**, 271

Miller, G., Heckmatt, J.Z. and Dubowitz, V. (1983) Drug treatment of juvenile dermatomyositis. *Archives of Disease in Childhood*, **158**, 445

Moosa, A. (1974) Muscular dystrophy in children. *Developmental Medicine and Child Neurology*, **16**, 97

Moosa, A. and Dubowitz, V. (1973) Spinal muscular atrophy in childhood: two clues to clinical diagnosis. *Archives of Disease in Childhood*, **48**, 386

Munsat, T.L. (1967) Therapy of myotonia. *Neurology*, **17**, 359

Munsat, T.L., Piper, D., Cancilla, P. and Mednick, I. (1972) Inflammatory myopathy with facio-scapulohumeral distribution. *Neurology*, **22**, 335

Newsom Davis, I. (1974) Myasthenia. *British Journal of Hospital Medicine*, **7**, 933

Newton, R. (1981) Plasma exchange in acute in post-infectious demyelination. *Developmental Medicine and Child Neurology*, **23**, 538

Niakan, E., Pitner, S.E., Whitiker, J.N. and Bertorini, T.E. (1980) Immunosuppressive agents in corticosteroid-refractory childhood dermatomyositis. *Neurology*, **30**, 286

Nicholson, G.A. Gardner-Medwin, D., Pennington, R.J.T. and Walton, J.N. (1979) Carrier detection in Duchenne muscular dystrophy: assessment of the effect of age on detection-rate with serum creatine kinase activity. *Lancet*, **i**, 692

Norman, A., Thomas, N., Coakley, J. and Harper, P. (1989) Distinction of Becker from limb-girdle muscular dystrophy by means of dystrophin cDNA probes. *Lancet*, **i**, 466

Pavone, L., Giullotta, F., Grasso, S. and Vannuchi, C. (1986) Hydrocephalus, lissencephaly, ocular abnormalities and congenital muscular dystrophy. A Warberg syndrome variant? *Neuropediatrics*, **17**, 266

Pearn, J. (1980) Classification of spinal muscular atrophies. *Lancet*, **i**, 919

Pearn, J. and Hudgson, P. (1978) Anterior-horn cell degeneration and gross calf hypertrophy with adolescent onset. *Lancet*, **i**, 1059

Pearse, R.R. and Höweler, C.T. (1979) Neonatal form of dystrophia myotonica. *Archives of Disease in Childhood*, **154**, 331

Pickard, N.A., Gruemar, H-D., Verrill, H.L. *et al.* (1978) Systemic membrane defect in proximal muscular dystrophies. *New England Journal of Medicine*, **299**, 841

Poll-Thé, B.T., Saudubray, J.M., Ogier, H. *et al.* (1986) Infantile Refsum's disease: biochemical findings suggesting multiple peroxisomal dysfunction. *Journal of Inherited Metabolic Disorders*, **9**, 169

Poskanzer, D.C. and Kerr, D.N.S. (1961) A third type of periodic paralysis with normokalaemia and favourable response to sodium chloride. *American Journal of Medicine*, **31**, 328

Prader, A. and Willi, H. (1963) Das Zyndrom von Imbezillitit, Adipositas, Muskelhypotonie, Hypogonadismus und Diabetes mellitus mit 'Myotonia-Anamnese'. In *2nd International Congress of Psychiatry and its Developments*, Vienna

Punnett, H.H. and Zakai, E.H. (1990) Old syndromes and new cytogenetics. *Developmental Medicine and Child Neurology*, **32**, 824–31

Ragab, A.H.M.F. (1971) Motor-end-plate changes in mouse muscular dystrophy. *Lancet*, **ii**, 815

Refsum, S. (1981) Heredopathia atactica polyneuridiformis; phytanic acid storage disease (Refsum's disease): a specific dietary treatment. *Archives of Neurology*, **38**, 605

Refsum, S., Solomonson, L. and Skatvedt, M. (1949) Heredopathia atactica polyneuritiformis in children. *Journal of Pediatrics*, **35**, 335

Richardson, A.T. and Barwick, D.D. (1969) Clinical electromyography. In *Disorders of Voluntary Muscles*, (ed. J.N. Walton), Churchill Livingstone, London

Ridley, A. (1969) The neuropathy of acute intermittent porphyria. *Quarterly Journal of Medicine*, **38**, 307

Riley, C.M., Day, R.L., Greeley, D. MeL. and Langford, W.S. (1949) Central autonomic dysfunction with defective lacrimation. *Pediatrics*, **3**, 468

Rowand, L.P. (1988) Clinical concepts of Duchenne muscular dystrophy. *Brain*, **111**, 479

Rowand, L.P., Lovelace, R.E., Schotland, D.L. *et al.* (1966) The clinical diagnosis of McArdle's disease. *Neurology*, **16**, 93

Satoyoshi, E. and Kowa, H. (1967) A myopathy due to glycolytic abnormality. *Archives of Neurology*, **17**, 248

Scadding, G.K. and Harvard, C.W.H. (1981) Pathogenesis and treatment of myasthenia gravis. *British Medical Journal*, **ii**, 1008

Scatpalezos, S. and Panayiotopoulos, C.P. (1973) Duchenne muscular dystrophy: reservations to the neurogenic hypothesis. *Lancet*, **ii**, 458

Schmid, R. and Mahler, R. (1959) Chronic progressive myopathy with myoglobinuria. Demonstration of glycogenolytic defect in the muscle. *Journal of Clinical Investigation*, **38**, 2044

Schwartz, M.S. and Moosa, A. (1977) Sensory nerve conduction in the spinal muscular atrophies. *Developmental Medicine and Child Neurology*, **19**, 50

Sen, S. and Das, P.K. (1978) Steroid-induced CPK estimation. A new diagnostic test for human muscular dystrophy and its carrier state. *Archives of Disease in Childhood*, **53**, 521

Shafiq, S.A., Dubowitz, V., Peterson, H. de C. and Milhorat, A.T. (1967) Nemaline myopathy: report of a fatal case with histochemical and electron microscopic studies. *Brain*, **90**, 817

Shy, G.M. and Magee, K.R. (1956) A new congenital non-progressive myopathy. *Brain*, **79**, 610

Shy, G.M., Gonatas, N. K. and Perez, M. (1966) Two childhood myopathies with abnormal mitochondria. I. Megaconial myopathy. II. Pleoconial myopathy. *Brain*, **89**, 133

Shy, G.M., Engel, W.K., Somers, I.E. and Wanko, T. (1963) Nemaline myopathy—a new congenital myopathy. *Brain*, **86**, 793

Sinclair, L. (1979) *Metabolic Disease in Childhood*, Blackwell Scientific, Oxford

Smit, L.M.E., Veldman, H., Jennekens, F.G.I. *et al.* (1986) A congenital myasthenic disorder with paucity of secondary synaptic clefts. Deficiency and altered distribution of acetylcholine receptors. *Annals of the New York Academy of Science*, **475**, 203

Sokoloff, M.C., Goldberg, L.S and Pearson, C.M. (1971) Treatment of corticosteroid-resistant polymyositis with methotrexate. *Lancet*, **i**, 14

Speer, A., Spiegler, A.W.J., Hanke, R. *et al.* (1989) Possibilities and limitation of prenatal diagnosis and carrier determination for Duchenne and Becker muscular dystrophy using cDNA probes. *Journal of Medical Genetics*, **26**, 1

Spiro, A.J., Shy, G.M. and Gonatas, N.K. (1966) Myotubular myopathy. *Archives of Neurology*, **14**, 1

Steinberg, D., Herdon, J.H., Uhtendorf, B.W. *et al.* (1967) Refsum's disease. Nature of the enzyme defect. *Science*, **156**, 1740

Steinbicker, V., von Roholen, L., Krebs, P. and Szibor, R. (1984) Duchenne muscular dystrophy: carrier detection by ultrasound. *Lancet*, **i**, 1463

Tanaka, K., Takishita, K. and Takita, M. (1981) Deoxycholic acid, a candidate for the maternal interuterine factor in early-onset myotonic dystrophy. *Lancet*, **i**, 1046

Towbin, A. (1969) Latent spinal cord and brain stem injury in newborn infants. *Developmental Medicine and Child Neurology*, **11**, 54

Trijbels, J., Sengers, R., Ruitenbeek, W. *et al.* (1988) Disorders of the mitochondrial respiratory chain: clinical manifestations and diagnostic approach. *European Journal of Pediatrics*, **148**, 92–7

Tsutsumi, A., Uchida, Y., Osawa, M. and Fukuyama, Y. (1989) Ocular findings in Fukuyama type congenital muscular dystrophy. *Brain and Development*, **11**, 413

Turnbull, D.M., Bartlett, K., Eyre, J.A. *et al.* (1988) Lipid storage myopathy due to glutaric aciduria type ii: treatment of a potentially fatal myopathy. *Developmental Medicine and Child Neurology*, **30** 1667

Turner, H.D., Brett, E.M., Gilbert, R.L. *et al.* (1978) Infant botulism in England. *Lancet*, **i**, 1277

Vanier, T.M. (1960) Dystrophia myotonica in childhood. *British Medical Journal*, **ii**, 1284

Viskoper, R.J. Wolf, E., Chaco, J. *et al.* (1975) McArdle's syndrome: the reaction to a fat-rich diet. *American Journal of Medical Science*, **269**, 217

Walton, J.N. (1961) The floppy infant. *Cerebral Palsy Bulletin*, **2**, 10

Walton, J.N. and Mastaglia, F.L. (1981) Muscle disease. In *Molecular Basis of Neuropathology* (eds. A.N. Davison and F.N.S. Thompson), Edward Arnold, London

Wang, P. and Clausen, T. (1976) Treatment of attacks in hyperkalaemic familial periodic paralysis by inhalation of salbutamol. *Lancet*, **i**, 221

Wijmenga, C., Frants, R.R., Brouwen, O.F. *et al.* (1990) Location of facioscapulohumeral muscular dystrophy gene on chromosome 4. *Lancet*, **336**, 651

Wiles, C.M. and Edwards, R.H.T. (1977) Weakness in myotonic syndromes. *Lancet*, **ii**, 598

Woolf, A.L. (1962) Muscle biopsy. In *Modern Trends in Neurology* (ed. D. Williams), Butterworth, London; Hoeber, New York

Woolf, A.L. (1969) Pathological anatomy of the intramuscular nerve endings. In *Disorders of Voluntary Muscles*, (ed. J.N. Walton), Churchill Livingstone, London

Wynne-Davies, R. and Lloyd-Roberts, G.C. (1976) Arthrogryposis multiplex congenita. *Archives of Disease in Childhood*, **51**, 618

Yoshioka, M., Okuno, T., Ito, M. *et al.* (1981) Congenital muscular dystrophy (Fukuyama type): repeated CT studies in 19 children. *Computer Tomography*, **5**, 81

8 Cerebral palsy

'Cerebral palsy' is a term that is used loosely for a group of chronic neurological conditions seen in childhood and characterized by impaired motor function with paresis, inco-ordination or involuntary movement. Obvious progressive disease of the nervous system is omitted. Most affected children will show improved motor performance with increasing age and maturation; deterioration is usually due to disuse, contractures and impaired maturation of the nervous system. The aetiology varies widely and includes disorders of cerebral development and cell migration, intra-uterine infections, prenatal and perinatal disturbances in nutrition and oxygen, as well as many postnatal causes of brain damage, such as kernicterus, meningitis and trauma. One source of confusion, especially to parents, is the tendency to refer to the spastic child as synonymous with the child with cerebral palsy, particularly as many of these children are hypotonic. The incidence of cerebral palsy has been estimated at around 2 per 1000 live births. There is evidence from some areas that this is dropping, due mainly to fewer children with cerebral diplegia (Hagberg, Hagberg and Olow, 1975). Conversely, because of better perinatal care, many more children are surviving who would previously have died.

Classification

The classifications used are based on clinical findings and not on aetiology. It is quite common for the various descriptive forms of cerebral palsy to overlap in one patient. The classification used here was introduced originally by Sigmund Freud, and subsequently modified by a number of people (Ingram, 1964). Ingram again discussed classification in 1984, under the following headings:

1. Hemiplegia
2. Double hemiplegia
3. Cerebral diplegia (hypotonic, dystonic, spastic, ataxic)
4. Ataxic cerebral palsy
5. Dysequilibrium syndrome
6. Dyskinetic cerebral palsy (dystonic, choreoid, athetoid, tension, tremor)
7. Mixed cerebral palsy

As with other conditions resulting in permanent brain damage, associated problems are common, and the main disadvantage of the various schemes that have been published is their almost total emphasis on the motor disability. However, it is important to have a framework on which to hang the many and varied problems which are included within the sphere of cerebral palsy, and also certain well-recognized terms which can be used as a means of communication between the many people who are involved in trying to solve these problems.

Most important of these is a range of cognitive problems which vary in severity from mild learning difficulties to global mental retardation. Seizures are frequent and usually take the form of tonic clonic seizures, but focal epilepsy with a cortical march also occurs at times. Speech difficulties are prominent, and many affected children have visual problems. Squints are especially common. Loss of hearing can be a severe handicap in children with choreo-athetosis. Disturbances of sensation are common, particularly in spastic cerebral palsy, and can affect limb function as markedly as the motor impairment does. Many children with cerebral palsy are dwarfed, particularly if the cerebral damage and the resultant clinical picture is gross. With hemiplegia, the dwarfing is unilateral and parallels the degree of handicap. Behavioural disturbances also occur and reflect the child's overall handicap, his or her ability to cope with life's frustrations, the degree of pressure to which he or she is exposed, and the support he or she is given both by the family and by his or her contacts in the schools and in the wider community. The various forms of cerebral palsy will be considered, followed by some of the associated disorders.

Hemiplegia

Aetiology

The perinatal histories of children with hemiplegia are often complicated, and abnormalities both of pregnancy and labour can occur together. These include ante-partum haemorrhage and pre-eclampsia, delay in the second stage of labour, and abnormalities of presentation, resulting in injury to the brain or impairment of its blood supply. Arterial occlusions can occur even before birth and recanalize relatively quickly in the first few months of life. Also, an embolus breaking off from a placental thrombus can block a major branch of the middle cerebral artery. This may be associated with the formation of porencephalic cysts. If the rest of the brain is unaffected and epilepsy is a major problem, this type of lesion can respond favourably to surgical treatment.

Hemiplegia also complicates postnatally acquired conditions, such as pyogenic or tuberculous meningitis, middle-ear infection, mastoiditis and cerebral abscess.

Another cause of acquired hemiplegia in infancy is status epilepticus complicating febrile illnesses. The reasons for this are probably multiple, but localized anoxia and metabolic changes are prominent (Falconer, 1974). It may follow trauma to the head, vascular thrombosis complicating dehydration and hyponatraemia, and virus infections causing a localized encephalitis. Acute disseminated encephalomyelitis or para-infectious encephalomyelitis often presents with the rapid onset of hemiplegia. There are many other causes, from carotid thrombosis following an injury to vascular malformations, but most of these are individually rare (Isler, 1971).

Clinical presentation

The arm
Characteristically, the arm is more severely affected than the leg (Fig. 8.1). The condition is not usually diagnosed in the first few weeks after birth, possibly because movements at this time of life are not so dependent on cortical function; but most

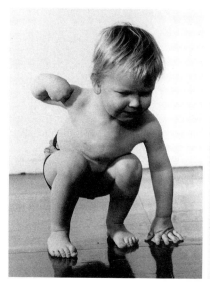

Figure 8.1   Child with hemiplegia.

Figure 8.2   Athetoid posture.

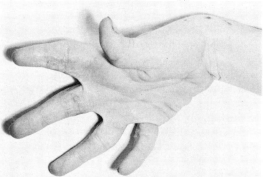

children with congenital hemiplegia are recognized in the first year of life because of neglect to use one hand or persistence of 'fisting', with the thumb clenched in the palm of the hand. Flexor tone and the tendon reflexes are accentuated. The increased flexor tone is customarily assessed by extending the elbow and stretching the biceps, but is most characteristically present in the pronators of the wrist, where it can easily be demonstrated even in mild cases by asking the patient to supinate the hand; the affected arm shows incomplete performance of this manoeuvre, and there is nearly always associated flexion of the elbow.

Voluntary movement is variably reduced and the affected side can be an effective assistant to the unimpaired hand in bimanual activity. Function can, however, be severely reduced and there is then often associated dwarfing of the limb and contractures. In its mildest form, contraction is limited to the wrist pronators, but it can involve the elbow, wrist flexors and shoulder adductors. Vasodilatation and cyanosis are frequently seen, and the limb is often colder than normal.

Any kind of exertion can precipitate associated involuntary movements of the athetoid type, which may result in grotesque hand and arm postures with hyperextension of the fingers and flexion of the wrist (Fig. 8.2). Hyperextension rarely involves the shoulder, and is then associated with internal rotation and extension of the elbow.

The leg

The mother may notice that her child kicks less well with one leg and that it is usually held extended at the knee. More often the disability is first observed when the child starts walking and does so on the toes of the affected side. Active dorsiflexion of the foot is difficult and, whilst the gastrocnemius and soleus spasm can be easily overcome in the first year of life, contracture soon results, and produces shortening of the tendo achillis. Clawing of the toes is occasionally a problem. Associated movements may also be seen and usually consist of flexion and adduction of the hip and plantar flexion of the foot. Dwarfing of the lower limbs is proportional to the degree of paralysis.

Walking will be delayed, but all children with hemiplegia will walk unless they are severely mentally handicapped (Crothers and Paine, 1959).

When the hemiplegia is acquired after birth, the mode of onset will be of significance, depending on the presence or absence of convulsions at this time. It has been shown that post-convulsive hemiplegia has a poor prognosis, with persistent epilepsy and mental handicap frequently being associated with the physical disability. Investigations usually show arterial occlusion only when there are no seizures at the beginning of the paralysis. It is suggested that the neurological lesion in the post-convulsive group may be, at least partly, the result of the fits whatever their cause may be (Aicardi, Amsili and Chevrie, 1969).

Double hemiplegia

Children with severe spasticity in all four extremities, which is more prominent in the arms than in the legs, are grouped under this heading. One side may be more affected than the other. Perinatal and postnatal cerebral injury are aetiologically important, although some cases may be due to developmental defects. In this and other forms of severe cerebral palsy the sequence of events may be interference with the development of the fetus *in utero*, which is then associated with premature birth and with various complications at birth for which the obstetrician may be unjustly blamed. The handicap is almost always the most severe of all forms of cerebral palsy. It is associated with a marked reduction in voluntary activity and only few developmental milestones are attained. Many of the patients never acquire independent sitting balance and some show persistence of primitive postural and feeding reflexes.

There may be a marked increase in the tone of all extremities and contractures can develop at the elbows, wrists, hips, knees and ankles. These children often assume a posture of generalized flexion, and asymmetries can contribute to the typical 'windswept' posture. It is suggested that this 'windswept' child syndrome (Fig. 8.3), seen among children with various types of cerebral palsy, is due to the effects of gravity on an immobile growing child, rather than spasticity or muscle imbalance. It should therefore be preventable (Fulford and Brown, 1976). Dwarfing of the whole body is common. Excessive irritability is a frequent feature, and feeding may be

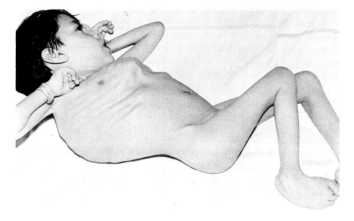

Figure 8.3   Gravitational wind-swept posture in very inactive child with cerebral palsy.

difficult because of a strong biting reflex and impaired chewing and swallowing. Drooling may be continuous, and aspiration of food and secretion results in recurrent chest infection. Sometimes aspiration leads to an allergic type of bronchitis and can be helped by giving a milk-free diet. Double hemiplegia is often accompanied by severe mental handicap and microcephaly, and by tonic clonic seizures (Ingram, 1964).

Cerebral diplegia

This clinical type of cerebral palsy was described in detail by Little and is frequently known as 'Little's disease', though the term 'diplegia', coined by Sigmund Freud, is in more common use. The spastic paralysis usually affects all four extremities and is of a particular type, involving the legs more than the arms.

Aetiology

There are, in all probability, many causes for this condition. Some children have congenital malformations in other systems, suggesting a cerebral developmental anomaly. Birth is sometimes preceded by a history of threatened abortion in the first trimester, and a few have had complications of late pregnancy and delivery. There is a particular association with premature delivery, especially when the clinical picture is a typical and uncomplicated one with severe spasticity of the legs and relatively little involvement of the arms. The production of this clinical picture by postnatal cerebral damage is rare, but does occur, for example from trauma, including trauma to the mother during pregnancy.

Clinical presentation

Diplegia in individuals of school age classically presents with a child who, when standing, assumes a posture with the body tilted forward, the hips and knees flexed and the weight taken on his or her toes. The legs are often internally rotated. Walking consists of short, staccato steps, with occasionally some body rotation to aid the leading foot. Balance is often precarious and the toecaps of shoes wear out very quickly. When sitting, the back is usually arched. One side of the body can be less severely affected than the other and, whilst some neurological deficit can nearly

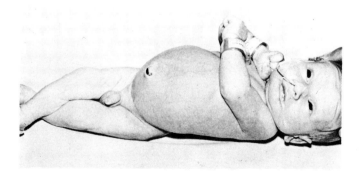

Figure 8.4 Typical abnormal posturing of the upper limbs and scissoring of the lower limbs in cerebral diplegia.

always be demonstrated, the arms are less severely involved and one upper limb may show almost normal function (diplegia with triplegic distribution). Affected limbs show an increase in flexor tone. The arms assume a posture of adduction at the shoulder, flexion at the elbow and pronation of the wrist. The legs, especially when the condition is severe take up the typical scissor position (Fig. 8.4). There is much reduction in voluntary movement, and associated movements of the dystonic type are frequently seen. In mild cases, resistance to passive wrist supination is one of the most sensitive indices of limb involvement. Increase in pronator tone will result in a rapid 'spring-back' on release. As mentioned, children with diplegia born prematurely often have almost normal arms, although the more carefully one looks for impairment of function the more likely it is to be found (diplegia with paraplegic distribution).

If an infant's progress is carefully observed from birth there may first be a stage of hypotonia. In spite of the baby's floppiness the tendon reflexes can be brisk, and if held in the vertical position there may be a suggestive tendency for the legs to cross. Then the mother may notice that when the baby is disturbed, for example while being dressed, there is a sudden excess of extensor tone in the trunk and limbs, and the development of the opisthotonic posture. This dystonic stage can last for a year or more and there may be a stage of rigidity affecting the extensor muscles before the spasticity and increase of flexor tone become apparent. Depending on the extent and severity of the lesion, this progress through various stages may halt, leaving the child with persistent hypotonia or dystonia. All tendon reflexes are increased, and ankle and patellar clonus can be elicited. There is a bilateral extensor plantar response. Contractures develop regularly and involve any muscle group which shows marked reduction in movement. Adductors of the thigh are often affected and contractures lead to limitation of abduction of the hips. This can be severe enough to cause dislocation of the hip joints. Gastrocnemius and soleus contractures cause shortening of the tendo achillis and permanent plantar flexion of the foot. Contractures also occur at elbows and wrists.

Ataxic diplegia

Patients with this mixed form of cerebral palsy show features of cerebellar involvement as well as diplegia, and this interesting subgroup has sufficient characteristics to warrant special consideration. Ataxic diplegia is frequently associated with low birth-weight, perinatal complications and hydrocephalus. In some instances there is a genetic aetiology, with occurrence in several members of the family. Both dominant and recessive pedigrees have been described.

In early infancy, hypotonia and reduced spontaneous motor activity are prominent features. The hypotonia improves slowly, and there is a considerable delay in attaining motor milestones. Cerebellar signs are not usually so prominent as in cases with pure ataxia, but intention tremor is always seen when children with this condition start grasping. Head and truncal ataxia may occur, especially if there is hydrocephalus. Signs of spasticity can be elicited quite early, but they are often not severe; these children usually walk on their toes with hip and knee flexion. The gait is broad-based and stamping, though adductor spasm is rare. The children often fall, though this lessens as balance improves.

As in most forms of cerebral palsy, advancing age brings functional improvement. Parental anxiety decreases once these children attain a steady gait. Inco-ordination is a particular problem when fine hand-skills, e.g. writing, are demanded. These children find it difficult to do things at speed and tend to fall behind at school. Not infrequently additional behavioural difficulties are then seen. Speech is often dysarthric and, for reasons that will be discussed under the heading ataxic cerebral palsy below, there is a frequent association of disorders of language development and low intelligence.

Ataxic cerebral palsy

This type of motor disorder is characterized by moderate to severe muscular hypotonia with generalized weakness, truncal and head ataxia, inco-ordinate movements and intention tremor.

Aetiology

The differential diagnosis is wide, and without investigations and a period of observation it is difficult to exclude the presence of a progressive disease, such as α-β-lipoproteinaemia and ataxia telangiectasia. Investigations may show a congenital malformation of the cerebellum, the cause of which is unknown, although cerebellar hypoplasia can occasionally be inherited as a recessive trait. The neurons of the cerebellum are particularly susceptible to lack of glucose and oxygen. A history of perinatal anoxia is not uncommon, and the brain-stem and cerebellum are liable to damage in breech births, with excessive longitudinal traction combined with flexion, hyperextension, or torsion of the spinal axis (Towbin, 1970). Lesny (1970) has described a bilateral cerebellar syndrome, characterized by ataxia, but almost always with an ability to walk unaided, an EEG showing bilateral slow wave activity blocked by eye opening, and a symmetrical hypoplasia of the cerebellum on neuroradiological investigation. The proven causes were more often prenatal; hereditary or teratogenic.

There is a well-defined group of children with inco-ordination of movements and defective balance who show evidence of arrested hydrocephalus. By the time the child is seen in the clinic the head may not be markedly out of proportion to the rest of the body, and the mother's description of the child's appearance in infancy is then of great importance. As stated previously, the ataxia is frequently associated with upper neuron lesions (ataxic diplegia). Although this type of cerebral palsy is often due mainly to an impairment of cerebellar function, the fact that so many of the causes, including perinatal factors and hydrocephalus, must involve other parts of the brain no doubt accounts for the frequency of epilepsy, disorders of language development and low intelligence in this group (Ingram, 1962).

Clinical presentation

Most patients present with muscular hypotonia in early infancy. Spontaneous movements tend to be reduced and motor milestones are delayed. The child is late in learning to sit and may show a coarse tremor of the head and trunk. Once he or she starts to grasp, an intention tremor of the arms and hand will be noticed; holding a cup will result in spilling.

Standing will accentuate the truncal tremor. The stance is always broad-based, with knees flexed and buttocks protruding. The knees may be adducted to improve stability without increased adductor tone. The arms are often raised to improve the balance. These children often fall, but balance and co-ordination improve with age and the ataxia becomes less obvious. The increasing demands for greater skills with advancing age will accentuate the inco-ordination again. Nystagmus is rare.

Dysequilibrium syndrome

Aetiology

One of the main justifications for separating this syndrome from ataxic cerebral palsy is the probability of an autosomal recessive mode of inheritance in a high proportion of cases (Sanner and Hagberg, 1974). Among children presenting with this syndrome the possibility of purine nucleoside phosphorylase deficiency with immunodeficiency should be considered (Soutar and Day, 1991).

Clinical presentation

There is difficulty in maintaining an upright body position and in experiencing the position of the body in space (Hagberg, Sanner and Steen, 1972). Motor development is severely retarded, and independent walking is rarely achieved before 9 years of age. Four developmental stages have been identified: floppy inactivity; crawling; standing; and walking. In this group, there is also often associated mental handicap, and sometimes spasticity. Impaired auditory and visual perception is particularly common. Families have been described with this syndrome combined with defective thymus dependent immunity (Graham-Pole *et al.*, 1975).

Dyskinetic cerebral palsy

This form of cerebral palsy is characterized by irregular and involuntary movements of some or all muscle groups of the body. These may be continuous, but are sometimes only present on movement. The group of dyskinetic cerebral palsies are colloquially referred to as 'athetoid', although the term 'athetosis' is best reserved for a more precise description of a certain type of movement disorder.

Aetiology

The association of damage to the central nervous system and, in particular, to the basal ganglia in conditions associated with hyperbilirubinaemia has been known for the past century. It was the discovery of the rhesus factor in 1939 that led to the understanding of the aetiological importance of erythroblastosis fetalis; and its eventual prevention first by exchange transfusion and, more recently, by the administration of anti-D serum to Rh-negative mothers immediately after parturition (Clarke, 1972). Severe jaundice with high levels of unconjugated bilirubin can also be seen in premature babies without evidence of Rhesus or ABO incompatibility. The unconjugated bilirubin is bound to albumin and when this is saturated by the bilirubin, or a competing drug, the bilirubin passes into the extravascular compartments and is bound to tissues with a high fat content. It has a particular affinity for the basal ganglia, and contributes to the pathological picture of kernicterus, with yellow staining of the basal ganglia. When severe anaemia accompanies the jaundice it is likely that brain damage will occur from anoxia as well as from the toxic effects of the jaundice. The present rarity of kernicterus due to blood group incompatibility is perhaps the best example of both the importance of the doctor's contribution to the prevention of brain damage, and how successful it can be. Other antibodies, such as Rh C, D, E, c and e, and Kell can produce the disease, but they are all rare (Whittle, 1992). Perinatal anoxia is also an important aetiological factor (Hagberg, Hagberg and Olow, 1975), and congenital malformations may occasionally also be implicated.

Dyskinesias do not usually cause the diagnostic difficulties mentioned in the group of ataxic cerebral palsies, but it may take time to exclude progressive conditions such as the Lesch-Nyhan syndrome, sudanophilic leucodystrophy (Pelizaeus-Merzbacher disease), ataxia telangiectasia, infantile neuroaxonal dystrophy, dystonia musculorum deformans and hepato-lenticular degeneration. These conditions will be considered in other chapters.

Clinical presentation

As in most other types of cerebral palsy, the classical picture of dyskinetic cerebral palsy in its various forms takes about 2 years to develop. As with cerebral diplegia, a number of stages are often recognized.

The postnatal period is frequently complicated by excessive irritability and occasionally by convulsions, hypertonicity, and even opisthotonus. This usually settles and is followed by hypotonia in infancy, which may be severe. There is greatly reduced tone in the muscles of the arms, legs, pelvic and shoulder girdles, but careful observation will always demonstrate some spontaneous motor activity and no true paralysis. Feeding problems are frequent, as are respiratory infections.

Involuntary movements are not obvious in the first few months of life, but grimacing and choreic hand movements will often be detected on careful observation, even at the age of 3 or 4 months. The sudden jerky movements of neonates are often unassociated with neurological abnormalities.

Dystonia gradually becomes more evident and usually takes the form of extensor spasms, particularly when the infant is startled or irritable. It is during this stage that persistence of the Moro response and the asymmetric tonic neck reflex is particularly obvious.

The final picture of dyskinetic cerebral palsy emerges after the age of two years, and

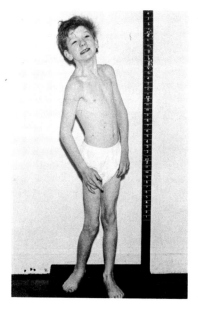

Figure 8.5 Dyskinetic cerebral palsy.

is determined by maturation and by attempts at voluntary control of movement and posture. In some children the hypotonia remains the predominant feature whilst others show rigid postures. Athetosis is the most common form of dyskinesia in cerebral palsy. The movements are slow and purposeless and both agonists and antagonists are involved without regard for their reciprocal use. They affect mainly the distal parts of the limbs, and are accentuated by voluntary movements (Fig. 8.5). During both passive and active movements a sudden excess of tone may occur, causing the whole limb to become stiff (the so-called 'tension athetosis'). This will cause an apparent arrest of movement.

Movements that are quick and jerky and tend to predominate in the proximal parts of the limbs are classified as choreic or choreo-athetoid. Slow, writhing movements affecting the muscles of the trunk are sometimes referred to as 'dystonia', but are rarely, if ever, present in the absence of athetoid movements of the limbs. Tremor is seldom a disability unless it is of the intention variety. The muscle tone is normal at rest and tendon reflexes are essentially normal, though they may be reinforced by tension. Overflow movements may be widespread, and secondary incoordination due to athetosis is common. Deformities and contractures are rare. Head control is poor and, even when the child has attained an independent sitting balance, the head often rolls forwards or backwards. Independent standing can take a long time to achieve.

Facial movements are exaggerated, and defective pharyngeal co-ordination will result in drooling, which the child controls only with difficulty over a number of years. Dysarthria is common and is due to involuntary movements of the lips and tongue, as well as the muscles of respiration. Phonation is consequently also defective, and speech is slow, monotonous and occasionally explosive. At times, the speech disturbance is severe enough to result in total absence of speech, although comprehension is frequently well preserved.

High-tone deafness is a frequent accompaniment of choreoathetosis due to kernicterus and anoxia, and accurate audiometry is mandatory. Paralysis of upward gaze is also seen in this form of choreoathetosis, and the teeth may show green discoloration and a tendency to early decay.

Progression and eventual functional status is very variable, and it is important to remember that of all individuals with cerebral palsy, those children with choreo-athetosis have the greatest preservation of intellect. Most are handicapped not only because of poor mobility and co-ordination but also because their appearance is ungainly and their speech difficult to understand. They have a greater barrier of acceptance to overcome than children with other forms of cerebral palsy, and less prospect of gaining employment than most. It is in this group that instances occur of individuals who are thought to be mentally backward but in fact, for example, are able to produce literature of a high standard.

Mixed cerebral palsy

This is the largest group, and though the clinical picture is usually dominated by one particular form of cerebral palsy it is not uncommon for children to present with neurological features of two or more types. Thus, some children with a spastic hemiplegia have associated athetoid movements; others may have a diplegia and show involuntary movements of various kinds. As has been stated, ataxic symptoms are quite frequent in the spastic forms of cerebral palsy. Almost any combination of motor disabilities can be found and must be taken into account when the child is assessed. This is of particular importance when determining orthopaedic treatment.

The results of operations on the legs of a child with uncomplicated spastic diplegia may be quite different when the disability is due in part to rigidity and dyskinesis.

Associated disabilities

The motor defects so far discussed may be of particular importance to the child's development and welfare, but these should not exclude the careful consideration of other disabilities.

Vision and hearing

Vision and hearing must be examined as a routine when a child is physically or mentally handicapped. They are more likely than normal children to suffer from squints, refractive errors and partial deafness. When these are combined with other disabilities they can have a proportionately greater effect and, if not diagnosed and corrected, may seriously impede the child's education. Anyone working in this field can give examples of children with mild cerebral palsy who failed to progress at school until given glasses for severe myopia, and others who were labelled as 'mentally backward' until found to have a high-tone deafness.

A squint is present in about 25% of children with hemiplegia. Some of the children in this group have a homonymous hemianopia which may cause particular problems from the educational point of view. Many children with cerebral diplegia have squints, severe refractive errors and impairment of visual acuity. The association of athetosis and high-tone deafness has already been mentioned.

Impaired sensation

Exteroceptive and proprioceptive sensation can be impaired in children with cerebral palsy. This is particularly true of the latter, especially in the presence of hemiplegia. As stated in Chapter 1 it is surprising how accurately stereognosis can be tested in very young children by making a game of it; for example, identifying toys by touch in a model of a railway tunnel, with suitable rewards for correct answers. The apparent reluctance of a child with hemiplegia to use the weak limbs, seeming to ignore them at times, may well be due to sensory loss so that the child really does not know where the limbs are.

Disorders of perception and of language development

Cerebral palsy is due to failure of brain development or damage to the brain, so that higher cerebral functions, such as language, are bound to suffer from the effects of the cerebral lesion, whether these are congenital or acquired; but there is more to the problem than that, which has been discussed when considering language function (Chapter 6). Children with physical handicaps are deprived; they cannot explore their environment and learn from their actions. The child's world may consist of one or two rooms at home and the classroom, and a special effort should be made to rectify this by taking the child into shops, on buses, into the countryside and so on. Such lack of experience is bound to limit the formation of concepts which is fundamental to perceptual and language function. Also, the diagnosis of physical and mental handicap influences the way people talk to such children, and this may deny them the richer experiences of language so essential to the early stages of development. There is usually the complicating factor of a dysarthria in the various types of cerebral palsy;

spastic, extra-pyramidal, and ataxic. The speech therapist can help the child with both dysphasia and dysarthria, and with drooling. The latter can also sometimes be improved with the use of benztropine (Camp-Bruno *et al.*, 1989), and other anticholinergic drugs, such as benzhexol hydrochloride.

As a result of brain damage and lack of experience, learning difficulties of all kinds are frequent among children with cerebral palsy. This has to be taken into account, particularly in schools for the physically handicapped, as some of the children will be affected by diseases, such as some myopathies, in which the CNS is unaffected. This has been used as an argument for educating children with cerebral palsy on their own in special schools. However, there seem to be greater advantages in mixing children with different types of disability, and providing for their individual needs by careful streaming within the school. Some children with cerebral palsy will manage remarkably well in a normal school, but some will not. If this is possible there is a greater chance of successful integration into the community, but a careful watch must be kept on the child's progress. It is all too easy for emotional disturbances to develop when the child feels he or she can no longer cope.

Intelligence

It has been stressed that children with severe cerebral palsy can be of average or above average intelligence and this possibility must not be forgotten even if the physical disability is severe. However, a realistic attitude to those with cerebral palsy must be taken, and about 75% of patients will be of below average intelligence. Also, the sum total of multiple disabilities always seems to add up to more than the contribution of each individual handicap. Even if a child with athetosis is of average intelligence, his or her education must be geared to the practical limitations of the child's physical potential. The aims of the educational programme must be to equip the individual to make the most of life's opportunities, whatever these may be. If not, it will not only be a waste of time and effort on the child's and teacher's part, but it will immeasurably add to the child's frustration as he or she grows older.

Epilepsy

The addition of epilepsy to any other disability causes an altogether new dimension. To a certain extent the problems are those of anyone with epilepsy, and range from the side-effects of anti-epileptic treatment to the prejudices against epilepsy that still exist in the community. The seizures may lead to difficulties of management at school and add greatly to parental anxiety; of all disabilities, epilepsy seems the one most likely to lead to emotional disorders. Epilepsy most frequently complicates hemiplegia, especially when it is of postnatal origin, and is also common among children with cerebral diplegia. It very rarely occurs among those with dyskinetic cerebral palsy (Crothers and Paine, 1959). The fits are usually generalized, but may be focal. The electroencephalogram is of limited value in the investigation of cerebral palsy. Abnormal records show some correlation with the severity of the physical handicap, but little correlation with the level of intelligence (Gordon, 1966).

Emotional Problems

Growing up, particularly during adolescence, requires continual adjustments in the personality of the normal child, and few escape entirely unscathed. The handicapped child has to try to come to terms with a physical disability as well. Emotional control takes time to develop, and the situation is complicated by the emotional immaturity so common among children with cerebral palsy. This immaturity also tends to make nonsense of educational planning for these children on a chronological basis, and they may be totally unsuited to leave school at 16 years of age and take part in a more adult-orientated environment.

Rutter, Graham and Yule (1970) have shown very clearly that, as might be expected, the risks of handicapped children developing behaviour disorders are considerably higher than among normal children, in fact a five-fold increase. One factor contributing to this may be the frustration resulting from the physical disability, and the increasing realization that so many of the pleasures enjoyed by their peers are denied to the handicapped child.

Depression can be a serious complication, and one that is easily missed among younger children. The child often becomes withdrawn and apathetic, and school performance deteriorates. Treatment may need the expert help of the child psychiatrist. Overactive behaviour can also be a problem among the less severely physically handicapped children, and can throw a considerable strain on the family.

There is no easy solution to the difficulties of adaptation, and sexual development presents particular problems. They may be so complex that it seems easier to ignore them and pretend they do not exist. If someone is prepared to discuss them with the child this alone may be beneficial, and even more so if this is combined with practical advice. More research is now being done on these problems, and parents groups and organizations such as the Sexual and Personal Relationships of the Disabled (Smyth, 1990), can often identify those experts who can give advice (ASBAH, 1983). Conversely, if nothing is done the emotional disturbance can become more of a problem than the physical handicap. The whole family will become involved, and attention must be paid to parental attitudes which can make or mar a child's progress. The doctor is not always the best person to advise the child and the family, unless he or she is very experienced. If the doctor is not prepared to give advice personally, he or she has a responsibility to ensure that social worker, teacher, therapist or parents will take part in these discussions. Many of the remarks made about counselling parents of mentally handicapped children apply equally to the families of the physically handicapped child.

Prevention

The effects of careful screening for blood group incompatabilities has already been mentioned as a major reason for the reduction in the incidence of dyskinetic cerebral palsy. Also, better obstetric and paediatric services for dysmature children has resulted in fewer cases of cerebral diplegia. This is probably due to a number of factors, such as the careful correction of acidosis, oxygen lack, abnormal temperature and hypoglycaemia. Hagberg, Hagberg and Olow (1976) have stressed that the cause of cerebral palsy is often multifactorial. It is important to point out again that fetal growth retardation and other disorders summarized in the term 'fetal deprivation of supply' are particularly important both in predisposing to and resulting in brain damage. The combination of 'fetal deprivation of supply', and asphyxia and cerebral haemorrhage at birth is common. The latter may only contribute to the child's disabilities, the primary important cause being of prenatal origin (Nelson and Ellenberg, 1986). When this is so, there are obvious implications both from the point of view of prevention and of litigation if the obstetrician is blamed for all that has happened (Hall, 1989). Studies on recent trends in cerebral palsy, particularly among low birth-weight infants suffering from diplegia, certainly favour an increased survival among these babies, although in the case of hemiplegia postnatal events may play a more important part (Pharoah *et al.*, 1990).

Much can still be done by good antenatal care and obstetrics and by educating mothers on the importance of adequate nutrition and on the dangers of smoking, alcohol, drugs and infections during pregnancy. The role of inborn errors of metabolism is more important in the prevention of severe mental handicap than cerebral palsy, but more information is required in the genetically determined syndromes, such as the dysequilibrium syndrome, if these are to be prevented by suitable advice to parents. The same applies to the ataxic form of cerebral palsy. Congenital hypothyroidism is also a preventable cause in this group which has been underestimated in the past (Sanner and Hagberg, 1974). The treatment of hydrocephalus significantly contributes to prevention in the ataxic diplegic group.

In the future, therefore, the prevention of cerebral palsy will depend on an attention to detail rather than concentrating on any single factor, whether this operates before, during or after birth. Hagberg and Hagberg (1984) have listed the prenatal, perinatal, and postnatal risks in the various types of cerebral palsy; and the need for advances in knowledge is most evident in the prenatal group where improvements have been relatively few (Stanley, 1984).

Assessment and management of cerebral palsy

Whilst the structural abnormality produced by aberrant development or damage to the central nervous system is permanent, functional improvement is seen in all but the most severe cases. Growing up is always accompanied by maturation, learning and adaptation to the environment. The approach to management involves individuals from many different professions who bring their own expertise to bear on the problem, and it is very important that they should co-ordinate and work as a team.

Assessment of children with cerebral palsy

After the initial analysis of the neurological disorder, it becomes imperative to assess the functional status of the child in detail and to relate it to the developmental norm expected for his or her age. This process takes time and is best spread over a number of days as the young child's tolerance to investigation is limited, and the child will usually only demonstrate the skills he or she has acquired in a relaxed setting in which he or she is encouraged to enjoy him or herself. Assessment must also be repeated so that the rate of progress can be determined and the training programme modified to suit the developmental level that has been reached.

It is important to remember that different aspects of development occur synchronously. No physiotherapist can work without using speech, and no occupational therapist can be effective without paying attention to motor control. Programmes must therefore be evolved together, and one therapist can often facilitate the work of the other.

Assessment of motor function

This is usually the easiest and most obvious to determine; to ascertain whether a child has attained good head control, stable sitting, supported or unsupported standing and a steady gait.

Hand function must be analysed and the degree of bi-manual competence assessed. Evidence of inco-ordination must be sought, and is best seen during play activities and during drawing. The determination of hand preference is important when planning remediation.

Assessment of motor function must be done with accuracy, because realistic planning for future education depends on it (Holt, 1965). Early integration into an appropriate educational setting is imperative for all children with motor handicaps, as this is by far the best way of ensuring that the child is exposed to a wide range of stimuli and learning situations. The paediatric neurologist who has no contact with his or her educational colleagues deprives him or herself of much therapeutic effectiveness.

Tests for vision

Vision must be checked carefully by a doctor who is used to dealing with young children and experienced in the techniques employed. Even serious defects are easily missed. Test material for visual acuity must be of a type that will evoke a measurable response from young children (Sheridan, 1973). Squints must be corrected where possible, refractive errors treated, and amblyopia prevented.

Tests for hearing

Every child with cerebral palsy should have his or her hearing tested, as deficits are common, particularly in children with dyskinesia. Accurate assessment is a skilled procedure and requires time and patience. The young infant is best tested with relatively unsophisticated test material, e.g. high frequency and low pitched rattles, paper, cup and spoon; as well as the human voice. Formal audiometry is rarely possible before the age of 4 years, but in view of the particular importance of peripheral hearing in the development of language among children who have already suffered cerebral damage the help of an expert using a variety of tests may have to be requested (Peterson, 1978). When a significant hearing loss has been found, a hearing aid should be provided if this is appropriate. The parents must be given advice, and the child is likely to need help from a teacher of the deaf.

Assessment of speech and language

Speech and language is essential to effective communication and integration into society. Many children with cerebral palsy have speech problems which require careful analysis and appropriate methods of corrective teaching and training, and all methods of communication must be included in the assessment. In helping a child to lead a tolerable life, communication is likely to be more important than locomotion. The role of the speech therapist in this assessment and some of the methods used are discussed in Chapter 6. There it will be seen that if there are multiple handicaps the correction of one may have a disproportionately beneficial effect.

Psychological testing

The complexity of the multiple disabilities of these children means that a battery of psychomotor tests may be needed to try to reach a meaningful assessment, and even then there are strict limitations in these methods. Many of the tests have been standardized on normal children, and constant allowances may have to be made for the difficulties of communicating with severely handicapped children.

Holt and Reynell (1967) have defined the aims of psychological assessment as an evaluation of present levels of functioning, an estimate of potentials for all aspects of development, and a suggestion of ways of helping this development to take place. They review tests available and also stress the need for reassessment, as the child's IQ level may vary with the years. The tests considered suitable for children under the age of 2 years are the Gessell, Cattell, Griffiths, and Bayley Scales. When the child has a severe impairment of hearing and speech, but has relatively intact vision and hand function, the Nebraska, Merrill-Palmer, and Columbia Mental Maturity Scales, and Raven's Matrices are used. With severely impaired vision but normal hearing and speech, the Williams Scale for the Blind and Partially Sighted and the Langan Adaptation of the Terman Merrill Scale for Blind Children are recommended. When there is no hand function or speech but no gross impairment of vision or hearing, the Peabody Picture Vocabulary Test, the Columbia Mental Maturity Scale, and Raven's Matrices can be helpful. Among school children with only mild sensory or motor impairment the Terman Merrill and Wechsler Intelligence Scale for Children may be adequate, but the examiner must be aware of the limitations of all these tests. Allowances will have to be made for difficulties in hand-eye coordination and in hand function when timed performances are used. Marked defects of speech and language are going to affect the results of virtually any test that is used to a greater or lesser extent. The deprivations, social and otherwise, imposed by physical handicap, which have already been mentioned, must also be taken into account.

A reasonable policy in assessing multiply handicapped children is: (1) to be prepared to give the child the benefit of the doubt as far as test results are concerned, and if necessary to observe the child's progress over a reasonable period of time, particularly in the teaching situation; (2) to maintain a realistic attitude to the child's potential. Although well-standardized tests will have predictive value, even among the severely handicapped, there will always be exceptions.

The results of these various assessments must be interpreted to the parents and their purpose carefully explained, as well as their defects. This inevitably takes time, but is time well spent and is likely to help the family function more satisfactorily and to increase the handicapped child's chances of achieving his or her full potential (Gordon, 1972).

Treatment of children with cerebral palsy

The younger the child with cerebral palsy the greater will be the medical contribution; but with increasing age the importance of education will steadily increase. Having said this, any hard and fast division between the two is to be avoided, and doctor and teacher should work together for the benefit of the child.

As with all handicaps, a major medical contribution to cerebral palsy must be to try to prevent brain damage occurring. Therefore every effort should be made to find a cause, as only in this way can knowledge of this condition be increased. This may necessitate a full investigation, sometimes including detailed neuro-radiological studies. Once brain damage has occurred, assessment should begin as early in life as possible, and a start made on ways in which the child can be helped.

Parent guidance

It must be accepted at the very beginning of the management process that parents play a central role in the successful habilitation of these children. As they are responsible for them and spend more time with them than any other adult, it is imperative to instruct and guide the parents in ways which are most likely to help their child. Inevitably, they are shocked and depressed by the information they have been given, to the extent that they are often unable to do as much for their handicapped child as they do for their normal offspring. The reverse can also occur, with concentration on the handicapped child leading to neglect of other children, who may then show behavioural disorders. Depression can best be helped by full discussion about the nature of the disabilities as they unfold, as well as instruction about learning methods and specific techniques directed towards solving individual problems. Parents are key figures in teaching the child the activities of daily living which are so important in gaining personal independence. It is often not stressed enough how important it is to give a handicapped child as much independence as possible, and it is easy for carers to limit this to an unnecessary extent as the child grows older. The process is a long one, and bringing up a child with cerebral palsy requires many times the effort devoted to a normal sibling. The ingenuity and experience of some parents often contributes to the well-being of their own and other handicapped children. If the mother is left with the whole responsibility for her disabled child, her energy for other activities may be sapped, so fathers must be encouraged to share the burden. Hospital or school staff will sometimes be willing to baby-sit so that parents of even a severely handicapped child can go out for the evening. Holiday facilities for the children may give parents a welcome break, and hospitals have to be prepared to admit patients when parents feel under excessive strain. A list of addresses of support groups in the UK for all types of handicap can be obtained from Ann Worthington, 10 Norman Road, Sale, M33 3DF (Worthington, 1990).

Physiotherapy

Claims have been made for the curative value of physiotherapy started in the first 6 months of life, but if all babies with abnormal neurological signs are treated at this age, there can be no doubt that in some these signs would have disappeared if no such treatment had been given Also, claims have been made for various methods of physiotherapy based on concepts of motor organization and control, as well as developmental sequence.

All methods of physiotherapy have their staunch supporters and their successes and failures. The best are solidly based in learning theory and utilize techniques which will motivate the child to improve his or her skills and advance up the developmental ladder. A hemiplegic child does not often have much problem in attaining the erect posture and walking. He or she can be trained to develop an improved gait and a wider range of hand function, thus lessening the risk of secondary complications such as contractures. A child with diplegia will have greater difficulty, but much can be done by correct posturing and, above all, by confidence building and by stretching the child so that success is never far away. Skills are learnt by repetition and by maintaining interest. The child with choreo-athetosis can be helped by reflex-inhibiting techniques, and major advances can be made by volitional, postural and movement control with graded exercises of increasing complexity.

It is surely arrogant to suggest that one particular method is the answer to all the problems of these children. Conversely it must be accepted that the enthusiasm generated by the followers of a particular method is in itself very valuable, and in planning treatment it is essential to have a structure around which the programme for a particular child can be organized.

Many physiotherapists will gain experience of several methods of treatment and take from these the items which seem likely to help a particular child and which also suit their own attitudes to such treatment. Examples of only some of these can be considered, but useful reviews of the various techniques have been given by Levitt (1975), and by Bleck (1987).

The Bobath method of treatment

Normal motor development is characterized by the development of postural reflexes, such as righting and equilibrium reflexes, and the appearance of postural tone; at the same time, primitive reflexes such as the total withdrawal response are gradually inhibited. In children with cerebral palsy there will be an inefficient development of the postural reflexes and inhibition of the primitive patterns of early childhood. Motor behaviour may be immature, with persistence of posture and movement present normally at an earlier age; or abnormal, if patterns (e.g. tonic reflexes producing abnormal postural tone) do not correspond to those found at any time of life (Bobath, 1980). The child is positioned in such a way that primitive and abnormal reflexes are inhibited and a more normal state of muscle tone is produced. Movements are then facilitated following normal developmental sequences, and postural reflexes can be stimulated to develop in a variety of ways. The child must be handled closely, and the therapists must know the reflex patterns which are integrated at various levels of the central nervous system, and the sequence in which they develop (Bobath and Bobath, 1964).

The Petö technique

The Petö technique was developed in Hungary. Like so many other techniques, it relies on a careful assessment of the child's needs and the creation of an 'educational' programme based on this. The programme is in charge of a 'conductor', and all therapists and teachers work under the conductor's direction and share in treatment. There is obviously much to be said for this close integration, and for the emphasis on the child's self-reliance so that he or she is taught to do something within his or her abilities, even if it takes a long time. Also, whatever the child does is with a verbal accompaniment so that even if the child cannot talk he or she will hear language in a very meaningful situation. There seems no reason why this method cannot be modified to local circumstances (Smith, 1970). The children are treated in groups, and as in many of these techniques it involves an all-day programme. It should be emphasized that the Petö method is only applicable to a certain group of handicapped children (Robinson, McCarthy and Little, 1989).

The Doman-Delacato method of treatment

This method is based on 'patterning', as originally suggested by Temple-Fay. It involves the passive movement of the body and limbs by a team of people in an ordered sequence based on normal motor development. It is obviously important to involve parents in the treatment of their handicapped child, but plans of this kind must be realistic and must not be to the detriment of other members of the family (MacKeith, 1973). The amount of attention given to the child and the experience of movement must be beneficial. It has yet to be proven that this treatment gives better results in the long term, rather than an initial acceleration of development, than other less dramatic methods.

There are other techniques, such as those of Rood, Kabat and Temple-Fay, but the boundaries between these have increasingly broken down.

Orthopaedic treatment

The various orthopaedic procedures and operations that can do so much to help children with the spastic forms of cerebral palsy cannot be considered in a book on paediatric neurology, and special texts must be consulted (Samilson, 1975; Bleck, 1987). Special footwear may help the gait and reduce wear. Aids such as calipers can be as much of a hindrance as a help and need evaluation for each affected child. There will always be debate how best to prevent and treat contractures and deformities of the limbs, and the decision will be an individual one applicable to a certain child at a particular stage of growth and development. The degree of disability is also of importance; for example, whether the foot can be dorsiflexed to a right angle at the ankle, to what extent this is interfering with walking, and whether there is less than 45° abduction of the hip. The timing of an operation is sometimes a difficult decision when further growth and development can so easily alter the situation.

Speech therapy and occupational therapy

It must be a constant theme that those trying to assist the handicapped child must work as a team. It has already been suggested that the speech therapist may have to help widen the handicapped child's experience of life, as well as deal with the various problems of speech and language which is his or her main role. Parents often need to be encouraged to speak to the child who is deaf, dysarthric or dysphasic.

The early work of the speech therapist frequently involves assessment and advice about feeding problems. The bite reflex which interferes with feeding can be fatigued by continuous oral stimulation prior to feeds. The use of the spoon and cup may replace the bottle at an early stage, and spoons are less likely to produce a bite reaction if they are of soft materials such as horn, rubber, plastic or wood. Children with chewing or swallowing difficulties cope best with semi-solids or purées.

The occupational therapist can help the child overcome some of his or her disabilities, both at school and at home, advising on suitable clothing, and on aids of all kinds from headguards to typewriters and toys. Help will be needed with all kinds of activities; for example swimming and horse riding can improve children's co-ordination and balance as well as enlarging their experience. Particular disabilities, such as defective vision or hearing, must be catered for with the use of noisy toys and objects of different texture.

Medicinal treatment

Apart from the treatment of epilepsy, drugs have a limited role to play in helping the child with cerebral palsy. If there is marked spasticity it is worth trying the effect of drugs, such as diazepam, in increasing doses, although the response is very variable and side-effects such as drowsiness may limit its use. Alternatives to diazepam are baclofen and dimethothiazine (Griffiths and Bowie, 1973). The treatment of athetoid movements is even more unpredictable. Any effect of diazepam on the involuntary movements may result from a reduction of tension and anxiety. This may also apply to tetrabenazine, although very occasionally it seems to have a more specific effect. If the athetosis is unilateral the possibility of a stereotactic operation on the basal ganglia can sometimes be considered, but rarely in generalized athetosis. Stereotaxic ablation of the cerebellar dentate nucleus (dentatotamy), bilateral if necessary, can reduce involuntary movements as well as spasticity (Gornall, Hitchcock and Kirkland, 1975).

Psychiatric treatment

Anxiety and depression can become very severe at times and may require urgent treatment. As stated the diagnosis can be difficult in the presence of severe physical handicap, but treatment can be of the utmost importance to the child's well-being and progress, and, if severe, the advice of the child psychiatrist will be needed.

The school-leaver

If there is still much to be done to help the child with cerebral palsy, the development of services for the severely physically handicapped school-leaver has, by comparison, hardly begun. What is the good of devoting a great deal of care and education to handicapped children if, when they reach adulthood, they are abandoned, and either have to live a life of inactivity and frustration at home or be admitted to a long-stay hospital for the rest of their lives? There is a great need for sheltered and specially designed workshops (Ingram *et al.*, 1964). These must be linked to hostel accommodation so that the services can be provided for rural as well as urban communities. Also, if such hostels can give short as well as long-stay accommodation there is no doubt that more of the severely handicapped will be able to live at home. Families can only tolerate a certain amount of strain, however loving they may be, and if this is unrelieved for even a single day for years on end it is not surprising that eventually it becomes intolerable, particularly as parents become older. A great deal more research is needed on the best kind of help to give to the handicapped young adult, by the medical, psychology and social services. These problems have been well reviewed by Thomas, Bax and Smyth (1989).

References

Aicardi, J., Amsili, J. and Chevrie, J.J. (1969) Acute hemiplegia in infancy and childhood. *Developmental Medicine and Child Neurology*, **11**, 162

ASBAH (1983) *Sex for Young People with Spina Bifida or Cerebral Palsy*, Association for Spina Bifida and Hydrocephalus with the co-operation of the Spastic Society, Scottish Spina Bifida Association and the Committee for Sexual and Personal Relationships of the Disabled, London

Bleck, E.E. (1987) *Orthopaedic Management in Cerebral Palsy*, Clinics in Developmental Medicine Nos. 99/100, Blackwell Scientific, Philadelphia

Bobath, K. (1980) *A Neurophysiological Basis for the Treatment of Cerebral Palsy*, Clinics in Developmental Medicine, No. 75. SIMP, William Heinemann, London

Bobath, K. and Bobath, B. (1964) The facilitation of normal postural reactions and movements in the treatment of cerebral palsy. *Physiotherapy*, **50**, 246

Camp-Bruno, J.A., Winsberg, B.G., Green-Parsons, A.R. and Abrams, J.P. (1989) Efficacy of benztropine therapy for drooling. *Developmental Medicine and Child Neurology*, **31**, 309

Clarke, C.A. (1972) Practical effects of blood group incompatibility between mother and fetus. *British Medical Journal*, **ii**, 90

Crothers, B. and Paine, R.S. (1959) *The Natural History of Cerebral Palsy*, Oxford University Press, London

Falconer, M.A. (1974) Mesial temporal (Ammon's horn) sclerosis as a common cause of epilepsy. *Lancet*, **ii**, 767

Fulford, G.E. and Brown, J.K. (1976) Position as a cause of deformity in children with cerebral palsy. *Developmental Medicine and Child Neurology*, **18**, 305

Gordon, N. (1966) The electroencephalogram in cerebral palsy. *Developmental Medicine and Child Neurology*, **8**, 216

Gordon, N. (1972) Parent counselling. *Developmental Medicine and Child Neurology*, **14**, 657

Gornall, P., Hitchcock, E. and Kirkland, I.S. (1975) Stereotaxic neurosurgery in the management of cerebral palsy. *Developmental Medicine and Child Neurology*, **17**, 279

Graham-Pole, J., Ferguson, A., Gibson, A.A.M. and Stephenson, J.B.P. (1975) Familial dysequilibrium-diplegia with T-lymphocyte deficiency. *Archives of Disease in Childhood*, **50**, 927

Griffiths, M.I. and Bowie, E.M. (1973) The use of Dimethothiazine in the treatment of childhood cerebral palsy. *Developmental Medicine and Child Neurology*, **15**, 24

Hagberg, B., Sanner, G. and Steen, M. (1972) The dysequilibrium syndrome in Cerebral palsy. *Acta Paediatrica Scandinavica*, Suppl. 226

Hagberg, B., Hagberg, G. and Olow, I. (1975) The changing panorama of cerebral palsy in Sweden, 1959–70. *Acta Paediatrica Scandinavica*, **64**, 187

Hagberg, B., Hagberg, G. and Olow, I. (1976) The changing panorama of cerebral palsy in Sweden 1954–70. The importance of fetal deprivation of supply. *Acta Paediatrica Scandinavia*, **65**, 800

Hagberg, B. and Hagberg, G. (1984) Prenatal and perinatal risk factors in a survey of 681 Swedish cases. In *The Epidemiology of the Cerebral Palsies* (eds. F. Stanley and E. Alberman), Blackwell Scientific, Oxford.

Hall, D.M.B. (1989) Birth asphyxia and cerebral palsy. *British Medical Journal*, **299**, 279

Holt, K.S. (1965) *Assessment of Cerebral Palsy I. Muscle Function. Locomotion and Hand Function*, Lloyd-Luke, London

Holt, K.S. and Reynell, J.K. (1967) *Assessment of Cerebral Palsy. II. Vision. Communication and Psychological Function*, Lloyd-Luke, London

Ingram, T.T.S. (1962) Congenital ataxic syndromes in cerebral palsy. *Acta Paediatrica Scandinavica*, **51**, 209

Ingram, T.T.S. (1964) *Paediatric Aspects of Cerebral Palsy*, Churchill Livingstone, Edinburgh

Ingram, T.T.S. (1984) A historical review of the definition and classification of the cerebral palsies. In *The Epidemiology of the Cerebral Palsies* (eds. F. Stanley and E. Alberman), Blackwell Scientific, Oxford

Ingram, T.T.S., Jameson, S., Errington, I. and Mitchell, R.G. (1964) *Living with Cerebral Palsy*, Clinics in Developmental Medicine, No. 14. SIMP, William Heinemann, London

lsler, W. (1971) *Acute Hemiplegias and Hemisyndromes in Childhood*, Clinics in Developmental Medicine, Nos. 41/42. SIMP, William Heinemann, London

Lesney, I. (1970) Symmetrical hypogenesis of the cerebellum. *Acta Neurologica Scandinavica*, **46**, 642

Levitt, S. (1975) Stimulation of movement. A review of therapeutic techniques. In *Movement and Child Development* (ed. K.S. Holt), Clinics in Developmental Medicine, No. 55, William Heinemann, London

MacKeith, R. (1973) What about Doman-Delacato? *Parents Voice*, **23**, 4

Nelson, K.B. and Ellenberg, J. (1986) Antecedents of cerebral palsy. Multivariate analysis of risk. *New England Journal of Medicine*, **315**, 81

Peterson, M.K. (1978) Impedence audiometry and the brain-damaged child. *Developmental Medicine and Child Neurology*, **20**, 800

Pharoah, P.O.D., Cooke, T., Cooke, R.W.I. and Rosenbloom, L. (1990) Birthweight specific trends in cerebral palsy. *Archives of Disease in Childhood*, **65**, 602

Robinson, R.O., McCarthy, G.T. and Little, T.M. (1989) Conductive education at the Petö Institute, Budapest. *British Medical Journal*, **299**, 1145–9

Rutter, M., Graham, P. and Yule, W. (1970) *A Neuropsychiatric Study in Childhood*. Clinics in Developmental Medicine, Nos. 35/36. SIMP, William Heinemann, London

Samilson, R.L. (1975) *Orthopaedic Aspects of Cerebral Palsy*. Clinics in Developmental Medicine, Nos. 52/53. SIMP, William Heinemann, London

Sanner, G. and Hagberg, B. (1974) 188 cases of non-progressive ataxic syndromes in childhood. Aspects of aetiology and classification. *Neuropädiatrie*, **5**, 224

Sheridan, M.D. (1973) The Stycar graded ball test. *Developmental Medicine and Child Neurology*, **15**, 423

Smith, A.V. (1970) The Bristol adaptation of the Hungarian method of conductive education for the cerebral palsied child. *Progress in Physical Therapy*, **1**, 254

Smyth, D.P.L. (1990) Care of severely handicapped children in the community. *Maternity and Child Health*, **15**, 366

Soutar, R.L. and Day, R.E. (1991) Dysequilibrium/ataxic diplegia with immunodeficiency. *Archives of Disease in Childhood*, **66**, 982–3

Stanley, F. (1984) Prenatal risk factors in the study of the cerebral palsies. In *The Epidemiology of the Cerebral Palsies* (eds. F. Stanley and E. Alberman), Blackwell Scientific, Oxford

Thomas, A.P., Bax, M.C.O. and Smyth, D.P.L. (1989) *The Health and Social Needs of Young Adults with Physical Disabilities*. Clinics in Developmental Medicine, No. 106. MacKeith Press, Oxford

Towbin, A. (1970) Central nervous system damage in the human fetus and newborn infant. Mechanical and hypoxic injury incurred in the fetal-neonatal period. *American Journal of Diseases of Children*, **119**, 529

Whittle, M.J. (1992) Rhesus haemolytic disease. *Archives of Disease in Childhood*, **67**, 65

Worthington, A (1990) *Useful Addresses for Parents with a Handicapped Child*, Worthington, Sale

9   Epilepsy

The aphorism that epilepsy is only a symptom needs to be repeated. Although it is a symptom which is sometimes difficult to identify it should not be given the diagnostic status of a disease entity. It is a symptom that some people are more liable to than others, just as some are more likely to suffer headaches. Cerebral lesions and metabolic disturbances of similar severity will cause epilepsy in only some of the affected people. Quite often the seizures occur for no apparent reason, when the threshold may be lowered by genetic rather than acquired factors, and a diagnosis of 'idiopathic epilepsy' is made. The reason for the varying liability to epileptic seizures is unknown, and a number of factors may be involved. The EEG has demonstrated that the end result in terms of electrical activity is the simultaneous discharge of large numbers of neurons. This hypersynchrony may be due to neurophysiological causes resulting from failure of inhibitory mechanisms, particularly in certain circumstances such as the abnormal sensitivity to photic stimulation. There may also be biochemical differences between individuals; for instance, in the concentration of gamma-aminobutyric acid in the brain; a substance which is known to have a synaptic inhibitory action (Aird, Masland and Woodburg, 1984). The occurrence of fits has to be viewed against this background of individual liability. If no remedial cause is found, treatment is given to protect the patient against the attacks by raising the threshold with drugs. Too little is known about the action of these drugs, and their beneficial effects are usually at a cost in terms of some aspect of cerebral function, or some disturbance of one or other of the body systems.

Some causes of epileptic seizures

Neonatal seizures

Fits at this age may take a number of forms different from the typical petit mal, partial seizure and grand mal of later life. Tonic fits often result from brain damage and have a bad prognosis. They are brief, but breathing may stop long enough to cause cyanosis. The back arches, the arms may extend or flex, and the legs stiffen (Brown, 1973). Clonic fits are more likely to be benign and to complicate metabolic disturbances, and, if these are caused by primary hypocalcaemia for example, they do not seem to upset the baby very much and he or she may continue feeding during them. They are often focal, with the clonus affecting various parts of the body at different times. Neonatal seizures can occasionally be very difficult to recognize, for instance when they consist of the sudden onset of nystagmus, autonomic phenomena such as flushing and sweating, and attacks of apnoea.

The incidence of fits at this time of life is around 12 per 1000 live births (Keen and Lee, 1973). The timing of the onset of the fits may give a clue to aetiology. When seizures occur in the first three days of life the cause is likely to be brain damage, particularly from conditions such as intrauterine anoxia. Hypoglycaemia can occasionally cause fits at this time of life. From the fifth to the eighth day of life the fits will more often be due to a primary disturbance of metabolism. Quite frequently no definite cause can be found for such seizures but then the condition is usually a benign one (Pryor, Don and Marcourt, 1981). After the eighth day brain damage again becomes a more frequent cause because of diseases such as septicaemia and meningitis.

Neurological abnormalities may occur in the presence of brain damage in the neonatal period, but tests will be needed to establish other aetiologies. When there are obvious signs of infection in an ill baby, blood cultures and examination of the cerebrospinal fluid are necessary, especially as signs of meningeal irritation are often absent. If there is likely to be a delay in obtaining the results of metabolic investigations it may be necessary to give emergency treatment with pyridoxine, magnesium, calcium and glucose, waiting a short interval between each injection to see if there is a response (Rose and Lombroso, 1970).

Hypoglycaemia occurring in the first few days of life can be a cause of brain damage as well as a result of it. Dysmature babies (small-for-dates) are particularly at risk as they are born with few, if any, reserves. Infants of diabetic mothers are also at considerable risk for other reasons. Neonatal hypoglycaemia is most often asymptomatic and then the baby's progress is almost always satisfactory; but serum levels must be monitored. If symptoms such as apnoea, cyanosis, jitteriness, twitching, convulsions and collapse occur, a high percentage of these babies will later on show evidence of brain damage (Creery, 1966). Therefore, even if the hypoglycaemia follows brain injury rather than vice versa, it is obviously a matter of urgency to diagnose it with the use of Dextrostix and other blood tests, and give the appropriate treatment in the form of a 10% glucose infusion, 65 ml/kg body weight/24 h. One interesting observation is that children who have shown low blood sugars in the neonatal period may be particularly liable to hypoglycaemia as they grow older. In some instances the child seems unable to withstand long periods of fasting due to failure of homoeostatic mechanisms mediated by the pituitary-adrenal complex, with a defective output of epinephrine in response to hypoglycaemia (Broberger, Junger and Zetterstrom, 1959).

Hypocalcaemia is a common cause of neonatal convulsions (Keen, 1969). It may occur in the first day or two of life as neonatal tetany, often associated with hypoglycaemia and evidence of brain damage. More commonly, the neonatal tetany is manifested towards the end of the first week of life among healthy, thriving babies. Although there are alternative explanations, it is suggested that this may be related to artificial feeding and the relatively large phosphorus load of cows' milk. This may temporarily overwhelm the homoeostatic mechanism of the parathyroids (Baum, Cooper and Davies, 1968). The infant's parathyroid glands may be underfunctioning due to hyperparathyroidism in the mother secondary to vitamin D deficiency. This could be explained by lack of sunlight and a poor diet, as neonatal tetanus is more common among babies born in late winter. It would also account for the enamel hypoplasia of the unerupted deciduous teeth (Roberts, Cohen and Forfar, 1973). The hypocalcaemia may sometimes be related to the water or osmolarity crisis of neonatal development which occurs between the third and eighth days of life. If the hypocalcaemia fails to respond to a change of diet and the giving of calcium, the possibility of *hypomagnesaemia* has to be considered (Friedman, Hatcher and Watson, 1967). This may also be due to the phosphorus load in cows' milk, and to functional hypoparathyroidism in the infant, and to factors such as magnesium deficiency in the mother and target unresponsiveness. A specific failure of magnesium absorption can occur, and there are a variety of other possible causes of hypomagnesaemia, including prolonged diarrhoea, malabsorption syndromes, renal tubular acidosis, and primary or secondary aldosteronism.

A 10% solution of calcium gluconate, 5–10 ml by mouth before feeds or 2–10 ml intravenously, can be given to correct hypocalcaemia, but the intravenous solution may cause dangerous slowing of the heart and its effect is quite short-lived. It has been shown that in many cases of hypocalcaemia there is hypomagnesaemia as well, and then it is better to give 0.2 ml/kg body weight of a 50% solution of magnesium sulphate intramuscularly, if necessary on two or three occasions at 12-hourly intervals. There is a slight risk of the magnesium causing a curare-like neuromuscular blocking action. The fact that magnesium sulphate can cure symptomatic neonatal tetany whether or not there is hypomagnesaemia may be related to improved calcium absorption, a reduction of muscle hyper-excitability or to a release of parathyroid hormone which mobilizes calcium from bone sites (Roberts, Cohen and Forfar (1973); Turner, Cockburn and Forfar, 1977).

Convulsions can occur with *hyponatraemia* and *hypernatraemia*. Water intoxication leading to hyponatraemia occurs with inappropriate secretion of antidiuretic hormone complicating neonatal asphyxia and severe infections, or when too much water is given in intravenous treatment. This can lead to central pontine myolinolysis.

One of the most common causes of hypernatraemia is gastroenteritis among children who are given too much sodium in artificial feeds. The brain shrinks, and bleeding can occur from traction on veins. Convulsions can also occur during the treatment of hypernatraemia if hypotonic fluids are given too rapidly. There is a delay of several hours before the level of sodium in the cerebrospinal fluid equals that in the serum, and cerebral oedema can result from the difference in osmotic pressures (Brown, 1973).

Although *kernicterus* is now a rare disorder it does occur in the presence of uncommon blood group incompatabilities or in premature babies with low serum albumen and acidosis.

There are rare instances of infants who respond immediately to large amounts of pyridoxine (200 mg or more a day) which prevents the incidence of convulsions, and the patient remains dependent on a maintenance dose. Such *pyridoxine dependency* should be borne in mind if any infant does not respond to conventional therapy and there is no apparent cause for this. Seizures may start *in utero* and then pyridoxine given to the mother can be beneficial. In most cases there appears to be no reason for the dependency, except for genetic factors. It is known that certain metabolic disorders may show evidence of pyridoxine dependency. Some patients with homocystinuria respond to treatment with pyridoxine alone, and pyridoxine therapy may also be effective in cystathioninuria. It seems possible that in these conditions the enzyme is present but is structurally defective, so that the normal binding power with the co-enzyme pyridoxine is incomplete unless in an environment saturated with it. If there are such known pyridoxine-dependent metabolic disorders, sometimes associated with epileptic seizures, there may be others. However, in the pyridoxine dependency syndrome it may be that in some instances there is an inability to maintain normal levels of pyridoxal phosphate in the body for any length of time. This could be due to an instability of a plasma pyridoxal phosphate-albumen complex, as transport of the vitamin into the brain in an inert form could be accomplished in this way (Heeley *et al.*, 1978). The most likely cause may be a deficiency of GABA due to a genetic defect at the pyridoxal posphate binding site of glutamate decarboxylase, the rate-limiting enzyme in GABA synthesis (Jaeken *et al.*, 1990) The diagnosis can be confirmed by normalization of the EEG when pyridoxine is given intravenously.

The tryptophan test has been found to be normal among babies with pyridoxine dependency, but may be abnormal when there is pyridoxine deficiency and among older children with pyridoxine responsiveness, when there seems to be clinical improvement on massive doses of pyridoxine (Meeuwisse, Gamstorp and Tryding, 1968). This suggests different underlying metabolic disorders in these conditions, although in the latter the improvement may be due to the large doses of pyridoxine lowering the level of the anti-epileptic drugs in the body, if they are causing toxic effects. However, fits of various types on different drugs may respond to pyridoxine, which raises problems of how to define the syndromes, but it may always be justifiable to give a trial of pyridoxine if fits are not responding to other forms of treatment (Stephenson and Byrne, 1983).

As might be expected, the prognosis is worse among babies with neonatal seizures who show evidence of brain damage than among those with uncomplicated metabolic disturbances (Brown, Cockburn and Forfar, 1972). There is an overlap between the brain-damaged and metabolic groups, and it may sometimes be difficult to apportion blame. As mentioned earlier, hypoglycaemia can result from brain injury, but can itself damage the cells of the brain, and this will be all too apparent on follow-up examination. Thus, in the absence of unequivocal evidence of birth trauma the exact cause of the injury remains in doubt. The primary or secondary role of metabolic disorders must, however, be taken into account when assessing prognosis. Hypocalcaemia occurs in both groups, but is most frequently due to metabolic causes. Hypomagnesaemia is uncommon in the brain-damaged group, but hypoglycaemia seems to be about twice as common in this group as in the metabolic one (Brown, Cockburn and Forfar, 1972).

In the neonatal period the EEG can be of prognostic significance, i.e. a normal record indicates a good prognosis. Rose and Lombroso (1970) found on follow-up that 86% of convulsing neonates with normal EEGs were progressing satisfactorily; only 11.8% of those with multifocal tracings were normal, and of those with isoelectric or paroxysmal records none were normal.

Apart from the management of the metabolic disorders already discussed, other aspects of treatment must be considered. If asphyxia has caused brain damage, attention must be paid to temperature regulation and correction of acidosis, and of metabolic disturbances including hypocalcaemia. Sometimes dexamethazone is indicated to reduce intracranial pressure, in a dose of 1 mg 4 hourly. This may also be given after birth injury. When intracranial haemorrhage occurs blood transfusion may be needed, as well as exchange transfusion, transfusion of specific factor extract or platelets, and the giving of vitamin K (Brown, 1973). If investigations indicate a remediable cause, appropriate action must be taken, and short-term anti-epileptic treatment may also be indicated, usually in the form of phenobarbitone. When the cause of the seizures cannot be completely removed, or if the aetiology is uncertain or unknown, long-term anti-epileptic treatment must be considered.

Types of epileptic seizures

Grand mal

The end result of an epileptic discharge in any part of the brain may be a major convulsion. The major fit sometimes starts with an aura or warning. This can give essential information on the site of origin of the epileptic discharge, and therefore of a possible focal lesion. Whether the hypersynchrony remains confined to one area, resulting in a focal fit, or spreads throughout the brain to cause a major convulsion depends presumably on the efficiency of mechanisms supposed to prevent propagation of the epileptic discharges. The convulsion may be the most dramatic manifestation of epilepsy, but it is the least informative from the medical point of view, particularly when there is no aura. Its importance lies in the dangers associated with any period of unconsciousness. Injury may occur if the onset is sudden, and aspiration is a possibility, especially if an attack happens during a meal. Recovery from a single attack will occur in an otherwise healthy person, as the anoxia and metabolic changes associated with the fit curtail the activity of discharging neurons. The most serious risks arise from a number of convulsions occurring in a short period of time.

Status epilepticus

If there is incomplete recovery between the convulsions the patient can be said to be in status epilepticus, and this is a medical emergency. If a number of fits have occurred before treatment is started, the child may never recover consciousness, even if the treatment eventually controls the seizures. This may be due to anoxic and metabolic factors, as autopsy may reveal evidence of cerebral oedema only. Animal studies suggest that removal of factors such as arterial hypotension and hyperpyrexia protect against cerebellar damage, but only to a slight extent against neocortical and hippocampal lesions. Sustained neuronal discharge with elevated metabolic rate may cause ischaemic changes in neurons by an accumulation of metabolites. A consequence of this is swelling of astrocytic end-feet, resulting in impaired transport of substrates and metabolites to and from active neurons (Meldrum, 1978). It has been shown that intracranial pressure rises during and after fits of any kind, even with minor seizures. These changes may often be related to increased cerebral blood flow, but when repeated major convulsions occur cerebral oedema may complicate the picture so that cerebral blood flow is impaired. Then treatment to reduce the pressure, with mannitol for example, may be of vital importance and is a strong argument for intracranial pressure monitoring in status epilepticus (Minns and Brown, 1978). Recovery will usually occur, but the incidence of subsequent brain damage among children is high if the status epilepticus has been prolonged, although the prognosis is not always bad. Urgent and energetic treatment is likely to prevent the morbidity and mortality. Status epilepticus may happen for no apparent reason, but is particularly liable to occur as a complication of acute infections and high fever, and after sudden stopping of anti-epileptic treatment. The frequency of status epilepticus, even as a presenting symptom, has been noted among patients with frontal lobe lesions (Rowan and Scott, 1970).

Febrile convulsions

There are a number of children aged between a few months and a few years who appear to be liable to convulsions when their temperatures rise above a certain level. The incidence is 3–5%. A rectal temperature of 38°C or more is usually accepted in the definition of this type of epilepsy. There is evidence that the liability is inherited as a dominant characteristic (Ounsted, Lindsay and Norman, 1966). Suggestions that the convulsions are precipitated by a specific infection, such as exanthema subitum, seems unlikely, but evidence of infections, particularly of the urinary tract, must always be sought; and it is certainly possible that some febrile convulsions could be due to invasion of the blood stream or CNS by a micro-organism, usually a virus (Lewis *et al.*, 1979). Some such seizures may be of a reflex anoxic type, emphasizing their possible heterogeneity (Stephenson, 1978a). After the first febrile convulsion there is a recurrence rate of about 37% within three years (Van den Berg, 1974), but most children who develop febrile convulsions cease to have fits as they grow older. Only 3–5 out of 200 such children studied in Denmark suffered from persistent epileptic seizures (Frantzen, Lennox-Buchthal and Nygard, 1968), and in a recent national population-based study, 9 out of 382 children had more than one afebrile seizure. The risk was greatest for those who had focal febrile convulsions (Verity and Golding, 1991), which may indicate previous brain damage. Parents can therefore be reassured that their child can lead a perfectly healthy life. However, in spite of this good prognosis, the condition does give rise to concern, and can be a cause of extreme worry to parents who, if they have never seen a fit before, may think that their child is dying (Baumer *et al.*, 1981). There may well be a risk of brain damage from status epilepticus, and, as Ounsted, Lindsay and Norman (1966) have shown, they may start life with one form of epilepsy and end it with another. Focal fits, particularly those arising in the temporal lobe, can result from such damage, quite apart from other symptoms such as mental retardation, hyperkinetic behaviour, and catastrophic rage, although the risk of complex partial seizures after febrile convulsions is slight, and may have been overestimated in the past due to different definitions used, and to such factors as ineffective treatment. Girls are more at risk of loss of intellectual attainments after febrile convulsions than boys, but both may show a higher incidence of learning difficulties than normal (Wallace and Cull, 1979). The EEG is usually normal between the seizures, but may show an excess of slow wave activity for a few days following a fit. After the age of 3 years, paroxysmal discharges of spike and wave complexes are more frequent, but do not seem to be of prognostic significance. In the past there have been doubts whether continuous prophylactic treatment prevents the seizures that occur under these special circumstances (Millichap, Aledort and Madsen, 1960). Present evidence sometimes justifies consideration of treatment if the fits start before the age of 13 months, or between 13 and 35 months if there is a family history of epilepsy of genetic origin, or if more than two episodes occur, as these are the children at greatest risk (Lennox-Buchthal, 1973). Wallace (1974) has also found an increased risk of recurrence of febrile convulsions if there are repeated seizures in the initial illness, an early onset especially among girls, among boys with a family history, persistent neurological abnormalities, and if the first fit is a complicated and unilateral one and lasts more than 30 minutes. The persistence of grand mal after febrile convulsions is largely determined by events preceding the initial fit, while temporal lobe seizures are related to prolonged, repeated and unilateral febrile convulsions and may therefore be prevented by adequate treatment (Wallace, 1977), although obviously this should not happen. Chevrie and Aicardi (1975) also emphasize that the expression of the first febrile convulsion depends upon multiple factors, such as age, sex, genetic predisposition, previous brain damage and the nature of the febrile illness. If there are no risk factors there is a recurrence rate of 12%. There is an increased risk of non-febrile seizures among these children which decreases with age, but by 26 years Wallace (1988) suggests that 7% of them are likely to have had at least two unprovoked fits. About 2 of every 3 children who have one non-febrile fit will have one or more subsequently (Wallace, 1988).

It has been claimed that the presence of one or more risk factors justifies treatment. The use of phenytoin sodium does not prevent febrile convulsions, although it may modify their severity (Melchior, Buchthal and Lennox-Buchthal, 1971). Another study from Denmark (Faero et al., 1972) suggests that phenobarbitone is effective if a constant serum level of 69.0 μmol/l (16 μg/ml) is obtained. The sedative effects of phenobarbitone can be largely avoided by giving the drug in the evening only and gradually increasing the dose up to 5 mg/kg body weight. In view of other side-effects, and because the role of phenobarbitone in the treatment of febrile fits has been questioned (Heckmatt et al., 1976), well-controlled trials of other drugs, such as sodium valproate, have been carried out. If the concentration of sodium valproate is 416.4 μmol/l (60 μg/ml) or more it can be as effective as phenobarbitone and is freer of side-effects, although some of these such as hepatitis are worrying (Wallace and Aldridge Smith, 1980). As an alternative to continuous prophylactic treatment, increased use is now being made of diazepam, given rectally to children at risk when their temperature rises, and in order to prevent prolonged convulsions. There seems to be no doubt that this is effective if given in time (Thorn, 1980); and continuous prophylactic treatment with sodium valproate or phenobarbitone may be unjustified, as it does not appear to reduce the risk of a recurrence of febrile convulsions (McKinlay and Newton, 1989). Also, the risks are greatest from the first febrile convulsion being a severe one, before prophylactic treatment can be considered.

As already mentioned, it is suggested that a significant number of children with febrile seizures are suffering from anoxic rather than epileptic attacks. This conclusion is based on the type of seizure, the family history, clinical and EEG findings and the response to the oculo-vagal or oculo-cardiac reflex. If confirmed, the management of these children will have to be re-examined (Stephenson, 1978a).

It is important to identify the children at risk and warn the parents that if the temperature rises certain precautions must be taken, and that if a convulsion occurs a doctor must be notified. If the height of the temperature is critical, it is obviously important not to shut the windows, put the fire on, or heap blankets on the bed. Tepid sponging, especially of the head, may well help to reduce the temperature, but shivering must be avoided. It seems reasonable to give antipyretics at the start of an illness, although there is no proof that they are effective. If a severe convulsion does occur in a child known to be at risk, parenteral therapy should be given without waiting to see if another one ensues. Paraldehyde may be the safest drug, but, if feasible, diazepam given intravenously, slowly, and in a dose appropriate to age, may be more effective (0.1–0.4 mg/kg body weight). In the case of selected parents, who are willing and able to co-operate, it is justifiable to supply them with rectal tubes containing 5 mg of diazepam ready to be administered. The dose is 0.25–0.5 mg/kg body weight as soon as a seizure occurs (Bower, 1978). The rate of absorption of diazepam from suppositories is variable and therefore unreliable except in prophylaxis (Agurell et al., 1975).

Partial or focal seizures

The description of the minor seizure, or of the aura of a major one, may indicate the area of the cortex primarily involved by the epileptic discharge. This can suggest the presence of a local lesion, although quite frequently not a progressive one. However, partial or focal fits and focal EEG findings are not a definite indication of a cortical lesion. The epileptic discharge may spread from some other more silent area of the brain, and from sub-cortical structures. This is particularly true of focal seizures in

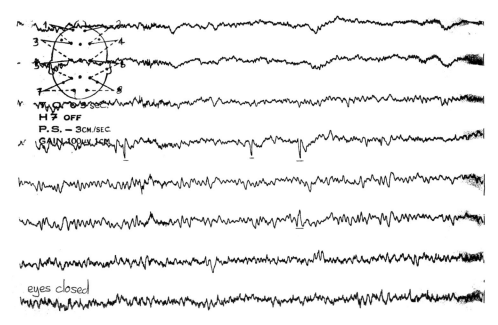

Figure 9.1   EEG in benign focal epilepsy of childhood.

young children; and among babies with metabolic disorders such attacks are quite common without indicating any structural lesion of the cerebrum.

There is a particular form of focal epilepsy starting in the first decade which has been designated *benign focal or partial epilepsy of childhood*. There may be a sensory aura, but typically they are focal motor seizures affecting the face and arm, with grunting, speech arrest and hypersalivation, and sometimes unpleasant feelings of suffocation. They often occur at night, and then are more likely to develop into a generalized convulsion. The EEG shows a centrotemporal spike focus and normal background activity (Fig. 9.1). The focal abnormalities may shift from side to side and are sometimes bilateral. The fits stop in the second decade and are not associated with a cerebral lesion (Lerman and Kivity, 1975). The good prognosis must influence the planning of investigations and treatment. This is a common form of epilepsy in childhood (Aicardi, 1979), but the presence of Rolandic spikes may not always be benign (Morikawa *et al.*, 1979). Other benign forms of epilepsy are now being described, such as 'atypical partial benign epilepsy of childhood' with certain features suggesting the Lennox-Gastaut syndrome, which emphasizes the importance of studying the natural history of epileptic seizures in all their forms (Aicardi and Chevrie, 1982; Aicardi, 1986).

The clinical manifestations of focal seizures will vary according to the area of the cortex involved, but always include both positive and negative features. For example, the positive features in the focal motor seizure are the clonic movements, perhaps initially involving the side of the face, the fingers and hand, and spreading up the arm. The negative features arise from the fact that no part of the brain occupied by epileptic activity can be used for normal function. Therefore, in a motor fit involving the arm, it will not be possible to move it during the attack and for a short period afterwards. The longer the paralysis (Todd's paralysis) lasts after a fit, the less likely is it to be a direct association, and other factors such as impaired blood supply to the part of the cortex involved have to be taken into account. This may be strong presumptive evidence of a local lesion. If it were possible to test sensation during a focal fit it is likely that the abnormal feelings involving various parts of the body would be accompanied by sensory impairment, and the crude visual hallucinations, typical of fits involving the occipital lobes, with hemianopia.

The prefrontal cortex is liable to damage from head injuries and infections spreading inwards from the frontal sinuses. If the lesion causes an epileptogenic focus the patient often drops suddenly in a major convulsion without warning, although sometimes the head and eyes turn to the opposite side. The explanation for this may be the ill-defined functions of this part of the brain, such as its role in ambition, planning, and the laying down of behaviour patterns in early life. To accomplish such integrative functions of this degree of complexity it must obviously have widespread connections with all other parts of the brain, which will facilitate the rapid spread of the epileptic discharge, and perhaps explains the relative frequency of status epilepticus among patients with frontal lobe lesions.

Seizures involving the temporal lobes: complex partial seizures

The only difference between fits arising in the temporal lobes and other focal fits is their varied and sometimes bizarre form. They are a relatively common type of epilepsy, probably comprising more than a third of any series of patients with frequent fits. They often start in childhood (Falconer, 1971), but the diagnosis can be difficult as the child cannot describe what is happening. The temporal lobe is a vulnerable part of the brain, being particularly liable to damage as a result of cerebral oedema. This may occur after such incidents as head injury, including birth injury, status epilepticus, and encephalopathies of various kinds. The swollen brain is forced down through the tentorial opening, and the inner surface of the temporal lobe is compressed. Local pressure and the cutting off of the blood supply will lead to an area of gliosis if the patient recovers. This in turn may result in an epileptogenic focus, sometimes after a long interval of time, although the mechanisms underlying these changes are unknown (Earle, Baldwin and Penfield, 1953). The damage to the temporal lobes often results in behaviour and personality disorders as well as fits, so that this form of epilepsy presents special problems. Also, the response to medical treatment is frequently unsatisfactory and surgical removal of the epileptic focus is sometimes considered. For these reasons, therefore, it is reasonable to keep the concept of 'temporal lobe epilepsy'.

The positive aspects of these fits, which, like the clonic movements of the motor seizures, can sometimes be elicited by the neurosurgeon at operation, usually take the form of some kind of sensory hallucination. The distortion of the sensation makes it difficult for the patient to describe in words, and this is often impossible for children. As a result, the attacks may present as a brief impairment of consciousness and can be difficult to distinguish from absences. A suggestive finding in these focal fits is the occurrence of fear which does not occur in absence attacks. Also, there can be no doubt that the temporal lobes are involved in both short-term and long-term memory processes. These features may account for some of the unusual sensations experienced by the patient and for the fact that much of the episode will not be recalled. Visual hallucinations can take the form of familiar scenes from the patient's past life, or of familiar faces, or occasionally of their own body. The patient may see animals, real or imaginary, and what is looked at may change in shape and size. Auditory hallucinations include music, often of a sentimental kind, voices, bells, and other sounds. Perhaps the best known hallucinations are the olfactory; the peculiar tastes and smells that often characterize seizures involving the uncinate part of the temporal lobe. Then there are the strange feelings which may occur on their own or in association with one or other of the sensory hallucinations already described. The most common is the sensation of familiarity, as if everything had happened before, the *déjà vu* phenomenon; others include feelings of strangeness and, as mentioned, of fear.

The negative aspects of these focal seizures constitute the efforts of the brain to work without that part of the temporal lobe involved by the epileptic discharge. This results in confused and automatic behaviour. The temporal lobe may subserve highly complex functions but does not appear to be necessary for those that have been performed many times before. This odd behaviour is referred to as 'epileptic automatism' or 'psychomotor epilepsy', and is indistinguishable from that complicating other types of epilepsy, particularly absences. The patient may talk in a confused way during these periods of automatism, but speech is likely to be affected more directly if the epilepsy involves the dominant hemisphere. As in any confused state, the patient's behaviour may be aggressive and difficult, but there will be nothing premeditated in this.

The idea of focal epilepsy affecting only the cortex is outmoded, and for this reason the term 'partial epilepsy' is used in order to denote that the discharge involves the subcortical structures as well, spreading to parts of the brain linked by well-developed tracts. For example, the limbic system includes the temporal lobes and parts of the diencephalon, which may account for some of the overlap between temporal lobe epilepsy and absence seizures.

Absence seizures (petit mal)

This term should be reserved for a special and relatively uncommon type of epilepsy, and the former is the better one, as petit mal is so often used to denote any kind of minor fit. The seizures are characterized by brief interruptions of consciousness, sometimes accompanied by flickering of the eyelids and deviation of the eyes. The epileptic activity involves the diencephalon, a part of the brain sometimes referred to as the 'seat of consciousness'. Certainly, if the afferent and efferent tracts relaying in this part of the brain are put out of action, unconsciousness will ensue. This will occur in the presence of epileptic activity, as already stated, and this will be the negative manifestation of these fits, although there may be no positive ones. The interference with cerebral function is sometimes incomplete and only inhibits projections to and from certain parts of the brain, particularly the temporal lobes, which results in automatisms as described in the previous section. There is also evidence that epileptic discharges can cause a disturbance of function of the subcortical structures unassociated with clinical fits or even EEG changes. This has been described as a state of bewilderment (Goldie and Green, 1961), and it may also be one of the reasons for the variable performance of these children. An impairment of immediate recall and of continuous performance can be correlated with generalized epileptic discharges in the EEG (Hutt and Lee, 1968) but, in addition, children with this form of epilepsy may state that on certain days they have great difficulties in attending, concentrating and memorizing, while on other days they are not aware of any impairment of function. Although other factors such as emotional disturbances and the toxic effects of drugs have to be taken into account, in some instances the cause may be due to prolonged epileptic activity in the absence of clinical seizures. Focal fits involving the cerebral cortex may last for days on end (epilepsia partialis continua), so there seems to be no reason why the same should not occur at a subcortical level. The automatisms that occur in association with absence seizures can cause confusion with those following focal fits arising in the temporal and frontal cortices, but the former are usually less complicated (Gordon and Aird, 1991).

Absences are most often seen among children, but occasionally among adults. The prognosis for the cessation of attacks is better if the minor seizures are not associated with convulsions. They stop frequently enough to justify a hopeful attitude in discussions with the parents (Gordon, 1965), although it has to be admitted that a certain number of children will continue to suffer from grand mal as they grow older, even if the minor seizures stop. Absences or petit mal are not a generalized form of epilepsy, but one confined to a particular system of neurons in the brain, which no doubt accounts for its unique response to certain drugs, as well as its genetic features (Aird, Masland and Woodbury, 1984).

Photosensitive epilepsy and other types of 'reflex' epilepsy

There are a number of people who are abnormally sensitive to flickering lights. When exposed to flashes of a certain frequency per second, usually around 12–20 Hz, they may develop fits, usually minor akin to absences, but occasionally major in type. If the patient is exposed to this stimulus while the EEG is being recorded, diffuse epileptic discharges of spikes and slow waves may occur which are not always associated with clinical changes. One situation in which the patient may be exposed to the risk of epileptic seizures if they are light-sensitive is in watching a black and white television screen when the picture is slipping. Some of these people may have seizures under other circumstances, and their management will be that of anyone else suffering from epilepsy. Others will never have a fit unless exposed to photic stimulation. In that case it seems best to avoid the precipitating factors rather than to give anti-epileptic drugs. For instance, in the case of television epilepsy, both the frequency of the flicker and the intensity of the illumination may be critical factors. It is also possible that in some cases it is a sensitivity to patterns rather than to flicker that is the precipitating factor in causing fits while looking at certain objects (Stefansson et al., 1977). The person should therefore be advised not to sit close to the set, particularly if it is not properly adjusted (Jeavons and Harding, 1975), and to avoid the flickering lights of computer games.

If the sensitivity is very marked, whether the seizures are precipitated by flickering light or by patterns, it is essential to consider treatment. Most anti-epileptic drugs are ineffective, but photosensitive fits can be abolished in more than 50% of affected patients by the use of sodium valproate (Harding et al., 1978). The fits do occur in response to a particular sensory stimulus, but only in that sense are they reflex. If medical treatment does fail it may be justifiable to try alternatives, such as the use of extinction techniques. These may consist of monocular photic stimulation or binocular stimulation with different light intensities (Forster et al., 1964), although covering one eye may be all that is required.

Similar methods have been used in the treatment of other types of 'reflex' epilepsy. In startle seizures precipitated by sudden noise, sounds are delivered to one ear so softly that they cannot be heard biaurally, and this may reduce the sensitivity. Sub-threshold biaural stimulation is sometimes necessary (Booker, Forster and Klove, 1965). Musicogenic epilepsy has also been modified by extinction techniques. Fits can sometimes be precipitated by touching the patient, especially if this is unexpected, and emotional stimuli can evoke epileptic activity. It may be possible to work out similar methods of treatment, for example with subliminal stimuli.

Rarely, patients may present with attacks of writhing movements of the limbs and trunk (Hudgins and Corbin, 1966). The seizures can be precipitated by sudden movements, and they are not associated with loss of consciousness. They are described under the term 'paroxysmal choreoathetosis', and there is sometimes a history of other members of the family being similarly affected (Lance, 1977). Although the exact relationship of paroxysmal choreoathetosis to epilepsy is unproven it seems possible that it can sometimes be included in the category of 'reflex' epilepsy. Treatment with phenytoin or carbamazepine is worth a trial.

Another rare but interesting condition which may have to be considered in the differential diagnosis of such abnormal movements is Sandifer's syndrome. This consists of torsion spasms and abnormal postures of the head and trunk associated with hiatus hernia and the discomfort caused by this (Sutcliffe, 1969).

Minor status

When epileptic activity involves the subcortical and cortical structures for a prolonged period (Fig. 9.2) the disturbance of function will be more profound than in the states of bewilderment already referred to. A child who has been developing normally becomes unsteady on his or her legs and clumsy in the movements of his or her arms. Myoclonic jerks may give an impression of ataxia, as sometimes the myoclonus is present only on voluntary movement or when a posture is maintained against gravity. Speech can become slurred or lost completely, and drooling of saliva is a prominent

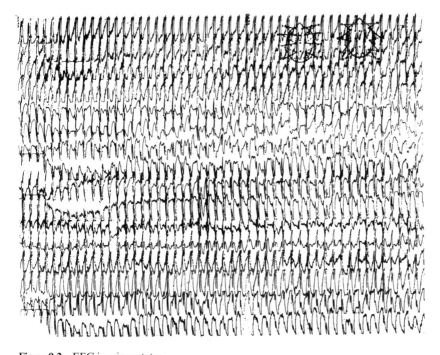

Figure 9.2   EEG in minor status.

feature. In this state a child commonly shows dulling of consciousness and responsiveness, and communication may become impossible. Like any other type of seizure, minor epileptic status is sometimes a symptom of progressive cerebral disease, such as a neurolipidosis (Brett, 1966). However, in many instances the condition is entirely reversible, often after treatment with intravenous diazepam, clonazepam or steroids; and the child may make a complete recovery even after a prolonged period of disability. However, this may not always be so, and there are dangers of brain damage from disturbances of neuronal energy metabolism, if the minor status does continue for any length of time (Doose and Völzke, 1979).

In absence attacks and in minor status there is no doubt that the epileptic activity involves the diencephalon, but almost certainly does not arise in this part of the brain. In fact, the diencephalon has to be intact for the propagation of the generalized discharges underlying both major or minor fits (Williams, 1965). Lesions of these central parts of the brain are not often associated with epilepsy, and it is claimed that stereotactic surgery on the diencephalon can decrease the incidence of such seizures.

Myoclonus

Myoclonus has been defined as 'a disturbance of neurological activity that gives rise to very sudden involuntary jerks which are asynergic and arrhythmic, involving portions of muscles, whole muscles or muscle groups' (Bradshaw, 1954). It can originate at any level of the nervous system, even as a symptom of a spinal lesion. It can occur on its own with no evidence of any other CNS disease, or in association with major seizures for which no definite cause has been found. However, there are a number of degenerative conditions of the nervous system, particularly some metabolic disorders and conditions affecting the cerebrum and cerebellum, such as the gangliosidoses and hereditary myoclonus epilepsy to be discussed in Chapter 11, which manifest themselves by myoclonus, convulsions and dementia, so that the sudden onset of myoclonus in a previously healthy child must always be viewed with concern.

However, myoclonus can be relatively benign, as in *juvenile myoclonic epilepsy* (Delgado-Escueta and Enrile-Bacsal, 1984). This form of epilepsy usually starts between the ages of 8 and 20 years with jerking of the shoulders and arms on awakening. After an interval, generalized tonic-clonic seizures may start, and although behaviour may be hyperactive there is usually no mental retardation. The EEG shows multiple spike-wave interictal discharges. There is often a positive family history, although the mode of inheritance is uncertain. There may be a linkage of juvenile myoclonic epilepsy to an abnormality on the short arm of chromosome 6. Diagnosis is often delayed because of lack of familiarity with the syndrome and failure to elicit a history of jerking. It responds to treatment with sodium valproate.

Rarely, a state of almost continuous myoclonus may occur for prolonged periods. *Myoclonic encephalopathy of infants* is characterized by irregular jerky movements of the limbs and eyes (dancing eyes) and is not associated with mental clouding. The EEG is normal. It may respond to treatment with corticosteroids (Kinsbourne, 1962). There is some doubt about the exact nature of the movements in this condition, but part of the dilemma seems to be due to the equating of myoclonus with epilepsy. If the involuntary jerks can result from disturbances of neurological activity at various levels of the CNS it may be misleading to include them all under the umbrella of epilepsy, or to maintain a rigid distinction between such movements resulting from disorders of the cerebral cortex, the extrapyramidal system, or the spinal cord. The syndrome is sometimes associated with a ganglioneuroblastoma, in which case there is often an increased excretion of catecholamines and their metabolites in the urine, and an abnormal reactivity to neuroblastoma antigens in the form of an inhibition of leucocyte migration (Stephenson *et al.*, 1976). It is suggested that even when no evidence of a neuroblastoma is found after a prolonged period of observation it may still be the causal factor, since there is evidence that these tumours spontaneously regress or mature into neural crest cells in early infancy (Brandt *et al.*, 1974). An excess of cystathionine may also be found in the urine (Von Studnitz, 1970).

Infantile spasms (West's syndrome)

This type of epilepsy is due to a variety of causes, but it is definitely related to the age of the patient. Its onset is usually between the ages of 3 and 9 months, presumably due to the level of cerebral maturation reached at that stage. The aetiology may be:

1. Prenatal, e.g. tuberose sclerosis, phenylketonuria, and interuterine infection with toxoplasmosis;
2. Perinatal, with insults such as haemorrhage or anoxia at birth or neonatal hypoglycaemia among dysmature babies; or
3. Postnatal, especially with diseases such as cytomegalic virus infection or other types of virus encephalitis.

The dermal manifestations of tuberous sclerosis must be sought carefully, as other CNS abnormalities may be absent in infancy. Computerized axial tomography can be helpful in diagnosis if it reveals evidence of intracranial calcification. Among babies who have developed normally before the onset of infantile or flexion spasms there will be the usual cryptogenic group without any certain aetiology, but some of these may have suffered from an allergic type of encephalitis, for example that related to triple vaccination. Jeavons and Bower (1964) found 16 out of 112 infants in whom the spasms had started within a few days of this immunization, and there was a very similar incidence in a group of 50 such patients studied at the Royal Manchester Children's Hospital (Gordon, 1970). Conversely, the relationship between infantile spasms and immunization against whooping cough may only be a time coincidence (Melchior, 1977), and other studies suggest that the risks of this and other serious neurological illnesses complicating pertussis immunization are very slight (Miller *et al.*, 1981).

There may be evidence of brain damage from birth, for instance microcephaly or a marked delay of motor development. However, if progress has been satisfactory before the onset of this type of epilepsy the history is often typical. The baby may be thought to have colic because of the flexion of the body and drawing up of the legs. This is often associated with a change in the baby's response to the environment, obvious to the observant mother. The baby ceases to recognize his or her mother and stops smiling. Development may cease and even regress. Follow-up studies have shown that mental retardation is likely to occur in more than 80% of cases. Although the aetiology is so varied the indications are that this type of epilepsy will occur only in the presence of extensive brain damage at a critical period of development, which is no doubt related to the poor prognosis. When the spasms suddenly affect a normal baby, it has been suggested that prompt treatment with steroids stands a chance of preventing subsequent mental handicap as well as controlling the seizures. A recent follow-up study (Jeavons, Harper and Bower, 1970) showed that there was no evidence that such treatment had any effect on intelligence, although is was beneficial as far as the spasms and EEG abnormalities were concerned. However, it may well be that the steroids must be started within a few days of the onset of the epilepsy if brain damage is to be prevented. Even though this is unproven, the possibility that this treatment may halt the spread of an allergic type of encephalitis cannot be ignored in the face of such a bad prognosis. Infantile spasms are a feature of the Aicardi syndrome described in Chapter 4.

The Lennox Gastaut syndrome (petit mal variant) and Otahara's syndrome (early infantile epileptic encephalopathy with suppression bursts)

The Lennox Gastaut syndrome is a somewhat unsatisfactory syndrome which, as with the other epileptic encephalopathies at this age, is based more on the EEG than the clinical findings. The EEG consists of irregular spike-wave complexes between 1.5 and 2.5 per second, and such a finding is likely to indicate a grave prognosis. The syndrome overlaps many others, as shown by Aicardi (1973), and, like West's syndrome, indicates a severe disorder of cerebral function but at an older age.

The age of onset is between 1 and 6 years. The seizures are varied, and include absences, myoclonus, tonic and focal fits. There is often evidence of mental handicap before the onset of the epilepsy. The aetiology varies from birth injury to acquired encephalopathies, but usually the cause is unknown. Treatment tends to be unsatisfactory, but ACTH, clonazepam, nitrazepam and vigobactrin can be tried.

A third encephalopathy has been described as *early infantile epileptic encephalopathy with suppression bursts (Otahara's syndrome)*. This describes the EEG findings among infants in the first few months of life who have suffered severe brain damage from a variety of causes. There is a close relationship between Otahara's, West's and the Lennox Gastaut syndromes which may evolve from one to the other, each being linked to the age of the patient and the severity of the brain damage (Otahara, 1984). The EEG findings in these epileptic encephalopathies are described later in this chapter.

Epileptic syndromes

There are advantages in collecting the varied manifestations of epilepsy into syndromes based on clinical and EEG findings, data on their evolution, and on aetiology when known (Roger *et al.*, 1985). A number of these have been considered, such as petit mal, benign focal epilepsy of childhood, the Lennox-Gastaut syndrome, juvenile myoclonic epilepsy, and others. They must not be regarded as definitive diagnoses which may stifle further research, but as possible entities which demand further study in order to elucidate their nature.

Differential diagnosis of epilepsy

The child who is brought to the clinic because of attacks of unconsciousness is more likely to be suffering from epilepsy than anything else, but it is unjustifiable to use the term unless there is no doubt about the nature of the episodes. In the case of minor seizures a period of observation may be necessary in the first instance. This caution is related as much to the social as the medical implications of labelling someone as suffering from epilepsy.

Syncope

Particularly in the case of teenagers, and especially girls, the diagnosis of syncope often has to be considered. Such girls usually have emotional problems and difficulties at school. It is suggested that the attacks may be precipitated by hyperventilation, of which the patient is quite unaware (Gillespie, 1954). Emotional stimuli, feelings of faintness, dizziness and symptoms indicating a disturbance of the autonomic nervous system, although suggestive, do not definitely distinguish syncope from epilepsy. Also, there are patients who may have typical faints in childhood and adolescence and who, as they grow older, start to suffer from undoubted epilepsy. A functional disturbance of the CNS may underlie both phenomena. Is it the failure of certain individuals to maintain consciousness in special circumstances that is the factor common to both fits and faints, even though syncope is not a special form of epilepsy? A longer period of unconsciousness followed by sleep, even if the patient remains limp throughout, favours a diagnosis of epilepsy. An onset while standing in a hot and stuffy atmosphere, giddiness and loss of vision before unconsciousness, pallor and sweating, suggest syncope. Very occasionally, syncope may be caused by an unduly sensitive carotid sinus.

Cardiac disorders

A number of cardiac abnormalities can present with syncope, and causes such as mitral valve prolapse, prolonged QT syndrome (including the Romano-Ward syndrome which is of dominant inheritance, sick sinus syndrome (Scott, Macartney and Deverall, 1976), congenital heart disease, cardiomyopathy and idiopathic ventricular tachycardia must be carefully excluded, especially as some of these conditions can be life-threatening. Ventricular arrhythmias can also be due to coronary heart disease, myocarditis or electrolyte imbalance (Radford, Izukawa and Rowe, 1977). Prolonged ECG recordings over 12 hours or more are valuable in diagnosis.

Breath-holding spells

These occur until the age of about 7 years. It has been suggested that they are due to syncope resulting from reflex respiratory arrest, although in some instances the anoxia resulting from the breath-holding may well precipitate an epileptic fit in an infant liable to such seizures. These cyanotic spells, which are related to apnoea, anger and frustration, are followed by crying and then loss of consciousness.

Reflex anoxic seizures

These pallid attacks are fairly common and characterized by the child experiencing usually unexpected pain or fear at the onset, without crying, and there may be evidence of cardiac arrest. They are often misdiagnosed as epileptic (Stephenson, 1980), and in the absence of a clear history, the oculo-cardiac reflex can be of value in diagnosis. Ocular compression is carried out for a period of 10 seconds by applying strong pressure with the thumbs, just below the supra-orbital ridges, over the closed eyelids of the child lying supine; and under EEG and ECG control. The diagnosis of a 'vagal attack' is strongly supported if asystole and an anoxic seizure is induced (Stephenson, 1978b). Anticonvulsant treatment is of no benefit when the attack is brought on in these ways, but in the case of reflex anoxic seizures, if the attacks are frequent and reassurance has not been beneficial, treatment with atropine methonitrate may be indicated (Stephenson, 1979). Sometimes an unusual form of epilepsy may simulate these attacks. Clusters of seizures occur with tonic, dystonic, or atonic components and involvement of autonomic functions. The interictal EEG is usually abnormal with epileptic activity but when the fits start the record becomes of low voltage, and for this reason they are referred to as *generalized cortical electrodecremental events*. These fits are not precipitated by factors such as unexpected pain and the patients show other neurological abnormalities (Fariello, Doro and Forster, 1979).

Benign paroxysmal vertigo of childhood

The attacks usually start between the ages of 3 and 8 years. They tend to be brief, rarely lasting for more than a few minutes. The child is often pale while the vertigo is present, and nystagmus may be seen. There may be associated sweating and vomiting. Consciousness remains unaltered and it is surprising how well even young children will describe their symptoms. Clinical examination between the attacks is negative, and hearing remains normal. Caloric tests show disordered vestibular function with varying degrees of canal paresis. As the attacks are brief, tend to occur at long intervals and cease spontaneously, no particular treatment is indicated, although sea-sickness remedies, such as dimenhydrinate, can be tried (Basser, 1964). The aetiology is unknown.

Gratification episodes

Masturbation in the young child tends to occur during periods of boredom. Apart from the rocking of the body there may be flushing of the face, tenseness of the muscles, overbreathing and lack of awareness.

Night terrors

During nightmares children can walk, talk and act as if terrified. Then the diagnosis from complex partial seizures can be difficult. A careful history can usually resolve the dilemma, but a period of observation may be necessary.

Pseudo-seizures

Quite apart from giving the wrong treatment it is surely of particular importance, as already stated, not to diagnose epilepsy if there is any question of doubt. Taylor (1982) has shown so well the problems that are raised by psychologically determined seizures, or pseudo-seizures, whether the child has epileptic fits in addition or not. The unravelling of the complex problems raised by such situations is obviously time-consuming, especially if the child does have both types of attacks, and needs special skills and attitudes on the part of the professionals involved. In discussing hysteria and epilepsy Taylor stresses that some people behave in a way that makes others wonder whether they may be having epileptic fits. These simulated attacks are not always easy to differentiate from genuine ones. Even if behaviour is bizarre, there is always the possibility of confusion with the abnormal behaviour associated with temporal lobe epilepsy.

The children must have a 'model'; either someone with epilepsy known to them, or themselves. If this pseudo-seizure is 'the language of human distress' which should have only token value as a signal for help, it may not be treated in the reassuring way it should be. Seizures are likely to evoke standard responses in doctors, revealing that physicians are not primarily orientated towards people who suffer sickness, but to the sicknesses people suffer. Their fail-safe strategy is to exclude disease rather explore predicament. This commits them to possible physical illness which necessarily reinforces that possibility. Treatment should consist of stopping all kinds of physical interference by drugs, regimes or investigations. This allows any physical process to declare itself, while at the same time it stops reinforcing illness behaviour. The patient must be provided with a means of recovery, and attempts made to alter the situation which has produced the distress (Taylor, 1982).

Fictitious epilepsy

Another difficult diagnosis in childhood is that of fictitious epilepsy, one of the most common manifestations of Munchausen's syndrome by proxy (Meadow, 1982). This is a condition caused by a carer, usually the mother, deliberately harming the child. The symptoms can imitate those of almost any system disorder, from faecal vomiting, to haematuria, to failure to thrive, but those of the CNS top the list. Recurrent episodes can be of loss of consciousness, ataxia or drowsiness. This form of child abuse can be among the most dangerous.

The 'illnesses' almost always occur at home and not in hospital, and are usually witnessed only by the mother. In the case of fictitious epilepsy (Meadow, 1984) the supposed attacks may only occur at night, or may be anoxic and caused by the parent. They most often affect young children but, particularly in the case of nocturnal episodes, the older child, as well as the doctor, may believe they are genuine. In this way the child is programmed into illness lasting into adult life.

The mother may have medical knowledge of some kind, and the father tends to be unsupportive. Warning signals include bizarre symptoms which are not compatible with the child's state of health, investigation results which are at variance with the clinical findings, an overattentive mother who refuses to leave her child alone and does not seem unduly worried about her child's ill-health. There can be a complete lack of response to treatment, in spite of many admissions to hospital; and the child will lead a life of many restrictions, with limited education.

If the child is to be rescued from this situation it must be while under paediatric care. After that it is almost certainly too late, and the victim remains an invalid for life; and may treat the next generation in the same way.

It may be necessary to arrange a 'place of safety' for the child, and to do everything possible in the way of rehabilitation. The mother may have no recognizable psychiatric disorder, and may refuse to accept the nature of her child's illness, but an attempt must be made to explain it to her.

Investigations

If it is decided that the patient is suffering from epilepsy it is then necessary to establish the origin of the epileptic discharge. The patient's description of the attack may provide this necessary information, especially when it is supplemented by the evidence of witnesses. However, some patients have no memory of the seizures or are unable to find words to describe their sensations, as stated. Particular difficulties can arise in differentiating absences from seizures arising in the temporal lobes, and such a differentiation is important from the point of view of prognosis and treatment.

Remembering that epilepsy is a symptom, it is often necessary to consider a number of tests, although this will depend on circumstances. The significance of an epileptic seizure will vary from patient to patient, depending on such factors as the frequency of the fits, associated symptoms and signs, and the patient's age. If the first fit occurs after the age of 40 years there is a definite possibility that it may be a symptom of cerebro-vascular disease or tumour. Conversely, if the first fit occurs early in life there is an equal possibility that it is a symptom of brain injury at birth or of a metabolic disorder.

An occasional seizure in an otherwise healthy person can indicate no more than an increased predisposition to such attacks. Certain routine investigations, such as an EEG, may be justifiable to make sure they are normal. Then the question of further investigations depends on the child's progress. If treatment is doing what is being asked of it and giving satisfactory protection, and no additional symptoms or signs develop, further tests are not indicated. Conversely, if the history or initial examination suggest an underlying cause, or the patient's progress is not satisfactory, a more detailed assessment will be needed.

In the neonatal period it is especially important to exclude infection, and, among other tests, this may indicate blood cultures and examination of the cerebrospinal fluid. The possibility of metabolic disorders must be considered whether there is evidence of brain damage or not, and serum levels of glucose, calcium and magnesium checked.

Examination of the urine by chromatography for amino acids; and for organic acids sugars and porphyrins, is a useful screening procedure. Many of the disorders of amino acid metabolism, such as phenylketonuria, homocystinuria and arginosuccinic aciduria are associated with epilepsy, and the diagnosis is not always indicated by the other symptoms and signs of these conditions. Metabolic disorders will also have to be considered among older children with seizures, for example the hypoglycaemia occasionally precipitated by ketosis. This may have to be investigated by trying to provoke hypoglycaemia with a ketogenic diet; 1200 calories, with 67% fat, 16% carbohydrate, and 17% protein, given for 24 hours. Failure of a blood glucose response to intramuscular glucagon when the patient is hypoglycaemic with ketonuria is a confirmatory test. It generally resolves after a few years. Treatment involves frequent small meals and avoidance of long fasts.

If the history, examinations, and preliminary investigations, such as the EEG, suggest a focal origin for epileptic seizures, or there is a possibility of a progressive lesion, further investigations will have to be planned. These will include computerized axial tomography, magnetic resonance imaging, and sometimes other special neurological techniques.

The electroencephalogram

Apart from identifying attacks as epileptic, there is the need to try establish the type of seizure from the point of view of prognosis and treatment. The EEG can help in both instances. However, it can only add to the pool of information, clinical and otherwise, on which such diagnoses are made. Much of the criticism of the EEG seems unfair. The implication is that the test is no good because it sometimes does not provide an exact answer to the problems raised. No one is likely to criticize radiological investigations on these grounds, and it seems unreasonable to apply different criteria to neurophysiological tests. It is not possible to discuss the technical aspects of this investigation in a book of this type, but, as far as the interpretation of the records of children is concerned, the main difficulty is the wide range of 'normality' and the changes that occur with increasing age. Also, epileptic seizures can occur with a normal EEG, and epileptic discharges may occur in the EEGs of people who have never had a fit.

The routine recording of the EEG during childhood does present certain technical difficulties, especially among infants to whom the test cannot be explained, but with the help of experienced staff a satisfactory record can almost always be obtained without the use of sedation. The younger the child the slower will be the dominant rhythm. Focal abnormalities in the very young may not have the significance of the same findings at a later age, although they can never be ignored. Spikes in the Rolandic areas are likely to be associated with a benign form of epilepsy in childhood. Single records may be of limited value, and the use of the EEG as a screening test is apt to be an unprofitable exercise. It seems better to formulate specific questions of the EEG and plan the investigation accordingly, making use of serial recordings and, if necessary, activating techniques.

Hyperventilation is usually performed as a routine at the end of the recording, and it is surprising how even very young children can be persuaded to over-breathe. This may precipitate epileptic discharges not present in the resting record. They are most often the generalized spike and wave discharges associated with petit mal epilepsy, and they may be accompanied by clinical changes. In fact, over-breathing is a useful diagnostic procedure during the clinical examination of any child suspected of having absences. The other routine activating technique is photic stimulation which may also cause epileptic discharges in the record (Fig. 9.3) and thus identify anyone who is

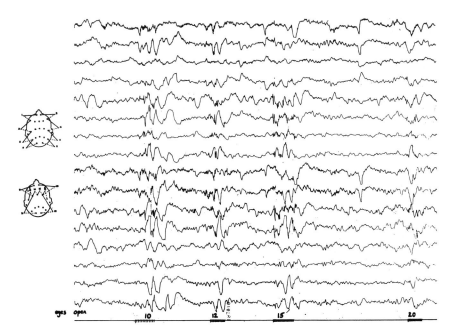

Figure 9.3 Abnormal sensitivity to photic stimulation.

abnormally sensitive to flickering light. The most critical flash frequencies lie between 12 and 20 Hz. If clinical seizures occur they usually take the form of myoclonic jerks or absences, although if there is a marked degree of sensitivity major seizures may be precipitated and due care must be taken to avoid this.

When the patient is suspected of having focal fits but the EEG taken with the patient awake fails to confirm the diagnosis it may well be helpful to repeat the test when the patient is asleep. This particularly applies to fits arising in the temporal lobes, when focal spikes often appear in the trace as drowsiness increases towards light sleep. This may correlate with the occasional history of minor seizures during the day and severe ones just after falling asleep or in the early morning sleep period, although it seems this is not as common as once thought (Currie *et al.*, 1971). These are times when there are normally rises of intracranial pressure which may be of significance (Minns and Brown, 1978). Occasionally, generalized discharges of the myoclonic and petit mal variant type may be accentuated during sleep. Lack of sleep can also increase the likelihood of epileptic activity in the EEG, but this procedure is more applicable to adults than children.

Other techniques, such as giving drugs like bemegride during the recording, can induce epileptic activity. Inserting special electrodes close to the under surface of the sphenoid bone may be used if, for instance, it is essential to identify the origin of the epileptic discharges prior to operations designed to remove an epileptic focus in the temporal lobe when other treatment has failed. Electrocorticography, by recording directly from the surface of the brain during the operation, also assists in identifying the affected tissue. Such complex investigations are rarely needed during childhood.

The typical EEG findings of absence seizures with generalized discharges of 3 per second spike and wave activity (Fig. 9.4), as opposed to the focal spikes seen in

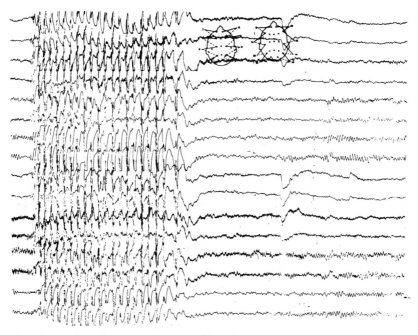

Figure 9.4   Spike and wave activity compatible with absence seizures.

temporal lobe epilepsy (Fig. 9.5), will usually help in diagnosis. Occasionally the differences may not be clear-cut. If the generalized discharges of spikes and slow waves are slightly atypical, for example with ill-formed complexes, asymmetries, and

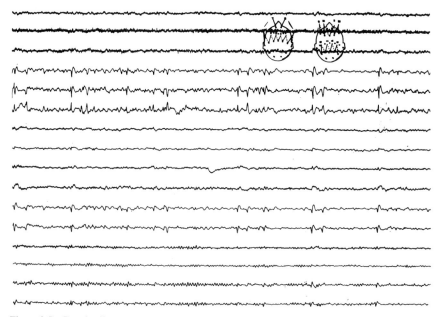

Figure 9.5   Focal spikes over the right temporal lobes.

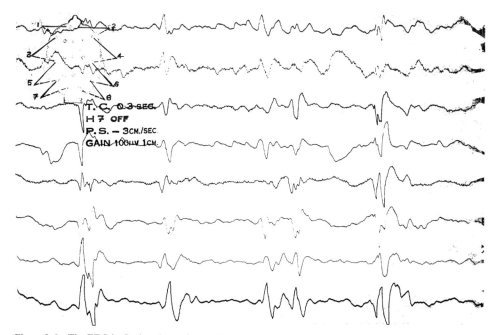

Figure 9.6   The EEG in Otahara's syndrome (suppression bursts).

variable frequencies, the possibility of secondary synchrony has to be considered. In this event the epileptic discharge will originate in a circumscribed area of one cerebral hemisphere, and, gaining entry into the neuronal circuits which involve the diencephalon, spread to involve the cortex on both sides.

Myoclonus is not always associated with EEG abnormalities. As with other types of epilepsy, the EEG changes, when they do occur, no doubt depend on such factors as the cause of the condition, the state of excitability of the cortex, and the level of the central nervous system primarily involved. The electrical equivalent of the myoclonic jerk when recorded at a cortical level consists of a brief generalized outburst of multiple spikes and sometimes slow waves, not occurring in definite complexes.

In Otohara's syndrome, or early infantile epileptic encephalopathy, the EEG pattern consist of burst of complex paroxsysmal activity, separated by periods of marked attenuation of the trace, or even of complete flattening (Fig. 9.6). In the case of infantile spasms the EEG frequently, but not always, shows the chaotic mixture of spikes and slow waves termed 'hypsarrhythmia' (Fig. 9.7). If there is a vestige of normal background activity the findings may be described as 'modified hypsar-rhythmia'. The importance of this EEG pattern is in confirming the diagnosis, especially among infants who have developed normally prior to the onset of the spasms, and may possibly respond favourably to treatment with steroids. However, it must be stressed that the association is not an invariable one. The EEG findings in other epileptic encephalopathies are also useful. The EEG in the Lennox-Gastaut syndrome is again of great importance in the diagnosis. The slow spike and wave complexes around 2 cycles per second, termed 'petit mal variant' (Fig. 9.8), have a poor prognostic significance, although this finding does not indicate any particular

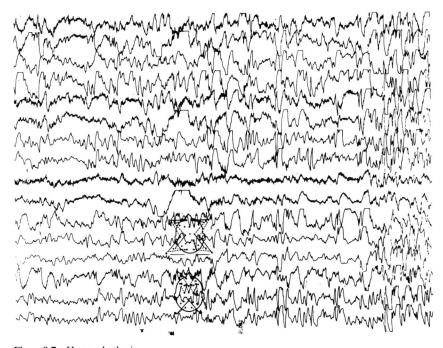

Figure 9.7 Hypsarrhythmia.

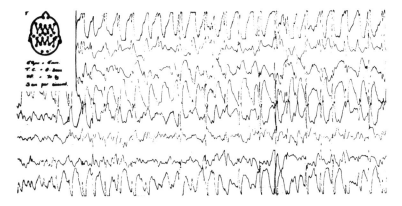

Figure 9.8   Petit mal variant, with slow spike-wave complexes.

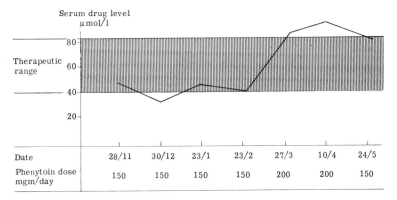

Figure 9.9   Serial phenytoin levels to show that an increase of 50 mg in the oral dose can raise the serum level from the bottom of the therapeutic range to a toxic level.

cause, other than a severe degree of cerebral dysfunction. This pattern characterizes the interictal record, although irregular fast spike-waves can also occur, and during the fits there can be the same diversity.

Apart from focal abnormalities in the EEG suggesting the presence of a local lesion, the findings may occasionally suggest some other underlying cause for the epilepsy. For instance, in subacute sclerosing pan-encephalitis the EEG frequently shows regularly occurring bursts of slow-wave complexes at intervals of about 8–10 seconds (Fig. 9.9). The complexes tend to be identical and are usually generalized, although they may be asymmetrical. They are often accompanied by myoclonic jerks. The EEG changes in this and other diffuse encephalopathies may well indicate the most likely cause of the cerebral degeneration (Gloor, Kalabay and Giard, 1968). When unusual attacks occur, and there are doubts if these are epileptic or not, a useful diagnostic aid is the cassette EEG monitor, which also includes an ECG channel. This allows the EEG to be recorded on magnetic tape for 24 hours or more, whatever the child is doing by day or by night. If any episode occurs it can then be checked if this is accompanied by any EEG or ECG changes (Duchowney and Bonis, 1985).

Table 9.1   Medical Treatment of Epilepsy (excluding newer drugs still on trial but mentioned in the text)

Types of epilepsy	Drugs to be used	Personal preference
Grand mal and focal (partial) seizures, including temporal lobe epilepsy	Carbamazepine	+ + + +
	Phenytoin	+ + +
	Sodium valproate	+ + +
	Primidone	+ +
	Phenobarbitone	+
		(Babies: + + +)
	Medium-chain triglyceride (MCT) diet	+
	Chlormethiazole	+
	Clonazepam	+
Absences (petit mal and other unclassified minor fits)	Sodium valproate	+ + + +
	Ethosuximide	+ + +
	Clonazepam	+ +
	Nitrazepam	+ +
	Acetazolamide	+ +
	Medium-chain triglyceride diet	+ +
	Troxidone	+
	Diazepam	+
	Chlormethiazole	+
Myoclonus	Nitrazepam	+ + + +
	Clonazepam	+ + +
	Sodium valproate	+ +
	Medium-chain triglyceride diet	+ +
	Primidone	+ +
	Acetazolamide	+
	Chlormethiazole	+
	Diazepam	+
	5 HTP + Carbidopa	+
	Propanolol	+
Infantile spasms	ACTH-if child normal before onset	+ + + +
	Nitrazepam	+ + + +
	Clonazepam—if marked neurological abnormalities present before onset	+ + + +
Febrile convulsions	Phenobarbitone	+ + + +
	Sodium valproate	+ + +
Major status	Intravenous diazepam (iv)	+ + + +
	Rectal diazepam	+ + +
	Paraldehyde (im)	+ +
	Chlormethiazole (iv)	+ +
	Clonazepam (iv)	+
	Phenytoin (iv)	+
	Barbiturates (iv)—if above fail	+ + +
Minor status	Diazepam (iv)	+ + + +
	Clonazepam (iv)	+ + + +
	ACTH	+ + +
Myoclonic status	ACTH	+ + + +
	Diazepam (iv)	+ + +
	Clonazepam (iv)	+ +

Drug treatment of epilepsy

The first step must be to try to identify the cause of the epileptic seizures. In many cases some specific form of treatment will be indicated, from the giving of glucose in hypoglycaemia to the removal of a cerebral tumour. This is of particular importance in the neonatal period. If investigations do not indicate a remedial cause, anti-epileptic drug therapy must be considered, although there are many problems related to the actions of these drugs, and their interactions; and much still to be learned about these (Eadie and Tyrer, 1980). Such treatment need not be started if only one or two seizures have occurred at intervals of 6–12 months, although there will be exceptions to this depending on various factors such as the severity of the fits, family history of epilepsy, the presence of neurological abnormalities, EEG findings, causal factors such as head injury, and if it believed that kindling occurs in humans and one fit makes a patient more liable to the next. The object of treatment will be to render the patient less liable to epileptic seizures or, if possible, free of them.

There are two main classes of drugs: those which help to control major and focal seizures and those which help to alleviate absences and myoclonus (Table 9.1). It may be important to check the serum levels of the drugs in certain circumstances, and the concept of a therapeutic range is useful, if not too rigidly applied. If the level is low and the fits are continuing, the drug may not have been taken as prescribed, or may be given in an inadequate dose, or may not be absorbed, or may be too rapidly metabolized. If the level is high, the drug may be having toxic effects, even if these are not obvious, perhaps increasing the liability to fits rather than vice versa. It has been shown that maintaining a drug within the therapeutic range will often ensure success with the use of one drug, and avoid polypharmacy (Reynolds, Chadwick and Galbraith, 1976). Calculating the dose of a drug according to the child's weight is the method most often used (Table 9.2). However, young children tend to metabolize anti-epileptic drugs more rapidly than adults do, and may require higher dosage in relation to body weight.

Treatment of grand mal and focal seizures

The three drugs most frequently used to control grand mal and focal seizures are carbamazepine, barbiturates and phenytoin sodium.

Carbamazepine is considered the drug of choice in the treatment of grand mal and partial epilepsies. Its effectiveness has been proven and it has relatively fewer side-

Table 9.2 Dose by Weight

Drug	Dose (mg/kg body weight)
Carbamazepine	10–20
Clonazepam	0.1–0.3
Ethosuximide	25
Nitrazepam	0.25–0.75
Phenobarbitone	5
Phenytoin	5
Primidone	20–30
Sodium valproate	20–40.

(Paraldehyde 0.2 ml/kg body weight)

effects than the other drugs. Sometimes the combination of carbamazepine and acetazolamide can be particularly useful (Forsythe, Owens and Toothill, 1981).

Phenobarbitone may be the drug of choice with which to start treatment in the very young, and occasionally in the older person, but is probably best avoided in the child of about 18 months to 10–12 years of age until alternatives have been tried. This is due to the tendency for barbiturates to cause overactive behaviour and irritability which will aggravate the difficulties of managing a child who is already hyperkinetic. Also, drowsiness may act as an activator of epilepsy. Although it is difficult to prove with absolute certainty, it seems reasonable to assume that primidone has anti-epileptic activity in addition to the effects of the phenobarbitone, which is one of its main metabolites. Other barbiturates, such as methylphenobarbitone and phenylmethyl-barbituric acid have no particular advantages and do not seem to be as active as phenobarbitone.

There is no doubt about the efficiency of the hydantoins, but, perhaps related to this, side effects are common. Phenytoin sodium can result in minor, if troublesome, toxic symptoms, such as hypertrophy of the gums, and hypertrichosis; or more severe ones, particularly ataxia and other kinds of encephalopathy. Ethotoin is said not to cause gum swelling, but it is a weak anticonvulsant. Methoin is a powerful drug, but because of its severe toxic effects, including blood dyscrasias and disseminated lupus erythematosus, its use should be postponed until safer drugs have been tried. Phenytoin sodium does have a long half-life, but is metabolized faster in children than adults and will often have to be given twice daily to children (Forsythe et al., 1979).

Sodium valproate is a useful addition to the anti-epileptic drugs. It may act by increasing the level of gamma-aminobutyric acid in the brain by inhibiting the enzyme responsible for its breakdown. As gamma aminobutyric acid (GABA) is a known inhibitor at certain synapses, this seems a logical approach. Doubt is now being cast on this theory and sodium valproate may effect membrane stability. It has been shown to be particularly useful in the treatment of minor and major attacks of centrencephalic type (Volzke and Doose, 1973; Jeavons and Clark, 1974). A fatal hepatotoxicity can occur from sodium valproate, but has become less frequent since it has been used on its own, and largely confined to children over the age of 2 years (O'Donohoe, 1991).

Newer drugs are now being assessed, of which vigabactrin is an example. This acts by binding to GABA amino-transferase and inhibiting the breakdown of GABA, and so increasing the concentrations at the synapse of this inhibitory transmitter. Patients with partial seizures, with or without secondary generalization, showed the best response, and it can be used in the treatment of the Lennox-Gastaut syndrome. It is given in an average dose of 3 g a day for an adult in two doses. Excitement and agitation are prominent side-effects in children (Reynolds, 1990). Another new drug is lamotrigine, which inhibits the release of excitatory amino acids at the synapse, such as glutamate. The exact role of these newer drugs in the treatment of children with epilepsy has still to be established.

It is rarely necessary to use more than two drugs, but, if it is, a careful watch must be kept for evidence of toxicity. (Reynolds, Chadwick and Galbraith, 1976; Shorven and Reynolds, 1977), and also for the effects of one drug on the metabolism of another.

Treatment of absences and myoclonus

In the treatment of absences (petit mal) the drugs of choice are sodium valproate and ethosuximide, which are frequently successful in stopping the minor seizures (Jeavons, Clark and Maheshward, 1977). Why they are not effective among some children, who are apparently indistinguishable on clinical and EEG grounds, has yet to be explained. When this does occur there may be a possibility of secondary synchrony, the fits being in fact of focal cortical origin with spread of the discharge to the subcortical areas. If the child has both major and minor seizures these drugs may have to be combined with others, such as carbamazepine or phenytoin sodium. Alternatives in treating absences may occasionally have to be considered. Troxidone has a reputation for severe toxic symptoms, especially blood dyscrasias and nephrosis. These have to be taken into account when prescribing this drug, but they do not preclude its use in certain cases. Other drugs which can be tried are clonazepam, nitrazepam, diazepam, chlormethiazole and acetazolamide, although they may only occasionally be effective. Sometimes it can be helpful to combined them with sodium valproate or ethosuximide.

Myoclonus is difficult to treat successfully, but the drugs most likely to be helpful are clonazepam, which raises the brain serotonin level, nitrazepam, sodium valproate, primidone and lamotrigine. Various forms of the ketogenic diet can be effective in the treatment of both petit mal and myoclonus. If such treatment fails in the case of myoclonus the reason may well be that the aetiology can be different from other types of epilepsy. Treatment with 5-hydroxytryptophan (20–100 mg a day), combined with carbidopa, a peripheral decarboxylase inhibitor (15 mg a day), has been used with effect in the treatment of post-anoxic action myoclonus in a boy of 4 years of age (Chadwick, Hallet and Harris, 1977; Nakano, Hayakawa and Shishikura, 1990). Propanolol, up to 120 mg a day, has also been tried in familial essential myoclonus (Ferro and Calhau, 1977), and in myoclonic encephalopathy (Fowler, 1976).

When a change of treatment is made it must be done gradually to minimize the risks of temporarily increasing the frequency and severity of the fits, one drug being reduced while the new one is increased to give the latter adequate time to reach a therapeutic level. Such changes are necessary if the treatment being given has been tried in adequate dosage and is not protecting the patient against the fits. If it proves necessary to give more than one antiepileptic drug this should not be continued if there is no satisfactory response.

Steroids in the treatment of epilepsy

There are special indications for the treatment of epilepsy with steroids. They may be of particular importance in the control of infantile spasms, minor status and myoclonic encephalopathy. It is obviously important to start reducing the dose as soon as there is evidence of a satisfactory response, and to stop it if there is no effect after a reasonable period.

Medium chain triglycerides in a ketogenic diet

Various types of ketogenic diets can be used in the treatment of epilepsy, and all of them may sometimes be helpful in the management of intractable fits. There are still arguments about which is the best form (Schwartz et al., 1989). It is certainly not that uncommon for epileptic seizures in childhood to fail to respond to drug treatment, especially in the case of minor motor fits. It is then justifiable to consider the use of a ketogenic diet, particularly if the child is under the age of 8 years and the fits are of a minor type. This does present certain management difficulties, such as the problems presented by having to avoid school lunches. Also the diet is expensive, and some children refuse to eat so much fat. The introduction of medium-chain triglycerides (MCT) has made the ketogenic diet a more practical proposition for some (Huttenlocher, Wilbornn and Signore, 1976). A normal energy intake for the child's age is given, and 50–70% of the calories are given as MCTs. MCTs can be used in cooking and can be given as an emulsion (Gordon, 1977). Extra vitamins are necessary and a watch must be kept on the haemoglobin level.

The presence of ketones in the urine is checked by the use of ketostix. These will appear as the MCT is gradually increased, and the diet has to be continued for several weeks with evidence of consistent ketosis before success or failure can be established. If successful, a sudden disappearance of the ketones in the urine is likely to result in an immediate return of the fits.

The effect of this treatment appears to be correlated with the plasma levels of acetoacetic acid and β-hydroxybutyrate, although the exact mechanism is unknown. It can help to estimate these levels, as with the levels of any anti-epileptic drug (Huttenlocher, 1976). If the fits stop with the addition of the diet it may be possible gradually to stop the drug treatment.

Treatment of status epilepticus

Treatment of status epilepticus is always a matter of urgency. The drug of choice is diazepam, except for during the neonatal period, when phenobarbitone in a dose of 5–10 mg/kg, given intravenously, is preferable (Volpe, 1973). The vehicle for the intravenous preparation of diazepam uncouples bilirubin from albumin. Diazepam given intramuscularly is unsatisfactory, because of the variable rate of absorption but, as discussed in the section on febrile convulsions, the intravenous preparation given rectally from specially prepared ampoules is a useful method of treatment, particularly in an emergency situation outside of hospital. If it is injected as a bolus the dose will be 0.1–0.4 mg/kg body weight. Although it is a respiratory depressant it is rare to encounter complications of this kind unless an excessive dosage is given too quickly. Nevertheless, facilities for supporting respiration should be available when it is used. As the effect of diazepam in bringing the status epilepticus to an end is likely to be either immediate or not at all, the best method of administration is by intravenous drip, 100 mg in 500 ml saline for the older child, and 50 mg in 500 ml saline for the younger one, the solution to be used within 6 hours. Another advantage of this method is that the rate of the drip can be varied in relation to the frequency of the fits. Clonazepam can also be given intravenously for the treatment of status epilepticus. For infants and children, the dose is 0.5 mg mixed with half an ampoule of the diluent by slow injection; this dose can be repeated but, if the fits continue, it is probably better to give an intravenous infusion of saline or dextrose, with up to 3 mg of clonazepam, in 250 ml used within 12 hours. Both intravenous diazepam and clonazepam are useful in the treatment of minor status epilepticus. Chlormethiazole given intravenously at rates up to 0.7 g per hour can be an effective alternative (Harvey, Higenbottom and Loh, 1975).

Paraldehyde can be used by intramuscular injection in a dose of 0.15 ml/kg body weight up to 6 ml or about 1 ml for each of the first 6 years of life (a dose of over 2 ml being given in two sites), but it has the obvious disadvantage of causing pain, an unpleasant smell, and the risk of producing sterile abscesses. Its merit is its relative safety, although it cannot be given in ever increasing quantities with impunity. It may be an advantage to combine the paraldehyde with hyaluronidase, 1 ml of sterile water being added to the phial and 0.1 ml of this solution being aspirated into the syringe syringe containing the paraldehyde. The paraldehyde can also be given rectally in a 10% solution. Phenytoin sodium by intravenous injection is often helpful and does not depress respiration. The rate of injection should not exceed 50 mg per minute. The dose for an adult in status epilepticus is 150–250 mg, and, if the fits do not stop, about half the original dose can be given after 30 minutes. As the drug is an anti-arrhythmic agent, cardiac resuscitation equipment should be at hand. Children appear to tolerate a relatively high dosage, 5 mg/kg body weight initially, reducing to 3 mg/kg body weight if a repeat injection is necessary.

Lignocaine has also been used by intravenous infusion in a dose of around 4 mg/kg body weight an hour, the dose being reduced after 24 hours. It may have a depressant effect on respiration, but not on the level of consciousness (Bohm, 1959). Unless the help of an anaesthetist is available, barbiturates given parenterally are probably best avoided because of their respiratory depressant action. Thiopentone is undoubtedly useful in the treatment of status epilepticus when other drugs have failed. After giving an initial dose of 25–100 mg intravenously, an intravenous drip of Ringer-lactate solution is started containing 1 g in 550 ml, given at a rate of 1 ml per minute, and when the patient has been free of fits for 30 minutes, reduced by half and continued for 24–48 hours (Brown and Horton, 1967). Thiopentone can be given to a young child in a single dose of 150 mg in 6 ml intravenously, or in double that dose as in enema. Monitoring serum levels of thiopentone is helpful.

Whatever treatment is chosen it seems pointless to continue it for too long if there is no response, but better to try another drug. Occasionally, if seizures continue in spite of intensive treatment it may be justifiable to place the patient on artificial ventilation and, after curarization, stop all drugs. In view of the evidence suggesting the likelihood of brain damage occurring after convulsions lasting more than 30 minutes perhaps this should be considered sooner rather than later (Simpson, Habel and George, 1977). If the seizures continue for any length of time there is evidence that raised intracranial pressure may complicate the patient's condition. If a craniotomy is carried out on a patient in status epilepticus the surgeon may comment on the pulseless dura until it is incised; and the impaired circulation is bound to aggravate the anoxia and cerebral oedema. The monitoring of intracranial pressure can contribute to a reduction in mortality and morbidity (Minns, 1977). Unexpectedly high levels can be found by this method, which may not have been accompanied by clinical changes. The treatment of the raised intracranial pressure is by simple methods, such as propping the patient up in bed; and, when due to cerebral oedema, by dexamethazone 1–4 mg i.m. 6-hourly or mannitol 5 ml/kg body weight as a 20% solution i.v. every 20–30 minutes as necessary. A trial of diuretics, such as frusemide and acetazolamide is also sometimes justifiable. Although cerebral oedema can undoubtedly play an adverse role in status epilepticus in the early stages the rise of intracranial pressure may well be in part the result of increased cerebral blood flow needed for the intense activity of the neurons if they are not to suffer damage, and the treatment with diazepam can interfere with this (Minns and Brown, 1978).

The success of treatment, as with any unconscious patient, will depend on scrupulous attention to such factors as maintaining adequate airway, the placing of the patient in the lateral semi-prone position, and fluid and electrolyte balance. Possible metabolic disturbances, which may be secondary to status epilepticus, such as hypoglycaemia and hypocalcaemia must be investigated and treated if necessary. Pyrexia must be reduced if this is a factor. Also, the cause of the status epilepticus must be investigated as soon as possible.

Toxic effects of drug treatment

Although space does not permit a detailed survey of drug dosage and toxic effects, it must be noted that too little attention has been paid to these in the past and that no anti-epileptic drug can be given without paying a price (Reynolds, 1975). Epilepsy should be treated as energetically as possible, but a constant watch must be kept for side-effects, or the patient's condition may be worsened unwittingly. Such a danger occurs with phenytoin therapy. An early sign of intoxication can be an increase in frequency of seizure (Troupin and Ogemann, 1975), and, unless the possibility of drug-induced encephalopathy is considered, the dosage may be increased rather than reduced. Patients with severe brain damage are particularly susceptible to phenytoin intoxication (Iivanaimen, Viukari and Helle, 1977). Reynolds and Shorven (1981) stress that this is very likely to occur with polytherapy, and that once this has been instituted it may become increasingly difficult to reduce the drugs because of withdrawal effects, including an exacerbation of the seizures. Also, a very small increase in the oral dose of phenytoin can cause a sharp rise in the serum level, sometimes from below the therapeutic range to a concentration which will cause toxic effects (Fig. 9.9). This is an example of non-linear kinetics, the relationship between the serum level and the oral dose being a curve which rises steeply as the oral dose increases, rather than being a straight line.

Although there is still a tendency to undertreat patients with epilepsy, enthusiasm must be tempered by realism. It is no good stopping a child's fits entirely if his or her teacher states that he or she spends most of the time in class half-asleep as a result. Toxic effects may be mild or severe, but even mild effects can be a matter of concern, especially among the very young. For example, the excess salivation and bronchial excretion caused by nitrazepam may be lethal in a small, debilitated baby, and gum hypertrophy and hirsutism due to phenytoin can be very distressing to an adolescent. The toxic effects can sometimes be of an unusual nature and cause considerable diagnostic difficulties; for example, phenytoin intoxication is sometimes manifested by choreo-athetoid movements, particularly affecting the tongue (Kooiker, 1974). Carbamazepine can be associated with water intoxication, possibly through potentiation of the action of antidiuretic hormone on the renal tubules (Ashton et al., 1977). If this occurs it is likely to cause additional fits. The EEG of anyone taking carbamazepine may deteriorate, but often without any associated clinical changes. This is possibly due to the fact that carbamazepine is structurally related to the tricyclic antidepressants, certain of which have a convulsant action (Jeavons, 1973). Even drugs such as sodium valproate, which are said to be relatively free of side-effects, may have unexpected dangers and, as has been mentioned, possibly cause hepatitis, and even more rarely pancreatitis (Willmore et al., 1978); and spina bifida in the offspring of mothers taking the drug (Lindhout and Meinardi, 1984). Quite apart from the more obvious side-effects of these drugs, there may be unknown long-term effects, although there is no doubt that the control of treatment by the estimation of the serum levels of the drugs used has helped to reduce intoxication. The role of folic-acid deficiency among patients taking barbiturates and hydantoins has still to be defined, and even the statement that giving large doses of folic acid may make the fits worse has yet to be proved (Reynolds, 1967). However, the possible effects of long-term folic acid deficiency, even if it is not enough to cause anaemia, cannot be ignored, especially in the growing child (Gordon, 1968). Perhaps some of the deterioration seen among patients with epilepsy is iatrogenic. Blood counts and folic acid and vitamin B12 levels should be checked from time to time when children are taking barbiturates and phenytoin, and 5 mg folic acid should be given daily if indicated.

Alkaline phosphatase levels are frequently raised during treatment with phenytoin, which is probably an example of enzyme induction. Occasionally, hypocalcaemia and osteomalacia also occur among these children (Dent *et al.*, 1970). The induction of enzymes which metabolize vitamin D may be partly responsible, but there are likely to be additional factors, such as inadequate diet and lack of sunlight; and the calcium level should also be estimated at regular intervals. Overt bone disease must be treated with 2000–10 000 units of calciferol (vitamin D2) per day. A maintenance dose of 1000–3000 units per day may be needed if precipitating factors cannot be modified, but there is insufficient evidence to support prophylactic treatment of all epileptic patients on drug therapy. Cholecalciferol (vitamin D3) 37.5–125 μg per week corrects the biochemical abnormalities more dramatically (Offerman, Pinto and Kruse, 1979), but may not be so effective in reversing the osteomalacia (Christiansen *et al.*, 1975). Treatment should be monitored by serum calcium and alkaline phosphatase levels and X-rays of the bones. The appearance of babies born of mothers taking phenytoin, and other drugs, may be altered (Hanson and Smith, 1975), and various other toxic effects can occur, such as haemorrhage in the infant. These are well reviewed by Meadow (1991), who also confirms that breast-feeding by mothers on treatment for epilepsy is not contraindicated.

Surgical treatment of epilepsy

Before operative treatment for epilepsy can be considered a number of criteria have to be fulfilled. Adequate medical treatment must have failed and, in the case of focal seizures, it must have been demonstrated that they are arising from a part of the brain the removal of which will not result in unacceptable disability. With careful selection there is no doubt that some people can be relieved of their seizures and enabled to lead a normal life. Those with temporal lobe epilepsy often respond well, as the anterior part of the lobe can be removed without great difficulty. If the operation is not performed until the patient's early adult life, he or she is likely to have missed a lot of schooling and also training for suitable jobs. A plea has therefore been made for a consideration of surgical treatment between the ages of 12 and 14 years (Davidson and Falconer, 1975). If this is successful, the patient will still have several years of schooling left.

When the epileptic discharges involve the central areas of the brain causing major and minor seizures, and they do not respond to medical treatment, it has been claimed that interrupting nerve tracts within the diencephalon by stereotactic surgery may bring relief. This is based on the surmise that this part of the brain has to be intact for this type of epilepsy to occur. A number of operations have also been devised which aim to separate one side of the brain from the other and thus prevent the spread of the epileptic discharge, and chronic cerebellar stimulation can reduce intractable seizures (Cooper and Upton, 1978).

Other methods of treatment of epilepsy

There is much more to the treatment of epilepsy than the prescribing drugs or the use of surgery, and Aird (1988) has analysed some of the alternative measures which may reduce the incidence of fits. These include the avoidance of tension states, lack of sleep and drowsiness. Drowsiness may be caused by drugs, and it should be remembered that it is used as a EEG activator. Other factors to be considered are emotional disturbances, water balance, toxic states and the cultivation of regular habits.

Ensuring more effective treatment in this way may prevent the overprotection by parents which may be understandable, but if allowed to grow into an obsession is bound to be to the detriment of the child. Once such attitudes have become firmly established it may be very difficult, if not impossible, to change them. It is obviously important to discuss problems of daily living so that parents and the child can be reassured, and common-sense reasons given if restrictions are imposed. When such seizure-inducing factors were given careful consideration, more than 20% of children with refractory epilepsy were greatly benefited, and in a further 14% the seizures were controlled.

Conclusions

The subject of epilepsy cannot be left on this depressing note, as there is so much that can be done to help those with epilepsy (O'Donohoe, 1979). There is no doubt that, with well-regulated treatment, the majority of people with epilepsy can and do lead normal lives. The estimation of anti-epileptic drug levels in the serum by various methods means that treatment can be less haphazard (Eadie and Tyrer, 1980). Routine use of these methods is not indicated, but can be helpful if the response to treatment is not satisfactory or there is suspicion of toxic side-effects. As has been stated such estimations can demonstrate levels outside the supposed therapeutic range, and the effects of adding one drug to another, for example sulthiame raising the serum level of phenytoin (Aird and Woodbury, 1974). Also, they will show if the serum level, and therefore the level of the drug within the brain, is too low, and that the particular drug in use has not been given an adequate trial. There are wide variations between individuals in the serum levels achieved for any given dose of anticonvulsant, but factors influencing these levels include compliance, age and body weight, genctic factors, absorption, liver and renal disease and the metabolism of the drug (Reynolds, 1978).

When the child has been free of fits for a year or two, and especially if the EEG is normal, it is justifiable to stop the treatment gradually, although there is always a chance that the seizures may return. This is a decision that must be taken on an individual basis, and will depend on the age of the child and the other factors which led to the start of treatment in the first place. On theoretical grounds it seems reasonable to start to begin reducing treatment sooner in children than adults, for instance after a fit-free period of 2 years (Gordon, 1982; Chadwick and Reynolds, 1985). If anti-epileptic treatment can only be taken at the cost of side-effects of one kind or another, then the sooner the treatment can be stopped the better; and surely it is preferable to risk the recurrence of fits in some children, when treatment can be immediately started again, than to treat a number of children unnecessarily; although it must be emphasized that the previous treatment is not always so successful on the second occasion. The very occasional fit occurring while treatment is being stopped is not necessarily a reason for abandoning this, as it may be a withdrawal seizure.

In childhood the brain is maturing, and this may include the development of biochemical or electrophysiological mechanisms controlling the spread of the hypersynchrony that results in the epileptic seizure. In adult life the changes are more likely to be degenerative.

It must be emphasized again that, apart from giving drugs, there is much more to be done to help the child. If he or she is under considerable stress, either at home or at school, the incidence of fits may increase regardless of whatever medical treatment is given. Problems at home are almost inevitable, and time must be given to discuss these with the parents. Although generalizations are to be avoided, common sense dictates that children with epilepsy must not be allowed to ride bicycles on busy roads, or to swim unless someone is watching them, although such people are more likely to drown in their bath than in the swimming pool. Also certain aspects of physical education, such as climbing ropes may present unacceptable risks. It is easy to forget to give simple practical advice, such as the fitting of fire-guards and of a gate at the top of a staircase and the removal of the bathroom lock, but these precautions can be of vital importance. However, unless restrictions are kept to a minimum, and the parents encouraged to accept certain risks, the child may well become resentful, particularly during adolescence.

Among any group of children with epilepsy there is likely to be a larger proportion than normal with below-average IQ or with specific learning difficulties. Those with focal epilepsy will tend to have defects of auditory learning and memory if the fits are arising in the left cerebral hemisphere, and of perceptual-motor functions if they occupy the right. In the case of generalized epilepsy involving the diencephalon, the disability will affect attention and recall (Stores, 1971). Preliminary studies have shown that, in the case of reading retardation, inattentiveness of various types, dependency, and certain behaviour disorders such as anxiety, social isolation and overactivity, the children at most risk are boys with left temporal lobe spike discharges (Stores, 1978). Children with epilepsy will also have to cope with the effects of their treatment and the attitudes of their teachers and peers. Under-achievement at school is common, as not enough is expected of children with epilepsy. Teachers may be frightened of putting them under any pressure in case a seizure occurs. Children and their parents are right to be worried about the diagnosis. In a follow-up of childhood seizures it has been shown that 10.1% had died, 11.2% were confined to institutions and 6.6% were invalids at home (Harrison and Taylor, 1976). There is obviously still much to be done from the medical point of view to improve the situation

The social implications of epilepsy must be given more attention, and though long-standing prejudices are gradually being broken down, the effects of labelling anyone as 'epileptic' are still far-reaching. Teachers can play a key role by their attitude to the child with epilepsy, but they can only do this successfully if they have an adequate knowledge of the subject. More knowledge about the cause of fits would go a long way towards solving these dilemmas, leading to more effective treatment and greater understanding.

References

Agurell, S., Berlin, A., Ferngren, H. and Hellstrom, B. (1975) Plasma levels of diazepam after parenteral and rectal administration in children. *Epilepsia*, **16**, 277

Aicardi, J. (1973) The problem of the Lennox syndrome. *Developmental Medicine and Child Neurology*, **15**, 77

Aicardi, J. (1979) Benign epilepsy of childhood with Rolandic spikes (BECRS). *Brain and Development*, **i**, 71

Aicardi, J. (1986) *Epilepsy in Childhood*, Raven Press, New York

Aicardi, J. and Chevrie, J.J. (1982) Atypical benign partial epilepsy of childhood. *Developmental Medicine and Child Neurology*, **24**, 281

Aird, R.B. (1988) The importance of seizure-inducing factors in youth. *Brain and Development*, **10**, 73

Aird, R.B. and Woodbury, D.M. (1974) *The Management of Epilepsy*, Charles C. Thomas, Springfield, Illinois

Aird, R.B., Masland, R.L. and Woodbury, D.M. (1984) *The Epilepsies. A Critical Review*, Raven Press, New York

Ashton, M.G., Ball, S. G., Thomas, T.H. and Lee, M.R. (1977) Water intoxication associated with carbamazepine treatment. *British Medical Journal*, **i**, 1134

Basser, L.S. (1964) Benign paroxysmal vertigo of childhood. A variety of vestibular neuronitis. *Brain*, **87**, 141

Baum, D., Cooper, L. and Davies, P.A. (1968) Hypocalcaemic fits in neonates. *Lancet*, **i**, 598

Baumer, J.H., David, T.J., Valentine, S.J. *et al.* (1981) Many parents think their child is dying when having a first febrile convulsion. *Developmental Medicine and Child Neurology*, **23**, 462

Bohm, E. (1959) Effect of intravenous lignocaine on epileptic seizures. *Nordisk Medicin*, **61**, 885

Booker, H.E., Forster, F.M. and Klove, H. (1965) Extinction factors in startle (acousticomotor) seizures. *Neurology*, **15**, 1095

Bower, B. (1978) The treatment of epilepsy in children. *British Journal of Hospital Medicine*, **19**, 8

Bradshaw, J.P.P. (1954) A study of myoclonus. *Brain*, **77**, 138

Brandt, S., Carlson, N., Glenting, P. and Helweg-Larsen, L. (1974) Encephalopathia myoclonica infantalis (Kinsbourne) and neuroblastoma in children. A report of three cases. *Developmental Medicine and Child Neurology*, **16**, 286

Brett, E.M. (1966) Minor epileptic status. *Journal of the Neurosciences*, **3**, 52

Broberger, O., Jungner, I. and Zetterstrom, R. (1959) Studies in spontaneous hypoglycaemia in childhood. *Journal of Pediatrics*, **55**, 713

Brown, A.S. and Horton, J.M. (1967) Status epilepticus treated by intravenous infusions of thiopentone sodium. *British Medical Journal*, **1**, 27

Brown, J.K. (1973) Convulsions in the newborn period. *Developmental Medicine and Child Neurology*, **15**, 823

Brown, J.K., Cockburn, F. and Forfar, J.O. (1972) Clinical and chemical correlates in convulsions of the newborn. *Lancet*, **i**, 135

Chadwick, D., Hallet, M., Harris, R. *et al.* (1977) Clinical, biochemical and physiological features distinguishing myoclonus responsive to 5-hydroxytryptophan, tryptophan with a monoamine oxidase inhibitor, and clonezapam. *Brain*, **100**, 445

Chadwick, D. and Reynolds, E.H. (1985) When do epileptic patients need treatment? Starting and stopping medication. *British Medical Journal*, **290**, 1888

Chevrie, J.J. and Aicardi, J. (1975) Duration and lateralisation of febrile convulsions. Etiological factors. *Epilepsia*, **16**, 781

Christiansen, C., Rodbro, P., Munck, O. and Munck, O. (1975) Actions of vitamins D2 and D3 and 25-OHD in anticonvulsant osteomalacia. *British Medical Journal*, **ii**, 363

Cooper, I.S. and Upton, A.R.M. (1978) Use of chronic cerebellar stimulation for disorders of disinhibition. *Lancet*, **i**, 595

Creery, R.D.G. (1966) Hypoglycaemia in the newborn: diagnosis, treatment and prognosis. *Developmental Medicine and Child Neurology*, **8**, 746

Currie, S., Heathfield, K.W.G., Henson, R.A. and Scott, D.F. (1971) Clinical course and prognosis of temporal lobe epilepsy. *Brain*, **94**, 173

Davidson, S. and Falconer, M.A. (1975) Outcome of surgery in 40 children with temporal lobe epilepsy. *Lancet*, **i**, 1260

Delgado-Escueta, A.V. and Enrile-Bacsal, F. (1984) Juvenile myoclonic epilepsy of Janz. *Neurology*, **34**, 285

Dent, C.E., Richens, A., Rowe, D.J.F. and Stamp, T.C.B. (1970) Osteomalacia with long-term anti-convulsant therapy in epilepsy. *British Medical Journal*, **iv**, 69

Doose, H. and Völzke, E. (1979) Petit mal status in early childhood and dementia. *Neuropädiatrie*, **10**, 10

Duchowny, M.S. and Bonis, I. (1985) Long term cassette EEG monitoring of childhood seizures. *Pediatric Neurology*, **1**, 38

Eadie, M.J. and Tyrer, J.H. (1980) *Anticonvulsant Therapy: Pharmacological Basis and Practice*, Churchill Livingstone, Edinburgh

Earle, K.M., Baldwin, M. and Penfield, W. (1953) Incisural sclerosis and temporal lobe seizures produced by hippocampal herniation at birth. *Archives of Neurology and Psychiatry*, **69**, 27

Faero, O., Kastrup, K.W., Lykkegaard Nielsen, E. *et al.* (1972) Successful prophylaxis of febrile convulsions with phenobarbitol. *Epilepsia*, **13**, 279

Falconer, M.A. (1971) Genetic and related aetiological factors in temporal lobe epilepsy. *Epilepsia*, **12**, 13

Fariello, R.G., Doro, J.M. and Forster, F.M. (1979) Generalised cortical electrodecremental event. Clinical and neurophysiological observations in patients with dystonic seizures. *Archives of Neurology*, **36**, 285

Ferro, J.M. and Calhau, E.S. (1977) Treatment of essential myoclonus with propanolol. *Lancet*, **ii**, 143

Forster, F.M., Ptacek, L.J., Peterson, W.G. *et al.* (1964) Stroboscopic-induced seizure discharges: modification by extinction techniques. *Archives of Neurology*, **11**, 603

Forsythe, W.I., Pendergrast, M.P., Toothill, C. and Broughton, P.M.G. (1979) Phenytoin serum levels in children with epilepsy: a micro immuno-assay technique. *Developmental Medicine and Child Neurology*, **21**, 448

Forsythe, W.I., Owens, J.R. and Toothill, C. (1981) Effectiveness of acetazolamide in the treatment carbamazepine-resistant epilepsy in children. *Developmental Medicine and Child Neurology*, **23**, 761

Fowler, G.W. (1976) Propanolol treatment of infantile polymyoclonia. *Neuropädiatrie*, **7**, 443

Frantzen, E., Lennox-Buchthal, M. and Nygard, A. (1968) Longitudinal EEG and clinical study of children with febrile convulsions. *Electroencephalography and Clinical Neurophysiology*, **24**, 197

Friedman, M., Hatcher, G. and Watson, L. (1967) Primary hypomagnesaemia with secondary hypocalcaemia in an infant. *Lancet*, **i**, 703

Gastaut, H. and Fischer-Williams, K. (1967) Electroencephalographic study of syncope. *Lancet*, **ii**, 1018

Gillespie, J.B. (1954) The hyperventilation syndrome in childhood. *Archives of Pediatrics*, **71**, 197

Gloor, P., Kalabay, O. and Giard, N. (1968) The electroencephalogram in diffuse encephalopathies: electroencephalographic correlates of grey and white matter lesions. *Brain*, **91**, 779

Goldie, L. and Green, J.M. (1961) Observations on episodes of bewilderment seen during a study of petit mal. *Epilepsia*, **2**, 306

Gordon, N. (1965) The natural history of petit mal epilepsy. *Developmental Medicine and Child Neurology*, **7**, 537

Gordon, N. (1968) Folic acid deficiency from anticonvulsant therapy. *Developmental Medicine and Child Neurology*, **10**, 497

Gordon, N. (1970) Reactions to triple immunisation. *Neuropädiatrie*, **2**, 119

Gordon, N. (1977) Medium chain triglycerides in a ketogenic diet. *Developmental Medicine and Child Neurology*, **19**, 535

Gordon, N. (1982) Duration of treatment for childhood epilepsy. *Developmental Medicine and Child Neurology*, **24**, 84

Gordon, N. and Aird, R.B. (1991) Idiopathic childhood absences, a system disorder: its diagnosis and differentiation. *Developmental Medicine and Child Neurology*, **33**, 744

Hanson, J.W. and Smith, D.W. (1975) The fetal hydantoin syndrome. *Journal of Pediatrics*, **87**, 287

Harding, G.F.A., Herrick, C.E. and Jeavons, P.M. (1978) A controlled study of the effect of sodium valproate on photosensitive epilepsy and its prognosis. *Epilepsia*, **19**, 555

Harrison, R.M. and Taylor, D.C. (1976) Childhood seizures: a 25 year follow-up. *Lancet*, **ii**, 948

Harvey, P.K.P., Higenbottom, T.W. and Loh, L. (1975) Chlormethiazole in treatment of status. *British Medical Journal*, **ii**, 603

Heckmatt, J.Z., Houston, A.B., Clow, D.J. (1976) Failure of phenobarbitone to prevent febrile convulsions. *British Medical Journal*, **i**, 559

Heely, A., Pugh, R.J.P., Clayton, B.E. *et al.* (1978) Pyridoxal metabolism in vitamin B6-responsive convulsions of early infancy. *Archives of Disease in Childhood*, **53**, 794

Hudgins, R.I. and Corbin, K B. (1966) An uncommon seizure disorder: familial paroxysmal choreoathetosis. *Brain*, **89**, 109

Hutt, S.J. and Lee, D. (1968) Some determinants of the amnesic phenomenon in a light-sensitive epileptic child. *Journal of Medical Science*, **6**, 155

Huttenlocher, P.R. (1976) Ketonemia and seizures: metabolic and anticonvulsant effects of two ketogenic diets in childhood epilepsy. *Paediatric Research*, **10**, 536

Huttenlocher, P.R., Wilbornn, A.J. and Signore, J.M. (1976) Medium-chain trigycerides as therapy for intractable childhood epilepsy. *Neurology*, **21**, 1097

Iivanaimen, M., Viukari, M. and Helle, E.P. (1977) Cerebellar atrophy in phenytoin-treated mentally retarded epileptics. *Epilepsia*, **18**, 375

Jaeken, J., Casaer, P., Haegele, K.D. and Schechter, P.J. (1990) Review: normal and abnormal central nervous system GABA metabolism in childhood. *Journal of Inherited Metabolic Disease*, **13**, 793

Jeavons, P.M., Harper, J.R. and Bower, B.D. (1970) Long-term prognosis in infantile spasms: a follow-up report on 112 cases. *Developmental Medicine and Child Neurology*, **12**, 413

Jeavons, P.M. and Bower, B.D (1964) *Infantile Spasms*. Clinics in Developmental Medicine, No.15. SIMP, William Heinemann, London

Jeavons, P.M. (1973) Carbamazepine and the EEG. In *Tegratol in Epilepsy* (ed. C.A.S. Wink), Nicholls, Manchester

Jeavons, P.M. and Clark, J.E (1974) Sodium valproate in treatment of epilepsy. *British Medical Journal*, **ii**, 584

Jeavons, P.M. and Harding, J.F.A. (1975) *Photosensitive Epilepsy*. Clinics in Developmental Medicine, No. 56. SIMP, William Heinemann, London

Jeavons, P.M., Clark, J.E. and Maheshward, M.C. (1977) Treatment of generalized epilepsies of childhood and adolescence with sodium valproate. *Developmental Medicine and Child Neurology*, **19**, 9

Keen, J.H. (1969) Significance of hypocalcaemia in neonatal convulsions. *Archives of Disease in Childhood*, **44**, 356

Keen, J.H. and Lee, D. (1973) Sequelae of neonatal convulsions. *Archives of Disease in Childhood*, **48**, 542

Kinsbourne, M. (1962) Myoclonic encephalopathy of infants. *Journal of Neurology, Neurosurgery and Psychiatry*, **25**, 271

Kooiker, J.C. (1974) Movement disorders as a manifestation of diphenylhydantoin intoxication. *Neurology*, **24**, 68

Lance, J.W. (1977) Familial paroxysmal dystonic choreoathetosis and its differentiation from related syndromes. *Annals of Neurology*, **2**, 285

Lennox-Buchthal, M.A. (1973) Febrile convulsions. A reappraisal. *Electroencephalography and Clinical Neurophysiology*, Suppl. 32,

Lerman, P. and Kivity, S. (1975) Benign focal epilepsy of childhood. *Archives of Neurology*, **32**, 261

Lewis, H.M., Parry, J.V., Davies, H.A. *et al.* (1979) Role of viruses in febrile convulsions. *Archives of Disease in Childhood*, **54**, 869

Lindhout, D. and Meinardi, H. (1984) Spina bifida and in-utero exposure to valproate. *Lancet*, **ii**, 396

Meadow, R. (1982) Munchausen's syndrome by proxy. *Archives of Disease in Childhood*, **57**, 92

Meadow, R. (1984) Fictitious epilepsy. *Lancet*, **ii**, 25

Meadow, R. (1991) Anticonvulsants in pregnancy. *Archives of Disease in Childhood*, **66**, 62

McKinlay, I. and Newton, R. (1989) Intention to treat febrile convulsions with rectal diazepam, valproate or phenobarbitone. *Developmental Medicine and Child Neurology*, **31**, 617

Meeuwisse, G., Gamstorp, I. and Tryding, N. (1968) Effect of phenytoin on the tryptophan load test. *Acta Paediatrica Scandinavica*, **57**, 115

Melchior, J.C. (1977) Infantile spasms and early immunisation against whooping cough. *Archives of Disease in Childhood*, **52**, 134

Melchior, J.C., Buchthal, F. and Lennox-Buchthal, M. (1971) The ineffectiveness of diphenylhydantoin in preventing febrile convulsions in the age of greatest risk, under three years. *Epilepsia*, **12**, 55

Meldrum, B. (1978) Physiological changes during prolonged seizures, and epileptic brain damage. *Neuropädiatrie*, **9**, 203

Miller, D.L., Ross, E.M., Alderslade, R. *et al.* (1981) Pertussis immunisation and serious acute neurological illness in children. *British Medical Journal*, **i**, 1595

Millichap, J.G., Aledort, L.M. and Madsen, J.A. (1960) A critical evaluation of therapy of febrile seizures. *Journal of Pediatrics*, **56**, 364

Minns, R.A. (1977) Clinical application of ventricular pressure monitoring in children. *Zeitschrift für Kinder Chirurgie*, **22**, 430

Minns, R.A. and Brown, J.K. (1978) Intracranial pressure changes associated with childhood seizures. *Developmental Medicine and Child Neurology*, **20**, 561

Morikawa, T., Osawa, T., Ishihara, T. and Seino, M. (1979) A reappraisal of benign epilepsy of children with centro-temporal EEG foci. *Brain and Development*, **1**, 257

Nakano, K., Hayakawa, T., Shishikura, K. *et al.* (1990) Improvement of action myoclonus by an administration of 5-hydroxytryptophan and carbidopa in a child with muscular subsarcolemmal hyperactivity. *Brain and Development*, **12**, 516

O'Donohoe, N.V. (1979) *Epilepsies in Childhood*, Butterworth, London

O'Donohoe, N.V. (1991) Use of antiepileptic drugs in childhood epilepsy. *Archives of Disease in Childhood*, **66**, 1173–9

Offerman, G., Pinto, V. and Kruse, R. (1979) Antiepileptic drugs and vitamin D supplementation. *Epilepsia*, **20**, 3

Otahara, S. (1984) Seizure disorders in infancy and childhood. *Brain and Development*, **6**, 509

Ounsted, C., Lindsay, J. and Norman, R. (1966) *Biological Factors in Temporal Lobe epilepsy*, Clinics in Developmental Medicine, No.22. SIMP, William Heinemann, London

Pryor, D.S., Don, D. and Marcourt, D.C. (1981) Fifth day fits: a syndrome of neonatal convulsions. *Archives of Disease of Childhood*, **56**, 753

Radford, D.J., Izukawa, T. and Rowe, R.D. (1977) Evaluation of children with ventricular arrhythmias. *Archives of Disease in Childhood*, **52**, 345

Reynolds, E.H. (1967) Effects of folic acid on the mental state and fit-frequency of drug-treated epileptic patients. *Lancet*, **i**, 1086

Reynolds, E.H. (1975) Chronic antiepileptic toxicity: a review. *Epilepsia*, **16**, 319

Reynolds, E.H. (1978) Drug treatment of epilepsy. *Lancet*, **ii**, 721

Reynolds, E.H. (1990) Vigabactrin. Rational treatment for chronic epilepsy. *British Medical Journal*, **300**, 277

Reynolds, E.H. and Shorven, S.D. (1981) Monotherapy or polytherapy for epilepsy. *Epilepsia*, **22**, 1

Reynolds, E.H., Chadwick, D. and Galbraith, A.W. (1976) One drug (phenytoin) in the treatment of epilepsy. *Lancet*, **i**, 923

Roberts, S.A., Cohen, M.D. and Forfar, J.O. (1973) Antenatal factors associated with neonatal hypocalcaemic convulsions. *Lancet*, **ii**, 809

Roger, J., Dravet, C., Bureau, M. *et al.* (1985) *Epileptic Syndromes in Infancy, Childhood and Adolescence*, John Libby, London and Paris

Rose, A.L. and Lombroso, C.T. (1970) Neonatal seizure states; a study of clinical pathological, and electroencephalographic features in 137 full-term babies with a long-term follow-up. *Pediatrics*, **45**, 404

Rowan, A.J. and Scott, D.F. (1970) Major status epilepticus. *Acta Neurologica Scandinavica*, **46**, 573

Schwartz, R.H., Eaton, J., Bower, D.B. and Aynsley-Green, A. (1989) Ketogenic diets in the treatment of epilepsy: short-term clinical effects. *Developmental Medicine and Child Neurology*, **31**, 145

Scott, O., Macartney, F.J. and Deverall, P.B. (1976) Sick sinus syndrome in children. *Archives of Disease in Childhood*, **51**, 100

Shorven, S.D. and, Reynolds, E.H. (1977) Unnecessary polypharmacy for epilepsy. *British Medical Journal*, **ii**, 1655

Simpson, H., Habel, A.H. and George, E.L. (1977) Cerebrospinal fluid acid-base status and lactate and pyruvate concentrations after convulsions of varied duration and aetiology in children. *Archives of Disease in Childhood*, **52**, 844

Stefansson, S.B., Darby, C.E., Wilkins, A.J. *et al.* (1977) Television epilepsy and pattern sensitivity. *British Medical Journal*, **ii**, 88

Stephenson, J.P.B. (1978a) Reflex seizures (white breath-holding): anoxic non-epileptic vagal attacks. *Archives of Disease in Childhood*, **53**, 193

Stephenson, J.B.P. (1978b) Two types of febrile seizure: anoxic (syncopal) and epileptic mechanisms differentiated by oculocardiac reflex. *British Medical Journal*, **ii**, 726

Stephenson, J.P.B. (1979) Atropine methonitrate in management of non-fatal reflex anoxic seizures. *Lancet*, **ii**, 955

Stephenson, J.P.B. (1980) Reflex anoic seizures and ocular compression. *Developmental Medicine and Child Neurology*, **22**, 380

Stephenson, J.P.B. and Byrne, K.E. (1983) Pyridoxine responsive epilepsy: expanded pyridoxine dependancy? *Archives of Disease in Childhood*, **58**, 1034

Stephenson, J.P.B., Graham-Pole, J., Ogg, L. and Cochran, A.J. (1976) Reactivity to neuroblastoma extracts in childhood cerebellar encephalopathy (Dancing Eyes syndrome). *Lancet*, **ii**, 975

Stores, G. (1971) Cognitive function in epilepsy. *British Journal of Hospital Medicine*, **6**, 207

Stores, G. (1978) School children with epilepsy at risk for learning and behaviour problems. *Developmental Medicine and Child Neurology*, **20**, 502

Sutcliffe, J.I. (1969) Torsion spasms and abnormal postures in children with hiatus hernia. *Progress in Peadiatric Radiology*, **2**, l00

Taylor, D.C. (1982) The components of sickness: diseases, illnesses and predicaments. In *One Child* (eds. J. Apley and C. Ounsted), Heinemann, Tadworth

Thorn, I. (1980) Prophylactic treatment of febrile convulsions phenobarbitol contra intermittent diazepam. *Developmental Medicine and Child Neurology*, **22**, 267

Troupin, A.S. and Ojemann, L.M. (1975) Paradoxical intoxication—a complication of anticonvulsant administration. *Epilepsia*, **16**, 753

Turner, T.L., Cockburn, F. and Forfar, J.O. (1977) Magnesium therapy in neonatal tetany. *Lancet*, **i**, 283

Van den Berg, B.J. (1974) Studies on convulsive disorders in young children. *Epilepsia*, **15**, 177

Verity, C.M. and Golding, J. (1991) Risk of epilepsy after febrile convulsions: a national cohort study. *British Medical Journal*, 303 1373–6

Volpe, J. (1973) Neonatal seizures. *New England Journal of Medicine*, **289**, 413

Volzke, E. and Doose, H. (1973) Dipropylacetate (Depakine, Ergenyl) in the treatment of epilepsy. *Epilepsia*, **14**, 185

Von Studnitz, W. (1970) Cystathioninuria in children with neuroblastoma with and without metastatis. *Acta Paediatrica Scandinavica*, **59**, 80

Wallace, S.J. (1974) Recurrence of febrile convulsions. *Archives of Disease in Childhood*, **49**, 763

Wallace, S.J. (1977) Spontaneous fits after convulsions with fever. *Archives of Disease in Childhood*, **52**, 192

Wallace, S.J. (1988) *The Child with Febrile Seizures*, Wright, London

Wallace, S.T. and Cull, A.M. (1979) Long-term psychological outlook, for children whose first fit occurs with fever. *Developmental Medicine and Child Neurology*, **21**, 28

Wallace, S.T. and Aldridge-Smith, J. (1980) Successful prophylaxis against febrile convulsions with valproic acid or phenobarbitone. *British Medical Journal*, **i**, 353

Williams, D. (1965) The thalamus and epilepsy. *Brain*, **88**, 539

Willmore, L.J., Wilder, B.J., Bruni, J. and Villarreal, H.J. (1978) Effect of valproic acid on hepatic function. *Neurology*, **28**, 961

10   Infections of the nervous system

The changes that have occurred in paediatrics in the past few years have been due largely to improved perinatal care, better hygiene and the advent of antibiotic therapy. This has resulted in the solving of many of the problems related to acute infections, so that more time and effort can be devoted to the long-term disabilities that affect so many children. Conversely, the availability of effective treatment for so many infections has made early and accurate diagnosis more important than it has ever been. The prognosis for mortality and morbidity is related to the speed with which appropriate treatment for infections is started. There can be no denying the importance of the subject and the enormous contribution that treatment has made to the health and welfare of children. The paediatric neurologist, however, is unlikely to be in the forefront of the battle against acute infections unless complications occur, such as subdural effusions developing during a pyrogenic meningitis; when he or she is likely to be involved in their treatment.

Meningitis

Acute meningitis

Meningitis due to bacterial infections is usually borne by the blood from septic foci in other parts of the body, but it can also gain access to the meninges through other channels; for example, from the nose via the perineural space of the olfactory nerves, or through sinuses in proximity to the spinal canal, usually the sacrum. Direct spread from sepsis in the middle-ear, the nasal sinuses, boils on the face, or infected injuries to the head are also possibilities. The suspicion that the infection is a meningitis will be confirmed by the presence of stiffness of the neck muscles, a positive Kernig's sign due to spasm of the hamstring muscles, and Burdzinski's sign, when flexion of the neck results in flexion of the hip, knee and ankle. These signs are not always present, especially if the child is comatose, and in babies. Co-existence of infections at other sites should not preclude a lumbar puncture prior to the start of antibiotic therapy when there are grounds for anxiety. Lumbar puncture should not be performed if there are signs of increased intracranial pressure with a risk of coning, evidence of coagulation defects and local infection. The organism may be identified by blood culture, by detection of its antigens, by Gram staining of the cerebrospinal fluid and by culture of the fluid (Robinson and Roberts, 1990a). As the fluid is needed as soon as possible for a culture, a CT scan when the patient's condition permits, may well resolve the situation.

Neonatal meningitis

The absence of specific signs of meningitis in newborn babies, especially if premature, is sufficiently common to justify routine examination of the cerebrospinal fluid to exclude this possibility in the presence of a suspected infection. The baby will be irritable, lethargic and hypotonic, and seizures may occur. Sucking is poor, and vomiting and diarrhoea may be present. The cry is often high-pitched, and the temperature is not always raised; in fact it may be below normal. The fontanelle is tense, except in the presence of dehydration. As has been stated, neck stiffness is often absent. At this time of life the meningitis is frequently due to Gram-negative organisms or to the group B streptococcus. Therefore, until the organism has been identified, treatment is with chloramphenicol, or gentamicin or other aminoglycoside, or a cephalosporin; usually in combination with a penicillin (de Louvois et al., 1991). The use of alternative drugs may be indicated once the organism has been identified, and sensitivities determined. These include cefotaxime or ceftazidime for Gram-negative infections, and co-trimoxazole which will reach effective levels in the cerebrospinal fluid when given systemically. Chloramphenicol doses which result in levels over 50 µg/ml may cause the grey baby syndrome and careful monitoring is necessary. A cephalosporin should not be used on its own in this age group until listeria infection has been excluded, since they are not effective against this.

Depending on the severity of the infection it may be necessary to give some drugs intravenously to start with, and then if possible intramuscularly for three weeks or more. Intrathecal treatment when indicated may have to be continued until four or five negative cerebrospinal fluid cultures have been obtained (Davies, 1978). If after 48–72 hours organisms can still be cultured from the fluid, ventriculitis is likely and ventricular puncture is indicated. If this diagnosis is confirmed, antibiotics will need to be instilled into the ventricular cerebrospinal fluid (Robinson and Roberts, 1990b). It must also be stressed that when, and if, treatment is indicated for meningitis complicating hydrocephalus and meningomyelocele, intrathecal treatment will be needed (Ceftazadime plus gentamicin is the most commonly used treatment for pseudomonas infections).

Apart from antibacterial therapy, other supportive measures will be of vital importance, including the treatment of acidosis, apnoea, hypoglycaemia, respiratory distress and fits (Davies, 1977).

Bacterial meningitis

At any age the treatment of acute meningitis will be governed by the identification of the causal organism and its sensitivity, if this can be done rapidly. Even before a bacterial diagnosis is made, treatment should be started with chloramphenicol, usually in combination with penicillin or ampicillin. Sometimes sulphonamides were added to the treatment regime (de Louvois et al., 1991). This can be modified as soon as the organism is known. Pneumococcal meningitis is a fairly common complication of chest infections in infancy, and will usually respond to this treatment. Meningococcal meningitis will be suggested when the signs of meningitis are associated with a petechial rash and other haemorrhages due to a meningococcal septicaemia; always a grave prognostic sign. The cerebrospinal fluid can be normal in the very early stages of the disease. The meningococcus is likely to be sensitive to ampicillin or penicillin G, 300 mg/kg body weight/day, given intravenously in 4 doses.

For those with evidence of anaphylaxis to penicillin a parenteral cephalosporin can be given instead. A low white blood count and a low platelet count are also of bad prognostic significance, as is a high antigen titre in the cerebrospinal fluid which persists for longer than 48 hours after the start of treatment, and a high titre in the serum present for more than 2 or 3 days. A particularly dangerous complication of a meningococcal septicaemia is the Waterhouse-Friderichsen syndrome, when haemorrhage or necrosis of the suprarenal glands results in sudden and dramatic circulatory failure. If there is adrenal insufficiency, hydrocortisone is given intravenously and intramuscularly, and norepinephrine can be used. Intravenous glucose saline, plasma or blood may have to be given. In the early stages of a consumption coagulopathy syndrome intravenous heparin is also indicated. The treatment of acute bacterial meningitis has been well reviewed by Bell and McGuinness (1985). The rapid diagnosis of meningococcal disease followed by early treatment is essential, and the polymerase chain reaction to detect meningococcal DNA in a culture-negative cerebrospinal fluid may well be useful (Kristiansen et al., 1991).

Although penicillin is almost invariably effective in systemic meningococcal infections, to eradicate the nasopharyngeal carrier state in the affected child and close family contacts rifampicin should be given (10 mg/kg body weight, 5 mg/kg body weight for children under the age of 1 year, twice daily for 2 days) (Venkat Raman, 1988).

Haemophilus influenzae meningitis is relatively common in childhood, often complicating upper respiratory tract and middle ear infections. There has recently been some controversy over treatment. Ampicillin is still the drug of choice, rather than chloramphenicol and sulphadiazine with their greater risks of toxic side-effects. To avoid failures, the dose of intravenous ampicillin has been raised to 300–400 mg/kg body weight per day, given in four to six divided doses. Deafness has been noted in a number of cases so treated, although an ototoxic effect of this drug has not been proven (Gamstorp and Klockhoff, 1974). It has been claimed that additional therapy with intrathecal ampicillin or chloramphenicol gives significantly better results (Lorber, 1974). Occasionally resistance to both chloramphenicol and ampicillin may be found. Then other drugs such as the cephalosporins will have to be used (Lorber, 1981). There is no doubt that the introduction of newer antibiotics, such as cefotaxime and ceftriaxone, has improved the prognosis, and reduced the incidence of hearing loss (Peltola, Anttila and Renkonen, 1989; Robinson and Roberts, 1990b). Rifampicin can also be used in the prophylaxis of Haemophilus influenzae type b; being given to the affected child and to close contacts if there is a sibling aged under 5 years; in a dose of 20 mg/kg once daily for 4 days. There is now a successful vaccine against Haemophilus influenzae type b (Booy and Moxon, 1991).

Whatever the type of meningitis, the risk of convulsions resulting in brain damage is sufficiently great to warrant the use of prophylactic anticonvulsant treatment as soon as such an infection is suspected, and convulsions occurring during the illness must be treated as an emergency (Ounsted, 1978). Fits should be treated with intravenous anti-epileptic drugs, especially phenytoin which does not depress the level of consciousness. The possibility of drug interactions between antibiotics and anticonvulsants must be considered and serum levels checked. For example the serum concentration of chloramphenicol may be influenced by anti-epileptic drugs, such as phenobarbitone or phenytoin, which are enzyme inducers. Fluid restriction for the first few days may help to prevent hyponatraemia, and may limit cerebral oedema. Giving corticosteroids is not yet justifiable for all patients, but in the case of Haemophilus influenzae, meningitis dexamethasone can be helpful.

Complications of acute meningitis

If the meningitis does not respond to appropriate antibiotic treatment, complications are likely to be present. The persistence of seizures in spite of treatment suggests intra- or extra-cerebral focal infection. The use of the CT scan has greatly helped the management of focal infection, subdural effusions and hydrocephalus.

Subdural effusions

These are particularly common in *Haemophilus influenzae* meningitis. The child does not recover completely and begins to develop signs of increased intracranial pressure, including bulging of the fontanelle in infancy, and there may also be focal neurological signs. The cerebrospinal fluid protein often remains raised. Subdural taps in the infant will reveal yellow or blood-tinged fluid which is sterile. Repeated taps will usually resolve this complication, and operation to remove a membrane is seldom necessary. Infection in the fluid to produce an empyema is fortunately very rare. When subdural puncture is indicated for any reason the site chosen is the lateral angle of the anterior fontanelle or just lateral to it in the coronal suture if it is small. It is best to displace the skin before puncturing it with a short bevelled needle with a stilette, then releasing it before advancing the needle caudally, laterally and obliquely until a sudden decrease in resistance is felt. This technique reduces subsequent leakage. The fluid is allowed to drain or is aspirated slowly, and not more than 20–40 ml must be removed at one time. Taps must always be done on both sides as bilateral subdural effusions are so common. Rapid aspiration causes cerebral displacement or venous engorgement with diminished venous return to the heart and resulting collapse of the infant.

Hydrocephalus

The possibility of hydrocephalus must also be kept in mind, for although it is sometimes of acute onset with headache and vomiting, it can be insidious. In the early stages of the illness thick exudate may obstruct the aqueduct or foramen in the roof of the fourth ventricle, and then spontaneous cure may occur. Later, adhesions form and can cause permanent obstruction to the flow of the cerebrospinal fluid at the roof of the fourth ventricle or at the tentorium, and necessitate by-pass operations of various kinds. Shunts, when these are used in the treatment of hydrocephalus, can cause problems due to infections. They should be suspected if the distal end of a ventriculo-peritoneal catheter becomes blocked, especially if a walled-off cyst develops. Removal of the shunt, combined with appropriate antibiotic cover is the most reliable treatment (Robinson and Roberts, 1990b). The diagnosis will be confirmed by cerebrospinal fluid cultures from the shunting system. A quicker method is to measure serum C-reactive protein (CRP), supplemented by coagulase-negative staphylococcus antibody testing in the cerebrospinal fluid (Bayston, 1989).

Cranial nerve palsies

The nerves most frequently damaged by infection as they cross the subarachnoid space are the oculomotor nerves and the eighth cranial nerve. Ocular palsies often disappear, but deafness can persist. It may be severe, but is often mild, and is then all too easy to miss if the child is not carefully examined at follow-up. With a slight degree of deafness a young child may respond quite normally to most sounds, but the disability can be highly significant in terms of language development and in the classroom. There is some evidence that endotoxin may be the cause of post-meningitic deafness, and that it may be possible to prevent this by pre-treatment with dexamethazone.

Chronic meningitis

There are a number of rare forms of meningitis which run a protracted course, caused by such organisms as the cryptococcus which can be treated with a combination of amphotericin B and 5-fluorocytosine (Polak and Wain, 1977) However, the most frequent diagnostic problem is between tuberculous meningitis and viral meningitis, although other causes of aseptic meningitis include leptospirosis, syphilis, brucellosis and the meningeal inflammation found in collagen diseases and malignancy. Partially treated bacterial meningitis must always be included in the differential diagnosis.

Tuberculous meningitis

The infection usually spreads to the meninges from the lungs or lymph glands. Tubercles form along the blood vessels of the cortex and then rupture into the subarachnoid space (Rich and McCordock, 1933).

The illness can be divided into three stages. In the first (prodromal) stage the child is 'off colour', but there does not seem to be anything specifically wrong. There is an obvious loss of energy and appetite. Headaches may start, and the child may have an intermittent high temperature. After a few days the child becomes more seriously ill, with headache, malaise, vomiting, and sometimes convulsions. A stiff neck and positive Kernig's sign will appear, suggesting the diagnosis of meningitis. The final stage should not be reached if an early diagnosis is made and appropriate treatment given. If it is not, there is an increasing likelihood of the child lapsing into coma and showing evidence of severe brain damage, for example a hemiplegia or signs of brain-stem involvement. This is presumably the result of vascular lesions, as the onset of these complications is usually sudden. Perhaps it is surprising that it does not happen more often in meningitis when the vessels at the base of the brain are bathed in pus. Acute communicating hydrocephalus may also contribute to the problem.

When the diagnosis of a more chronic form of meningitis is first suspected and a lumbar puncture is done, the cerebrospinal fluid is likely to be clear and colourless. There may be a spider-web clot and a slight increase of mononuclear cells and protein. Biochemical analysis, however, can be normal, even the sugar showing no definite reduction. Then, as has been stressed, the diagnostic dilemma is between tuberculous and viral meningitis, and the former must be treated immediately if a good prognosis is to be assured. Occasionally the diagnosis is made on general examination, by finding evidence of pulmonary tuberculosis or the presence of a choroidal tubercle in the retina. Dermal tests should always be done to aid the diagnosis, but can be negative. The longer that acid-fast bacilli are searched for in the centrifuged deposit of the cerebrospinal fluid the more likely they are to be found, and it may be possible to make a rapid diagnosis by using the enzyme-linked immunoabsorbent assay (ELISA) and latex particle agglutination detection of mycobacterial antigen (IgG and IgM). Sometimes anti-tuberculous treatment has to be started before a definite diagnosis has been made, and then reviewed in the light of subsequent events. Some methods of diagnosis for viral meningitis such as C-reactive protein (CRP) and lactic acid levels are rarely worthwhile (Robinson and Roberts, 1990a). Once the diagnosis is proven, it is essential to track down its origin, as other children within the family, or at school, may be at risk.

Treatment is with a combination of drugs, for example isoniazid (INAH) in a dose of 15–20 kg body weight per day as a single dose (maximum 500 mg), with rifampicin up to 20 mg/kg body weight per day in one dose (maximum 600 mg daily) and pyrazinamide 20 mg/kg body weight/day in three divided doses. The treatment may have to be continued for at least a year. A combination of isoniazid, rifampicin and ethambutol, 35 mg/kg body weight per day as a single daily dose for up to 3 months, may be preferred, as both the latter drugs enter the cerebrospinal fluid more adequately than streptomycin does, even when the meninges are inflamed. Rifampicin can effect liver function, although asymptomatic enlargement of the liver with normal liver function tests does not necessarily mean that this treatment must be stopped, as long as the situation is constantly reviewed. Ethambutol can cause loss of vision due to optic neuritis, usually with gradual recovery when the drug is stopped. When isoniazid is given, pyridoxine, 10 mg a day, should be added to prevent a neuropathy developing. If there is not a rapid response to specific treatment it can help to add steroids, systemically and intrathecally, to reduce cerebral oedema and to suppress some of the inflammatory effects of the infection, especially adhesions within the subarachnoid space. Hydrocephalus used to be a fairly common complication of tuberculous meningitis before the use of such treatment. Inappropriate secretion of antidiuretic hormone may occur and the resulting disturbance of fluid balance can effect the level of consciousness, and also the level of chloride in the cerebrospinal fluid. Treatment with fluid restriction and with demedocycline, which reduces urinary concentrating ability (600 mg daily) is worth considering (Perks, Mohr and Liversedge, 1976).

Virus meningitis (aseptic meningitis)

The onset of virus meningitis can be acute, and there is nothing diagnostic in the symptomatology. Recovery is usually rapid, i.e. within a matter of days, and complications do not occur unless there is a meningo-encephalitis. The cerebrospinal fluid shows a raised cell count, usually of mononuclear cells, but occasionally of polynuclear cells. The protein may or may not be raised, and culture is sterile. Coxsackie, echo and myxoviruses are most commonly involved, and can be cultured from throat swabs, urine and faeces; but the diagnosis is usually made by a rise in the specific antibody titre in the serum during, and for the few weeks after, the onset of the illness, except in the case of the echovirus, as no serological test is available. The antibodies which develop in response to infections of any kind are associated with the IgG and IgM fractions of the serum immunoglobulins. IgG antibodies persist for very long periods, so unless a marked increase can be demonstrated in the convalescent phase of the illness, their presence may only indicate a past infection or vaccination. IgM antibodies, however, usually appear only during the course of the primary infection. The viruses of mumps, coxsackie B, echovirus and lymphocytic chorio-meningitis can be relatively easily cultured from the cerebrospinal fluid. There are now an increasing number of antiviral agents, which are therapeutically effective (Booth, 1991), so that the diagnosis of viral meningitis and encephalitis is becoming more and more urgent. These include acyclovir (herpes simplex and zoster viruses), ganciclovir (cytomegalovirus), azidothymidine (immunodeficiency viruses), and ribavirin (respiratory syncytial virus).

Recurrent meningitis

If several attacks of bacterial meningitis occur there may be focal or systemic reasons for this. Any history of trauma or chronic infection could mean that the dura has been perforated in relation to a nasal sinus or the middle ear, and X-rays of the base of the skull are important. An infected dural sinus must be sought in the cervical and sacral regions. When such causes cannot be found it may be a question of an increased liability to infections, for example from an immune deficiency state.

Non-infective meningitis

Acute infections, especially pneumonia, are occasionally accompanied by the signs of meningitis (meningism), but the cerebrospinal fluid is found to be normal. Subarachnoid haemorrhage, although rare in childhood, can mimic infectious meningitis. Meningeal leukaemia usually occurs in a phase of haematogical remission, but does not often cause diagnostic problems, as the diagnosis of leukaemia will usually have already been made. The diagnosis of a neoplastic meningitis can prove much more difficult, especially as there may be a low sugar content in the cerebrospinal fluid. Repeated searches may be needed to identify malignant cells in the fluid.

Encephalitis

Prenatal infections

The effects of virus encephalitis can start before birth, and there can be no doubt that such prenatal infections make a significant contribution to the number of children physically and mentally handicapped as a result of brain damage. It has been estimated that 1% of infants are congenitally infected with cytomegalic inclusion disease, and that the virus causes significant brain damage in at least 10% of those infected (Krech, Jung and Jung, 1971). Congenital rubella and toxoplasmosis have been the cause of about 2–3% of all cases of mental deficiency.

Rubella

Infection of the mother with rubella in the first trimester of pregnancy is a well-known cause of mental retardation with microcephaly, cataract (Fig. 10.1), deafness, congenital heart disease, hepatosplenomegaly and other anomalies. Rubella embryo-

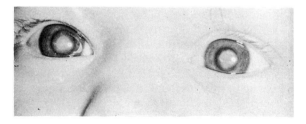

Figure 10.1   Congenital rubella cataracts.

pathy can cause sensorineural deafness as its sole manifestation (Peckham *et al.*, 1979). The fact that it causes not only an encephalitis but affects so many other organs emphasizes how often a virus infection is widespread throughout the body, even if it involves mainly one part. The diagnosis can be established by isolating the virus from the urine, the nasopharynx and cerebrospinal fluid. The excretion of the virus in the urine for months after birth can constitute a risk to the nursing staff.

Immunization programmes can now protect young women from the risks of acquiring rubella in the first three months of pregnancy. It is hoped that recent vaccination programmes may eliminate the disease altogether.

Cytomegalovirus

Recently, interuterine infection by the cytomegalovirus has received increasing attention, especially when it occurs in the first two trimesters. Such congenital infection occurs in 0.3–0.4% of live births in the UK and results from both primary and recurrent maternal infection. It has been related to stillbirths and prematurity. Fewer than 10% of congenitally infected infants have clinical manifestations of cytomegalovirus infection at birth, but most of these will have serious mental and physical handicaps. About 5% of those who have no symptoms at birth will develop disabilities related to the infection, such as hydrocephalus, or a meningo-encephalitis with motor and mental retardation. The affected child may suffer from specific learning disorders, epilepsy and a spastic quadriplegia and is sometimes deaf and blind. Sensorineural deafness may not become apparent for several years (MacDonald and Towbin, 1978), and infection with cytomegalovirus may account for 12% of children with bilateral sensorineural hearing loss (Peckham, 1989). Chorioretinitis is occasionally found, but the lesions are more peripheral than those of toxoplasmosis; and there may be optic atrophy. Also, there may be microcephaly and microphthalmia. The clinical picture in the neonatal period may be similar to that of haemorrhagic disease of the newborn with anaemia, purpura, jaundice, thrombocytopenia, and enlargement of the liver and spleen. X-ray of the skull can show intracerebral calcification (Fig. 10.2).

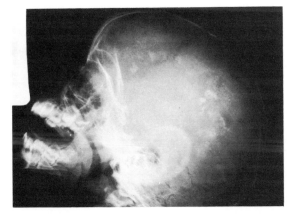

Figure 10.2   Intracerebral calcification in cytomegalic inclusion disease.

Symptoms and signs usually appear at birth, but can be delayed for several months. The diagnosis is from congenital toxoplasmosis, haemorrhagic disease of the newborn, neonatal sepsis and other virus infections, such as rubella. After primary infection of the mothers during pregnancy (often a mononucleosis-like syndrome) the incidence of fetal infection is about 30%, and is often more severe than after recurrent maternal infection. Of these, 10% or less may suffer severe brain damage (Stern and Tucker, 1973), but as many as 85% can show evidence of some CNS abnormalities on long-term follow-up (Hanshaw and Dudgeon, 1978). Another study has confirmed that congenital infection can follow both primary maternal infection in all three trimesters of pregnancy, and recurrent maternal infection. A total of 10% had appreciable deafness, neurological defects, or both, and a further 5% had minor handicaps, such as unilateral deafness (Preece, Pearle and Peckham, 1984). A recent follow-up of neonates with symptomatic congenital cytomegalovirus infection showed that the prognosis is better than previously reported (Ramsay, Miller and Peckham, 1991). Prevention is possible by the identification and termination of pregnancies at risk. Women who transmit the virus to the fetus may have a defective immunological response, and in the future a genetically engineered vaccine may be of help (Stern et al., 1986). This virus can also continue to be excreted in the urine for prolonged periods after birth, but the affected child need not be isolated, and nursing and teaching staff need only be extra careful with personal hygiene (Tookey and Peckham, 1991). Most asymptomatic virus excretors grow normally, but 10–20% can later develop physical and mental handicaps, especially if they have had transient hepatitis or purpura (Dudgeon, 1976). Evidence does not suggest that routine screening of pregnant women to detect primary infection is likely to be helpful, and most children with no obvious manifestations of this infection develop normally (Peckham et al., 1983).

The acquisition of cytomegalovirus infection after birth usually occurs early in life. The mother's serological status is of importance, and also the question of breast-feeding, as the virus can be passed in the mother's milk. Another possible source is transfusion of cytomegalovirus positive blood to a mother who is seronegative. Unless cytomegalovirus is detected in the urine within three weeks of birth, congenital and acquired infection cannot be distinguished, even when clinical problems suggestive of congenital infection are present (Peckham, 1989). The treatment of cytomegalovirus infection is now possible with dihydroxy-2-propoxy-methyl-guanidine, but not in congenital or neonatal infections (Barton and Gazzard, 1989).

Herpes simplex and varicella

Herpes simplex is known to cause teratogenic infections. The resulting microcephaly and intracerebral calcification can mimic cytomegalovirus infection (Kristenssen, Olssen and Sourander, 1974). Also, herpes infection can be acquired during birth from the mother's infected genitalia, the illness on average appearing six days later. Many organs can be affected, and involvement of the brain leads to convulsions and coma. The estimated frequency of neonatal herpetic infection varies from 1 in 3500 to 1 in 30 000 deliveries (Nahmias, Alford and Korones, 1970). Varicella infection of the mother in the first trimester causing congenital defects has been reported (McKendry and Bailey, 1973). Mental retardation, chorioretinitis and cataracts are typically present; and if a mother develops chicken-pox within a few days of delivery, passive immunization with antivaricella zoster immunoglobulin can be given to the baby as soon as possible after birth.

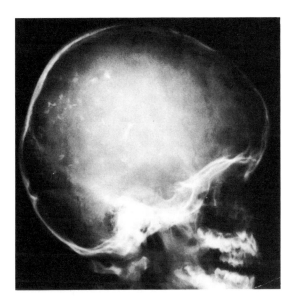

Figure 10.3   Cerebral calcification in toxoplasmosis.

Congenital toxoplasmosis

In congenital toxoplasmosis the *Toxoplasma gondii* presumably passes through the placenta and spreads widely throughout the body of the fetus. If this occurs early in pregnancy, abortion often results. Amongst the survivors the most common manifestations are internal hydrocephalus, microcephaly, chorioretinitis and signs of cerebral damage, including cerebral calcification (Fig. 10.3). Infection towards the end of pregnancy results in a clinical picture similar to haemorrhagic disease of the newborn.

It is suggested that the fetus may be affected from either an acute or chronic infection of the mother. The former can only be diagnosed for certain if a significant rise in the mother's dye test titre can be shown. It is claimed that such a high titre will protect the fetus in a future pregnancy, while in chronic infections with a low titre the toxoplasmosis may be passed on in successive pregnancies (Beattie, 1957). When tests for toxoplasmosis antibody are found to be positive during pregnancy (dye test titre of more than 1:512 with toxoplasma-specific IgM at any titre) termination should be considered before the twentieth week. The alternative is treatment with spiramycin 100 mg/kg body weight a day orally for 30 days, or pyrimethamine, 1 mg/kg body weight a day orally for 30 days, with sulphadiazine, 100 mg/kg body weight a day orally, and folic acid, 5 mg a day (Fleck, 1981). However the effectiveness of this treatment is still uncertain, and as the risks to the fetus are low it may be better to concentrate on health education, with advice against eating undercooked meat and unwashed raw fruit and vegetables, and against contact with cats and or litter. The incidence is very low, so that the argument for screening is correspondingly weak.

Congenital infection with *Listeria* is uncommon, but can cause death of the baby soon after birth, or septicaemia or meningitis. Treatment is with ampicillin and an aminoglycoside.

Diagnosis of prenatal infections

In the newborn infant, congenital infection with either rubella virus or cytomegalovirus can usually be confirmed by the isolation of the respective agent from products of conception, urine, saliva or throat swab. In some instances, biopsy material may be subjected to cultural procedures. The isolation of cytomegalovirus in tissue culture usually poses few problems, but the low excretion rate and difficulties at the technical level make the isolation of rubella virus problematical. In both cases the diagnosis can also be achieved by noting high levels of antibody at birth. The antibody does not decay, as would be expected with the loss of passive immunity of maternal origin, but persists well into the first year of life, and beyond. The presence of high levels of IgM in the newborn child is very suggestive of infection, and, if rubella-specific or cytomegalovirus-specific antibody can be detected in this immunoglobulin fraction, the diagnosis of congenital infection with one or other of the agents is confirmed.

As the majority of infections with herpes simplex virus in neonates are acquired from the infected birth passage of the mother, the diagnostic procedures should include a close examination of the cervix, vagina and vulva of the mother, as well as the isolation of the virus from skin vesicles in the child. At the earliest stages of infection in the baby the virus can usually be isolated from a throat swab, well before the appearance of cutaneous lesions. Serological tests are of little value in the diagnosis of neonatal herpes, except perhaps retrospectively in survivors. Congenital toxoplasmosis is diagnosed serologically. Positive toxoplasma-specific IgM in the young infant establishes the diagnosis of congenital infection, and is no longer technically that difficult (which also applies to tests for specific IgM in rubella and CMV infections). High levels of antibody in the child, as found by the less demanding Dye test, can also help in the diagnosis (Karim and Ludlam, 1975). Rubella IgM is almost always present in the neonate, but negative results do occur in CMV and toxoplasma infections, and following the decay of IgG is therefore necessary in IgM-negative patients.

Acute virus encephalitis in infancy and childhood

Encephalitis during the course of a virus infection may be more common than is thought. For example, it is possible that the EEG changes often found among children with measles (Pampiglione, 1964) may indicate cerebral involvement, even when this is not suspected on clinical grounds.

The spread of the virus to the brain may be via the blood or by the cranial or peripheral nerves. The younger the child the greater is the risk of brain damage, due possibly to a relative lack of antibodies and low interferon production. Defects of the blood-brain barrier also have to be considered (Kristenssen, Olson and Sourander, 1974). Diagnostic procedures include the examination of brain biopsy material and immunological tests on cerebrospinal fluid and serum (Longson and Bailey, 1978).

Herpes simplex encephalitis

A number of different viruses may directly invade the brain during infancy and childhood, and only a few examples of these can be considered. It is now realized that the herpes simplex virus is amongst the most common causes of encephalitis in temperate climates.

There will be symptoms related to a generalized infection, such as headache, fever, malaise, nausea, vomiting, abdominal pain and diarrhoea. Then symptoms and signs of CNS involvement occur. Liversedge (1973) has classified these manifestations into four types.

The meningo-encephalitic type is characterized by stupor, convulsions and a meningeal reaction with up to 200 lymphocytes per mm^3 in the cerebrospinal fluid. In the prolonged type, an acute attack lasting 10–14 days is followed by spontaneous improvement and then by a relapse 6–8 weeks later. The neurosurgical type has raised most interest in the past few years. It presents as a temporal lobe, space-occupying lesion, often with a hemiplegia. The EEG shows focal abnormalities over the temporal lobe, and neuro-radiological investigations can confirm the presence of a local lesion. The prognosis of these three types is poor, but in the fourth type (an encephalitis with coma, convulsions and paralyses) spontaneous recovery can occur, although the patient is likely to remain disabled. It may be that the presence of focal signs has been over-emphasized. Published series of patients with a herpes simplex infection, proven by examination of cortical biopsy material, have often come from neurosurgical departments, particularly if a cerebral abscess or tumour has been suspected. This may have led to a selection of those patients with herpes simplex encephalitis of focal type.

Symptomatology may vary considerably. Prodromal symptoms, such as headache, can occasionally persist for several weeks, although the onset is usually acute. Confusion, disorientation, bizarre behaviour and sometimes severe dysphasia can occur. The destructive lesions found at autopsy have in the past been described under the term 'acute necrotizing encephalitis'. The prognosis is grave, with a mortality of more than 50%.

In view of the possibility of anti-viral treatment, an exact diagnosis is of increasing importance. The clinical picture can certainly be suggestive, and occasionally the EEG gives supportive evidence. There is usually a generalized excess of slow-wave activity, especially in the frontal and temporal areas. There may be periodic complexes of sharp and slow waves, but these tend to be transient. Repetitive sharp waves and bursts of rhythmic slow waves in the temporal areas are other features of the record. When there are focal neurological signs, the EEG almost always shows abnormalities over the relevant part of the cerebrum. Sometimes these focal features are present in the absence of a hemiplegia and they can be of a shifting type (Upton and Gumpert, 1970). The cerebrospinal fluid cell count and protein level are often raised, although there may be exceptions to this; and the polymerase chain reaction assay of the fluid may offer a quick means of diagnosis (Aurelius *et al.*, 1991). Brain scans may show evidence of a focal lesion, usually in the temporal lobe. The differential diagnosis is from conditions such as brain abscess, venous sinus thrombosis, tubercular meningitis, neoplasms and other types of virus encephalitis.

However, an exact diagnosis can be made only by a positive identification of the infection by the herpes simplex virus, and this must be made rapidly so that treatment can be considered. It can be done by growing the virus in tissue culture or by using fluorescent antibody staining, when tissue has been obtained by a cortical biopsy (Fig. 10.4). The latter can give a diagnosis within four hours of the patient being anaesthetized (Longson, 1973). More sensitive assays for serum and cerebrospinal fluid IgG antibodies against herpes simplex may enable an early diagnosis to be made by these methods, rather than by brain biopsy (Klapper, Laing and Longson, 1981).

Although the evidence is not yet conclusive, the results of treatment are sufficiently encouraging to make diagnosis a matter of urgency; for if treatment is going to

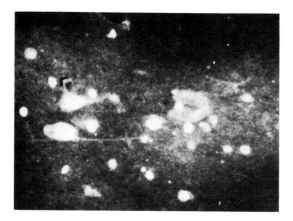

Figure 10.4   Fluorescent antibody staining in herpes simplex encephalitis (cortical biopsy).

prevent brain damage it must obviously be given as soon after the start of the illness as possible. This damage may be caused by cerebral oedema, an antigen-antibody reaction, or by the direct action of the virus on the brain cells. The oedema can be treated by medical or surgical decompression, and intracranial pressure monitoring can be of obvious help. The former is usually accomplished by giving intravenous infusions of urea or mannitol, or a course of dexamethasone. Steroids may also reduce the inflammatory reaction, which at certain times may have a deleterious effect. It seems likely that the effect of steroids may depend on the stage of the disease during which they are given. During some phases of the virus infection they may do harm by inhibiting natural protective mechanisms, whilst at other times they may prevent them getting out of hand; but there is no way of knowing when is the optimum time to start treatment with steroids.

Specific therapy is now a possibility in a number of viral infections by the use of inhibitors of DNA-containing viruses. In the case of herpes virus, cytosine arabinoside has superseded idoxuridine, and it is claimed that adenosine arabinoside is less toxic. More recently, more promising antiviral agents, such as acyclovir, given intravenously, have been developed which accumulate only in virus-infected cells and affect the metabolism of the virus(Field and Wildy, 1981), and is now the treatment of choice. The dose is 10 mg/kg body weight every 8 hours for 10 days (Whitley, 1988). Relapses of herpes simplex encephalitis can occur, which may be due to inadequate treatment or to a para-infectious demyelination (Pike *et al.*, 1991).

If a significant proportion of neurological disabilities among handicapped children are due to virus infections the discovery of an increasing number of anti-viral agents is likely to make a major contribution to the prevention of these conditions.

Coxsackie B encephalitis

Other direct virus infections of the brain which are relatively common during childhood include coxsackie B and mumps. The former usually causes a mild illness with meningeal irritation, but there may be a severe and even fatal encephalitis. Also, coxsackie and ECHO virus can cause paralysis, which is clinically indistinguishable from poliomyelitis. Occasionally, the coxsackie B virus affects newborn babies, but usually not until the third to sixth day of life, and it is most probably a postnatal infection. The heart, liver and CNS are involved, with myocarditis, hepatitis and a meningo-encephalitis.

Mumps encephalitis

Meningo-encephalitis complicating mumps is estimated to occur in about 10% of infections, but usually presents as a relatively mild condition. There may be only an aseptic meningitis with headache and neck stiffness. Sometimes a severe encephalitis particularly affecting the brain-stem may occur before, or in the absence of, swelling of the parotid glands. Other neurological complications include myelitis similar to poliomyelitis, facial palsy, and sensori-neural deafness. The diagnosis is confirmed by a rise in the titre of complement-fixing antibodies.

Acquired toxoplasmosis

A meningo-encephalitis can occur from toxoplasmosis, and there is nothing unusual in the symptoms. There will be an increase in cell count and protein content of the cerebrospinal fluid, which will be sterile on culture. The diagnosis may be suggested by an associated choroidoretinitis, and is confirmed by the dye test which identifies antibody present in the serum, or by haemagglutination, latex agglutination and fluorescence antibody tests. As in tuberculous meningitis a rapid diagnosis can be made by using the enzyme-linked immunoabsorbent assay (ELISA) and latex particle agglutination detection of antigen (IgM).

Treatment is with sulphadiazine in a dose of 1 g 6-hourly, and pyrimethamine in a dose of 25 mg daily, the former for 6 weeks and the latter for 3 weeks. Folic acid levels must be checked during this time. An alternative is spiramycin, 2–3 g per day in four doses for up to 6 weeks (Beverley, 1975). These are adult doses and must be adjusted accordingly for age. It is difficult to know whether these drugs have any significant effect.

Myalgic encephalomyelitis

This syndrome is referred to by a number of different names, including the post-viral fatigue syndrome. There has been much controversy on the nature of the condition, and whether it is due to an organic or functional disorder. There are many recorded symptoms, but the most characteristic one is fatiguability. Signs can be equally varied, and tests are of limited use, although in some there can be evidence of a virus infection, particularly an enterovirus, and of a disturbance of immune mechanisms.

The differential diagnosis therefore covers a wide range of possibilities, such as demyelinating disorders and psychiatric ones. Children can be affected, especially girls, and if they are living in groups as in a secondary school.

If, as frequently happens, tests are negative, it is no good telling the patient and parents there is nothing wrong. There obviously is, and those affected are in need of help. Management must be geared to the individual sufferer, and will be largely symptomatic, linked to a programme of rehabilitation.

The lesson to be learnt from all the controversy over the past decades is surely that this condition does exist as an entity, although sometimes it is difficult to define and to diagnose, and it contains several components some of which are organic and some of which are not; and both have to be assessed (Gordon, 1988).

Acute focal infections

Brain abscess

When a child becomes acutely ill, with an obvious infection and evidence of brain damage, the diagnosis lies between a pyogenic brain abscess or an acute viral encephalitis, although the diagnostic difficulties do not always present in this dramatic way. Once the possibility of a brain abscess is considered, it is the doctor's duty to exclude it by any investigations that may be deemed necessary.

The infection can reach the brain from a focus in some other part of the body, for example the lungs or heart. In the case of children with atrial or ventricular septal defects, the possibility of paradoxical bacterial embolism has to be considered, the embolus gaining direct access to the systemic arterial system from the systemic venous system. Infection may spread more directly from an otitis media or sinusitis. The former will most often cause an abscess in the temporal lobe or cerebellum, and the latter a frontal lobe abscess. The inadequate treatment of a middle-ear infection is a particular reason for the more insidious development of a brain abscess.

The symptoms and signs are of three types:

1. those due to any infection, such as malaise and temperature;
2. those resulting from the inevitable increased intracranial pressure, including vomiting, headache and papilloedema; and
3. the evidence of a space-occupying lesion in the cerebrum or cerebellum.

The latter can often be minimal or absent, especially if there is a gradual onset and the lesion is in a 'silent' area of the brain, such as the temporal lobe of the non-dominant hemisphere.

Diagnosis can be difficult, particularly when there has been prior treatment of an infection with antibiotics. The EEG can be particularly helpful (Fig. 10.5). It almost always shows well-marked focal abnormalities consisting of high voltage slow waves.

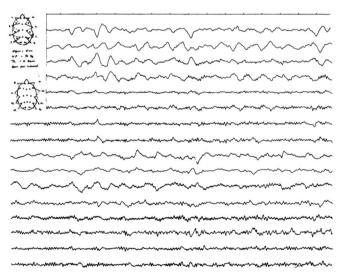

Figure 10.5   EEG in left frontal brain abscess.

These may sometimes be obscured by the severity of a generalized dysrhythmia, for example when there is an associated meningitis. The brain scans will also reveal the presence of a focal lesion, but, if these are not available, arteriography is the neuroradiological investigation of choice. The organisms involved include many types of bacteria and fungi. Aerobic and anaerobic organisms can be found; and the presence of mixed organisms is relatively common, especially when the abscess follows sinusitis or otitis media.

Treatment will be with the appropriate antibiotics, and surgical drainage of the abscess. Antibiotics must be given in massive doses, and before the organisms have been identified should include drugs such as intravenous penicillin G, chloramphenicol and metronidazole to combat both aerobic and anaerobic infections. If the walls of the abscess cavity are not rigid, cure may be possible with needle drainage of the abscess and the installation of the antibiotic into the cavity, as well as giving systemic therapy. Radio-opaque material injected into the cavity will also enable a check to be kept on its diminishing size. Surgical excision of the cavity is often needed to eradicate the infection.

Sinus thrombosis

Infection may spread to the dural sinuses, especially from the middle ear, but this is a difficult diagnosis to establish and to differentiate from conditions such as subdural empyema and cerebral abscess which require immediate surgical treatment. The thrombosis may be the result of the infection, of dehydration, or both.

If the superior saggital sinus is affected, convulsions and hemiplegia can develop. Raised intracranial pressure and hydrocephalus are not likely to occur unless the thrombosis spreads to the lateral sinuses.

In cavernous sinus thrombosis, apart from the symptoms of any infection, there will be pain around the eyes, oedema and ecchymosis of the orbital tissues and proptosis. There may be papilloedema, ptosis, and other paralyses of the oculomotor nerves.

The diagnosis is confirmed by angiography, and treatment is by correction of dehydration and by giving the appropriate antibiotic, or a wide-spectrum one if the organism cannot be identified. Dose-adjusted intravenous heparin is also an effective treatment (Einhäupl *et al.*, 1991).

Spinal abscess

Although spinal abscesses are rare, it must be remembered that they are potentially lethal unless they are operated on at an early stage. The infection usually spreads from a local source, such as an osteomyelitis, occasionally tuberculous, but may be blood-borne. The pus may be extradural or subdural.

The onset can be acute or chronic, with pain in the back, root pains, and signs resembling a radiculitis, followed by transverse myelitis. The latter will be an irreversible condition, so the diagnosis must be made when there are symptoms and no signs. X-ray examination of the spine and myelography is most likely to produce the correct diagnosis, and treatment depends on surgical drainage of the pus.

Spinal virus infections

Certain viruses have a greater affinity for nerve cells in the spinal cord and posterior root ganglia than for those in the brain.

Poliomyelitis

Fortunately, due to inoculation programmes, this disease is now very rare in most countries, but it does form part of the differential diagnosis of more common conditions. Isolated instances of paralytic poliomyelitis still occur, for example among travellers, and there is always a danger that parents will cease to have their children protected in the belief that there is no longer a danger.

There is usually an asymmetrical involvement of anterior horn cells, and although this is often widespread, occasionally one or two muscles only are affected. The weakness is normally preceded by muscle tenderness and spasm. There seems to be some association between the severity of the paralysis and the amount of exercise taken just before its onset. The brain-stem type of infection is particularly dangerous because of the effect on respiration.

The virus enters the body via the alimentary tract and spreads to the nervous system via the blood, or occasionally along nerve pathways. The bulbar form causes more diagnostic difficulty than the spinal form of poliomyelitis, but in either type the diagnosis is mainly from other virus infections. In polyneuritis the weakness is symmetrical, and the cerebrospinal fluid will often show a raised protein and normal cell count; while in poliomyelitis the cell count will be markedly raised with only a moderate elevation of the protein. Also, there are often relapses in polyneuritis, but in poliomyelitis, once the weakness has reached a peak and begun to improve, this will continue except in areas where there has been death of the anterior horn cells.

A polio-like condition (Hopkins' syndrome) has been described in association with asthma. A few days after the onset of wheezing, pain and weakness develops in a limb, usually an arm. The cerebrospinal fluid may show an increase in cells and protein and electrophysiological tests indicate an anterior horn cell or motor root lesion. Although no definite virus infection has been identified, the findings suggest an interaction between some neurotropic agent and an altered immunological state. There is usually severe permanent residual weakness (Manson and Thong, 1980).

Herpes zoster

Shingles is rarer in childhood than among the elderly. The virus affects the nerve cells in the posterior root ganglia, and is closely allied to, if not identical with, the chicken-pox virus. The first symptom is the pain that occurs in the distribution of whichever posterior root ganglia are affected, usually in the lower dorsal or upper lumbar area. This is followed by a vesicular eruption in the same distribution. It may occasionally affect the distribution of the trigeminal nerve, and then there is a considerable risk of a keratitis and scarring of the cornea. The infection can occasionally spread to the anterior horn cells and cause a lower motor neuron paralysis, or even more rarely result in a transverse myelitis or an encephalitis.

The typical clinical picture makes the diagnosis. The pain should be adequately controlled in the acute stage, and it is now possible to treat the infection with acyclovir, and the vesicular rash with the topical application of idoxuridine.

Slow virus infections

There can be no doubt about the seriousness of acute encephalitis, and it is equally disturbing to know that some viruses can invade the brain and occupy cells in a state of symbiosis for a number of years, only to ultimately cause their destruction. This may result in sub-acute encephalopathies of a degenerative type, like Kuru or Creutzfeld–Jacob disease, or of an inflammatory kind, such as multifocal leuco-encephalopathy or sub-acute sclerosing panencephalitis (SSPE).

Progressive multifocal leucoencephalopathy

This condition complicates severe wasting diseases, such as cancer (notably reticuloses), and immunodeficiency states; and has been mentioned among the degenerative cerebral diseases. A papovavirus, or the JC virus may invade the glial cells, cause nuclear abnormalities, and indirectly demyelination (Zu Rhein and Chou, 1965). Serological tests for antibodies to the JC virus are possible.

Subacute sclerosing panencephalitis

SSPE seems, in most cases, to be related to infection with the measles virus in early life, often before the age of 18 months. This disease will be discussed in detail in Chapter 11, as it often has to be considered in the differential diagnosis of degenerative conditions. It may have an acute onset, sometimes even with evidence of raised intracranial pressure. Conversely, it may begin so insidiously that it is impossible to know exactly when the child has ceased to progress normally. There is progressive deterioration, both physical and mental, associated with epileptic seizures, particularly myoclonus. The cerebrospinal fluid shows a paretic colloidal gold curve, and the EEG finding of repetitive outbursts of slow and sharp waves is highly suggestive. Serological tests confirm high levels of specific anti-measles antibodies in the serum and cerebrospinal fluid, with a diminished serum/cerebro-spinal fluid ratio. There is no specific treatment.

Progressive rubella panencephalitis

Examples have been described of children with congenital rubella who begin to suffer from seizures with intellectual deterioration in the second decade. Spasticity and ataxia are the main findings on examination. The EEG shows an excess of slow wave activity with polyspike complexes which may be related to myoclonic jerks, and the cerebrospinal fluid cell count and protein level may be raised. There will be high antibody titres to rubella virus in the serum and cerebrospinal fluid (Townsend et al., 1975). These reports raise the possibility that other viruses may persist in the body to cause damage several years after the initial infection.

Para-infectious demyelination

Another type of 'encephalopathy' related to virus infections is the acute disseminated encephalomyelitis which may complicate infectious fevers. This condition can also occur in relation to infections with mycoplasma pneumoniae. It is a demyelinating disorder which is probably not due to a direct invasion of the brain by the virus, but to an allergic type of response on the part of the cerebral tissues. It most often complicates measles, rubella, chicken-pox and infectious mononucleosis, and may follow smallpox vaccination. Sometimes it occurs without any previous illness. The demyelination is perivascular, and there is phagocytosis of lipid breakdown products by microglia. The pathological findings are not unlike those of multiple sclerosis, except for the marked perivascular distribution. For the time being it seems to be justifiable to classify these diseases in a separate group, although further research may include some with obvious anaphylactic reactions like serum sickness, and others with slow virus infections.

In the mild forms, the patient has headache, fever, drowsiness and weakness which may be limited to one limb, and sometimes involvement of one or two cranial nerves. If severe, there will be deepening coma, widespread paralysis, and evidence of damage to the brain-stem with derangement of the vital centres. Episodes of decerebrate rigidity can occur. Optic neuritis is common and is often bilateral, and then impaired pupillary reactions to light will differentiate the swelling from papilloedema resulting from raised intracranial pressure.

Acute haemorrhagic leucoencephalitis probably represents a fulminating form of acute disseminated encephalomyelitis, and, as might be expected, there is a high mortality.

Acute cerebellar ataxia

Para-infectious demyelination sometimes affects principally the cerebellum. There may be no preceding infection, but there is usually a history of an exanthem, particularly chicken-pox. Such an acute inflammation of the cerebellum may occur in as many as 3 per 1000 cases of chicken-pox. The symptoms usually start 1–3 weeks after the infection. There is truncal ataxia, inco-ordination of limb movements and an intention tremor. Speech is slurred, and nystagmus is usually present. Recovery may take several months, and defective balance, abnormal speech and learning difficulties can sometimes persist for a long time. Diagnosis is usually easy, but the possibility of a cerebellar abscess or neoplasm has to be considered. The cerebrospinal fluid in these acute disseminated encephalomyelitides shows a slight pleocytosis and raised protein. The EEG is diffusely abnormal. Acute cerebellar ataxia can be associated with mycoplasma pneumoniae infection, which can also affect the cerebral hemispheres and spinal cord. Serological evidence of active infection may be found, but it is uncertain if the symptoms are due to a direct infection of the CNS or occur as a post-infection phenomenon (Steele et al., 1972).

Treatment

There is some evidence of a favourable response to treatment with corticotrophin and adrenal steroids, so it is important to consider this diagnosis at an early stage. If a mistaken diagnosis is made and there is a direct invasion of the brain by a virus there is a possibility of interfering with immunity responses and allowing the virus to spread, but this may be a more theoretical than a practical risk when the steroids are given for only a short period, apart from the importance of their role in preventing damage from excessive antigen-antibody reactions. Other forms of immunomodulatory treatment can be used.

Infectious polyneuritis (Guillain Barré syndrome)

This condition, and neuralgic amyotrophy, are considered in Chapter 7 in the section on peripheral neuropathies. It seems possible that there are allergic types of reaction to infections at various levels of the nervous system. There is the acute disseminated encephalomyelitis in which the brain and spinal cord are affected. The term 'myelo-radiculitis' has been used when there is evidence of damage to the spinal cord and nerve roots. In infectious polyneuritis a similar kind of pathology may affect the nerve roots and peripheral nerves. Finally, nerve roots and peripheral nerves can be affected individually or in groups, as in neuralgic amyotrophy.

References

Aurelius, E., Johansson, B., Skoldenberg, B. *et al.* (1991) Rapid diagnosis of herpes simplex encephalitis by nested polymerase chain reaction assay of cerebrospinal fluid. *Lancet*, **337**, 189

Barton, S.E. and Gazzard, B.G. (1989) The treatment of cytomegalovirus disease in AIDS. *Maternal and Child Health*, **14**, 181

Bayston, R. (1989) *Hydrocephalus Shunt Infections*, Chapman and Hall, London

Beattie, L.P. (1957) Clinical and epidemiological aspects of toxoplasmosis. *Transactions of the Royal Society of Tropical Medicine and Hygiene*, **51**, 96

Bell, W.E. (1985) Current therapy of acute bacterial meningitis in children: Part 1. *Pediatric Neurology*, **1**, 5

Bell, W. E. and McGuinness, G.A. (1985) Current therapy of acute bacterial meningitis in children: Part 2. *Pediatric Neurology*, **1**, 201

Beverley, J.K.A. (1975) Toxoplasmosis. *Medicine*, **3**, 132

Booth, J.C. (1991) Antiviral agents. *Maternal and Child Health*, **16**, 376–9

Booy, R. and Moxon, E.R. (1991) Immunisation of infants against Haemophilus influenzae type B in the UK. *Archives of Disease in Childhood*, **66**, 1251–4

Davies, P.A. (1977) Meningitis. Neonatal bacterial meningitis. *British Journal of Hospital Medicine*, **18**, 425

Davies, P.A. (1978) Use of antibiotics. Treatment of neonatal bacterial infection. *British Medical Journal*, **ii**, 676

De Louvois, J., Blackbourn, J., Hurley, R. and Harvey, D. (1991) Infantile meningitis in England and Wales: a two year study. *Archives of Disease in Childhood*, **66**, 603

Dudgeon. J.A. (1976) Infective causes of human malformations. *British Medical Bulletin*, **32**, 77

Einhäupl, K.M., Villringer, A., Meister *et al.* (1991) Heparin treatment in sinus venous thrombosis. *Lancet*, **338**, 597–600

Field, H.J. and Wildy, P. (1981) Recurrent herpes simplex: the outlook for systemic antiviral agents. *British Medical Journal*, **i**, 1821

Fleck, D.G. (1981) Toxoplasmosis. *Archives of Disease in Childhood*, **56**, 494

Gamstorp, I. and Klockhoff, I. (1974) Bilateral, severe, sensorineural hearing loss after haemophilus influenzae meningitis in childhood. *Neuropädiatrie*, **5**, 121

Gordon, N. (1988) Myalgic encephalomyelitis. *Developmental Medicine and Child Neurology*, **30**, 677

Hanshaw, J.B. and Dudgeon, J.A. (1978) *Viral Diseases of the Fetus and Newborn*, W.B. Saunders, London

Karim, K.A. and Ludlam, G.B. (1975) Serological diagnosis of congenital toxoplasmosis. *Journal of Clinical Pathology*, **28**, 383

Klapper, P.E., Laing, I. and Longson, M. (1981) Rapid non-invasive diagnosis of herpes encephalitis. *Lancet*, **ii**, 607

Krech, U.H., Jung, M. and Jung, F. (1971) *Cytomegalovirus Infections of Man*, Karger, Basel

Kristiansen, B-E., Ask, E., Jenkins, A. *et al.* (1991) Rapid diagnosis of meningococcal meningitis by polymerase chain reaction. *Lancet*, **337**, 1568–9

Kristenssen, K., Olssen, Y. and Sourander, P. (1974) Virus encephalitis pathogenesis in the immature brain. *Developmental Medicine and Child Neurology*, **16**, 382

Liversedge, L.A. (1973) The clinical features of herpes simplex encephalitis (acute necrotising encephalitis). *Postgraduate Medical Journal*, **49**, 383

Longson, M. (1973) Immunofluorescence in the diagnosis of herpes encephalitis. *Postgraduate Medical Journal*, **49**, 403

Longson, M. and Bailey, A.S. (1978) Early diagnosis and treatment of virus infections of the nervous system. *The Practitioner*, **221**, 47

Lorber, J. (1974) Personal method of the treatment of haemophilus influenza meningitis in children. *Neuropädiatrie*, **5**, 353

Lorber, J. (1981) Antibiotic treatment of haemophilus influenzal type B meningitis: the problem of bacterial resistance. *Developmental Medicine and Child Neurology*, **23**, 531

MacDonald, H. and Towbin, J. O'H. (1978) Congenital cytomegalovirus infection: a collaborative study in epidemiological, clinical and laboratory findings. *Developmental Medicine and Child Neurology*, **20**, 471

Manson, J.I. and Thong, Y.H. (1980) Immunological abnormalities in the syndrome of poliomyelitis-like illness associated with acute bronchial asthma (Hopkins' syndrome). *Archives of Disease in Childhood*, **55**, 26

McKendry, J.B.J. and Bailey, J.D. (1973) Congenital varicella associated with multiple defects. *Canadian Medical Association Journal*, **108**, 66

Nahmias, A.J., Alford, C.A. and Korones, S.B. (1970) Infection of the newborn with herpes virus hominis. *Advances in Paediatrics*, **17**, 185

Ounsted, C. (1978) Preventing febrile convulsions. *Developmental Medicine and Child Neurology*, **20**, 799

Pampiglione, G. (1964) Prodromal phase of measles: some neurophysiological studies. *British Medical Journal*, **ii**, 1296

Peckham, C.S. (1989) Cytomegalovirus in the neonate. *Journal of Antimicrobial Chemotherapy*, **23**, Suppl. E, 17–21

Peckham, C.S., Martin, J.A.M., Marshall, W.C. and Dudgeon, J.A. (1979) Congenital rubellar deafness: a preventable disease. *Lancet*, **i**, 258

Peckham, C.S., Coleman, J.C., Hurley, R. *et al.* (1983) Cytomegalovirus infection in pregnancy: preliminary findings from a prospective study. *Lancet*, **i**, 1352

Peltola, H., Anttila, M. and Renkonen, O. (1989) Randomised comparison of chloramphenicol, ampicillin, cefotaxime, and ceftriaxone for childhood bacterial meningitis. *Lancet*, **i**, 1281

Perks, W.H., Mohr, P. and Liversedge, L.A. (1976) Demeclocycline in appropriate ADH syndrome. *Lancet*, **ii**, 1414

Pike, M.G., Kennedy, C.R., Neville, B.G.R. and Levin, M. (1991) Herpes simplex encephalitis with relapse. *Archives of Disease in Childhood*, **66**, 1242–4

Polak, A. and Wain, W.H. (1977) The influence of 5-fluorocytosine on nucleic acid synthesis in Candida albicans, Cryptococcus neoformans and Aspergillus fumigatus. *Chemotherapy*, **23**, 243

Preece, P.M., Pearle, K.N. and Peckham, C.S. (1984) Congenital cytomegalovirus infection. *Developmental Medicine and Child Neurology*, **59**, 1120

Ramsay, M.E.B., Miller, E. and Peckham, C.S. (1991) Outcome of confirmed symptomatic congenital cytomegalovirus infection. *Archives of Disease in Childhood*, **66**, 1068–9

Rich, A.T. and McCordock, H.A. (1933) The pathogenesis of tubercular meningitis. *Bulletin of the Johns Hopkins Hospital*, **52**, 5

Robinson, R.O. and Roberts, N. (1990a) Acute bacterial meningitis. I; diagnosis. *Developmental Medicine and Child Neurology*, **32**, 83

Robinson, R.O. and Roberts, N. (1990b) Acute bacterial meningitis. II; treatment. *Developmental Medicine and Child Neurology*, **32**, 174

Steele, J.C., Gladstone, R.M., Thanasophon, S. and Fleming, P.C. (1972) Acute cerebellar ataxia and concomitant infection with mycoplasma pneumoniae. *Journal of Pediatrics*, **80**, 467

Stern, H. and Tucker, S.M. (1973) Prospective study of cytomegalovirus infection in pregnancy. *British Medical Journal*, **ii**, 268

Stern, H., Hannington, G., Booth, J. and Moncrieff, D. (1986) An early marker of fetal infection after primary cytomegalovirus infection in pregnancy. *British Medical Journal*, **292**, 718

Tookey, P. and Peckham, C.S. (1991) Does cytomegalovirus present an occupational risk? *Archives of Disease in Childhood*, **66**, 1009–10

Townsend, J.J., Baringer, R.B., Wolinsky, J.S. *et al.* (1975) Progressive rubella panencephalitis. *New England Journal of Medicine*, **292**, 990

Upton, A. and Gumpert, J. (1970) Electroencephalography in diagnosis of herpes-simplex encephalitis. *Lancet*, **i**, 650

Venkat Raman, G. (1988) Meningococcal septicaemia and meningitis: a rising tide. *British Medical Journal*, **296**, 1141

Whitley, R.J. (1988) The frustrations of treating herpes simplex virus infections of the central nervous system. *Journal of the American Medical Association*, **259**, 1067

Whitley, R.J., Soong, S., Dolin, R. *et al.* (1977) Adenine arabinoside therapy of biopsy-proved herpes simplex encephalitis. *New England Journal of Medicine*, **297**, 289

Zu Rhein, G.M. and Chou, S.M. (1965) Particles resembling papova viruses in human cerebral demyelinating disease. *Science*, **148**, 1477

11   Degenerative cerebral diseases

The problem of a child suffering from a condition causing progressive mental and physical deterioration is fortunately rare, and for many such conditions there are no accurate estimates of frequency. But when a deteriorating condition does occur it is of supreme importance to the family involved. The process of establishing a definite diagnosis may be fraught with difficulty. Investigations will help to exclude treatable conditions, e.g. infections, space-occupying lesions and certain metabolic disorders, the last sometimes being identified by screening tests, such as amino acid chromatography. When these preliminary investigations are negative and the deterioration is pursuing a relentless course there are disorders of three main types that have to be considered: (1) the neuronal 'storage' diseases, in which substances accumulate in the neurons and destroy them; (2) the diseases which mainly affect myelin; and (3) 'encephalopathies', a group of conditions of doubtful or unknown aetiology.

The details of the clinical history can only be suggestive: frequent epileptic seizures, especially myoclonus, will favour a storage disease; the gradual development of spasticity, and of dementia, affecting visual and auditory perception and language function in particular, is sometimes the presenting feature of leucodystrophies; while certain encephalopathies, such as subacute sclerosing leucoencephalitis may start with psychiatric symptoms.

The clinical examination of the child may direct the investigations along certain lines; for example, the appearance of the child suggesting a disorder of mucopolysaccharide metabolism, abnormalities of the retina, a gangliosidosis, and hepato-splenomegaly, a form of Niemann-Pick or Gaucher's disease.

The EEG can also be helpful (Gloor, Kalabay and Giard, 1968). There is a definite relationship between bilaterally synchronous paroxysmal discharges and diffuse cortical and subcortical grey matter disease. In diseases involving the white matter the EEG may show continuous non-paroxysmal slow-wave activity, and when both grey and white matter are affected there is likely to be bilaterally synchronous paroxysmal discharges, as well as a marked increase of slow-wave activity.

As will be seen, a number of simple tests, such as raised acid phosphatase level in the neurological form of Gaucher's disease, vacuolated lymphocytes in the gangliosidoses, and metachromatic granules sometimes found in the cells from urinary deposits among those with leucodystrophy may suggest the diagnosis of these conditions.

It has now become possible to identify the lack of an increasing number of enzymes in leucocytes and cultured fibroblasts from patients with suspected cerebral diseases and thus prove the diagnosis. These include: β-galactosidase (Gm_1 gangliosidosis); hexosaminidase (Gm_2 gangliosidosis); glucocerebrosidase (Gaucher's disease); sphingomyelinase (Niemann-Pick disease); arylsulphatase A (metachromatic leuco-

Table 11.1   Degenerative cerebral diseases

Disease	Suggestive symptoms and signs	Main diagnostic tests
Gangliosidoses	Epilepsy, especially myoclonus, an early symptom Cherry red spot at macula Neurological deterioration usually rapid Abnormal appearance suggesting Hurler's syndrome in Gm_1 gangliosidosis	Blood-various enzyme deficiencies in peripheral leucocytes
Neuronal ceroid lipofuscinosis (Batten's disease)	Major and minor (myoclonic) epileptic seizures responding poorly to treatment Neurological deterioration variable in rate Visual symptoms first in juvenile type Pigmentary retinal changes	Blood-vacuolated lymphocytes common but non-specific finding Ultrastuctural changes may be typical EEG-infantile type rapidly becomes flat Late infantile type—photosensitivity to very slow rate of flicker Cortical biopsy—neurons distended by granules staining for ceroid and lipofuscin
Metachromatic leucodystrophy	Most frequent age of onset—late infancy Tendon reflexes may be absent	Urine-metachromatic granules in deposit Blood-deficiency of arylsulphatase A in peripheral leucocytes CSF-markedly raised protein level Nerve conduction studies—delayed conduction
Gaucher's disease	Enlarged liver and spleen with neurological abnormalities	Blood-increased level of acid phosphatase suggestive Deficiency of glucocerebrosidase in peripheral leucocytes
Niemann-Pick's disease	Enlarged liver and spleen with neurological abnormalities	Blood-deficiency of sphingomyelinase in peripheral leucocytes in acute infantile form Bone marrow—abnormal cells Biopsy-brain and viscera—accumulation of sphingomyelin and cholesterol
Mucopolysaccharidoses	Abnormal appearance of the child and progressive deterioration Corneal clouding, kyphosis, hepatomegaly in Hurler-Hunter syndrome	Urine-excess excretion of various mucopolysaccharides X-rays of bones-typical abnormalities Cultured fibroblasts—enzyme deficiencies

Table 11.1   Degenerative cerebral diseases (*continued*)

Disease	Suggestive symptoms and signs	Main diagnostic tests
Schilder's disease (diffuse cerebral sclerosis) to include adrenoleucodystrophy	Central blindness or deafness Bronzing of skin in adrenoleucodystrophy (Addison Schilder's disease)	EEG-dominated by excess slow wave activity No diagnostic test apart from CT scan, MRI and conjunctival biopsy, and in adrenoleucodystrophy tests of adrenal function and increased plasma levels of very long chain fatty acids
Globoid cell leucodystrophy-Krabbe's disease	Onset in first few months of life Bouts of fever and screening Upper motor neuron lesion, but absent tendon jerks	Blood-deficiency of galactocerebroside β-galactosidase in peripheral leucocytes Cerebrospinal fluid-protein level markedly raised Nerve conduction studies delayed conduction
Spongy sclerosis Canavan's disease	Enlargement of head Progressive deterioration	Raised plasma levels and increased excretion of *n*-asetylaspartic acid. CT scan and ultrasonography
Fibrinoid leucodystrophy-Alexander type	Enlargement of head Progressive deterioration	No diagnostic test apart from cerebral biopsy, CT scan and MRI
Pelizaeus-Mertzbacher's disease	Sex-linked inheritance Nystagmus an early sign	No diagnostic test apart from cerebral biopsy, CT scan and MRI
Reye's syndrome	Evidence of cerebral and hepatic involvement at the same time	No definite diagnostic tests, but hypoglycaemia and raised blood ammonia level suggestive
Subacute necrotizing encephalomyelopathy of Leigh	Evidence of brain-stem involvement Respiratory symptoms Fluctuating course	Urine-inhibitory factor to thiamine triphosphate Blood-raised levels of pyruvate and lactate suggestive Fibroblast culture—sometimes deficiency of pyruvate dehydrogenase Liver biopsy-sometimes deficiency of pyruvate carboxylase
Subacute sclerosing pan-encephalitis	Myoclonus Extrapyramidal syndromes Measles often contracted before the age of 18 months	Blood and CSF-high antibody titres against measles CSF-paretic Lange curve EEG-periodic discharges of slow and sharp waves

dystrophy); and galacto-cerebroside-β galactosidase (Krabbe's disease). Also, a deficiency of such enzymes in cells from the amniotic fluid may enable a prenatal diagnosis to be made, resulting, if necessary, in a termination of the pregnancy. This test cannot be performed before the 14th to 16th week of gestation, but with the use of the recently introduced chorionic villus sampling information can be obtained during the 8th and 12th week of gestation (Kingston, 1989).

Occasionally an exact diagnosis can be made only by examining biopsy material, but this is rarely necessary now that enzyme estimations are possible. Skin, muscle and rectal biopsies can be used in the diagnosis of a number of cerebral diseases, including the various types of neuronal ceroid lipofuscinosis, infantile neuroaxonal dystrophy, Lafora's disease (muscle fibres contain PAS and peroxidase positive granules), and the Kearns-Sayre's syndrome (ragged red fibres) and Canavan's disease (Brett and Lake, 1975; Carpenter *et al.*, 1977). Particular attention is now being paid to conjunctival biopsies because of their rich content of nerves (Libert *et al.*, 1977). A cortical biopsy very rarely has to be considered, except in situations such as suspected herpes simplex encephalitis and a possible demyelinating disorder. When examined histologically (especially with the electron microscope) and biochemically, biopsies will enable a diagnosis to be made in a high percentage of a variety of diseases (Cumings, 1960). Advising this investigation needs very careful consideration and is always an individual problem. The test may enable an exact diagnosis to be made, but, with very few exceptions (e.g. herpes simplex encephalitis), does not lead to treatment. However, if further advances are to be made in this field exact diagnoses are essential; they may make the distress of the parents a little easier for them to bear if the actual cause is known; and they often do enable genetic advice to be given. This is essential when advising parents whose child has developed such a serious illness as those about to be described; the inheritance in so many instances being of an autosomal recessive type. These biopsies very rarely cause complications of any kind, and if the patients are carefully selected for this investigation mainly on the basis of a definite deterioration of their condition and after other tests have proved negative, it may well yield positive information (Wilson, 1972).

Even after the most detailed investigations there will be some conditions, such as Hallervorden-Spatz disease and dystonia musculorum deformans, in which the diagnosis remains a clinical one, only to be confirmed at *post mortem* examination. Table 11.1 lists some of the diseases considered in this chapter, their symptoms, signs and diagnostic tests.

Neuronal storage diseases

In the neuronal storage diseases a disorder of metabolism due to deficient enzyme activity results in the neurons being unable to get rid of certain substances, which thus accumulate in the cells and destroy them. As most of the diseases manifest themselves, not at birth, but after a few years of normal development, there must presumably be an enzyme deficiency rather than a complete lack (Table 11.2). The mode of inheritance is autosomal recessive.

The classification of the various types of so-called amaurotic family idiocy on an age-dependent basis was never satisfactory. The use of eponyms may have been necessary when these conditions were first being described, and knowledge was confined to clinical and histological descriptions. Now that the biochemistry of these disorders is beginning to be elicited it is possible to start with a more sensible method

Table 11.2

Disease	Alternative title	Enzyme deficiency
Gm$_1$ gangliosidosis	Pseudo-Hurler's disease	Type 1 β-galactosidase ABC Type 2 β-galactosidase BC
Gm$_2$ gangliosidosis	Tay-Sachs' disease Sandhoff's disease Juvenile Gm$_2$ gangliosidosis Juvenile Sandhoff's disease	Type 1 hexosaminidase A Type 2 hexosaminidase A and B Type 3 partial deficiency Hexosaminidase A Type 4 hexosaminidase B and partial deficiency Hexosaminidase A
Gm$_3$ gangliosidosis	—	Acetylgalactosaminyl transferase
Neuronal ceroid lipofuscinosis	Batten's disease	Peroxidase (as yet unproven)
Metachromatic leucodystrophy	Sulphatide lipidosis	Cerebroside sulphatase (arylsulphatase A)
Gaucher's disease	—	Glucocerebrosidase
Niemann-Pick's disease	four sub-groups	Sphingomyelinase

of classification. The clinical manifestations of these conditions may vary slightly from one to another, and the factor of age will also play a part, but the differences are not sufficient to separate them on these grounds alone. The dementia is usually, but not always, progressive, and in some patients personality changes may predominate. Motor disturbances include dystonia, involuntary movements, ataxia and spastic quadraplegia. Visual symptoms and signs are not always present, and can vary, even within a single disease. Seizures are common, and are usually of a myoclonic or grand mal type.

The gangliosidoses

Among the sphingolipidoses, one of the most commonest types is *Gm$_2$ gangliosidosis type 1*, or *Tay-Sachs' disease*. The onset is in infancy, and the disease is due to a deficiency of the isoenzyme hexosaminidase A (Okada and O'Brien, 1969), resulting in an accumulation of Gm$_2$ ganglioside in the cells. The lack of this enzyme may enable a prenatal diagnosis to be made on cells collected by amniocentesis or chorionic villus sampling (Schneck *et al.*, 1970). Also, the condition can sometimes be related to an absence of both hexosaminidase A and B, *Gm$_2$ gangliosidosis type 2 (Sandhoff's disease)*. There are usually no clinical distinctions, but an aminoglycolipid known as 'globoside' accumulates in the peripheral tissues (Sandhoff, Andreae and Jatzkewitz, 1968). Many of the affected children with the Type 1 disease are of Ashkenazi Jewish descent, but not those with the Type 2 disease. The baby ceases to develop, becomes increasingly inactive, and begins to show signs of pyramidal and extrapyramidal lesions. Epileptic seizures become increasingly frequent and vision is impaired. The cherry red spot at the macula is a frequent finding. At the margins of the fovea the ganglion cells are reduced in number and are mixed with large phagocytes, while the

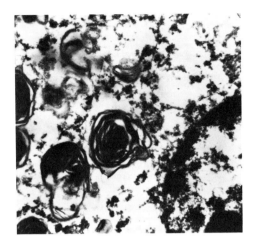

Figure 11.1   Gm$_2$ gangliosidosis: electron microscopy showing membranous cytoplasmic bodies.

inner and outer nuclear layers are unaffected. This results in the normal colour of the fovea being accentuated by a white flare. This whitish ring is caused by the increased opacity of the tissues due to lipid infiltration. The thinning of the nerve cell layer around the fovea may also make the red of the choriocapillary layer more evident. Physical and mental deterioration is progressive, and it is not long before the child is completely helpless. Atypical cases of juvenile Sandhoff's disease presenting with ataxia have been reported (MacCleod *et al.*, 1977).

At autopsy the brain tends to be larger than normal due to oedema of the white matter. The histology of biopsy material or of the brain *post mortem* is characterized by marked distension of most of the ganglion cells of the brain and spinal cord. The oedematous white matter may show evidence of demyelination. The appearances on electron microscopy are also typical, especially the membranous cytoplasmic bodies (Fig. 11.1). These are made up of concentric dark and pale bands, probably of myelin structure (Gonatas, Cambetti and Baird, 1968).

Gm$_2$ gangliosidosis includes many of the group described as 'infantile amaurotic idiocy'. A probable example of *juvenile Gm$_2$ gangliosidosis type 3* has now been reported (Suzuki *et al.*, 1970). The patient developed personality changes and dementia at about the age of 6 years, and this was followed by seizures, and cerebellar, extrapyramidal and pyramidal signs. The chemical abnormalities were qualitatively identical to those of Tay-Sachs' disease, although quantitatively milder. The total ganglioside content in the grey matter was twice normal. It is not known whether this patient represents a new disease or merely a variant of the infantile form with the same enzymatic defect. Examples of late infantile and juvenile Sandhoff's disease have also been described (Felding and Hultberg, 1978). The deterioration of these children has not been so rapid as in Gm$_2$ gangliosidosis, so it seems possible that this, and the later age of onset, may be due to a lesser degree of enzyme deficiency; a partial deficiency of hexosaminidase A in juvenile Gm$_2$ gangliosidosis, and a partial deficiency of hexosaminidase A and an absence of hexosaminidase B in juvenile Sandoff's disease. Also a type of Gm$_2$ gangliosidosis in Ashkenazi Jews which resembles Friedreich's ataxia has been described (Willner *et al.*, 1981).

Gm$_3$ gangliosidosis has also been identified, with rapidly progressive mental and motor retardation starting in the second year of life (Raine, 1970). The appearance of the infant is suggestive of gargoylism, and death occurs at around 3 years of age, with an accumulation of Gm_3 ganglioside in the liver and brain. It is suggested that there is a defect of ganglioside biosynthesis, sugar moieties not being added to Gm_3 to synthesize larger gangliosides. Acetylgalactosaminyl transferase has been found to be absent (Max *et al.*, 1974).

Mucolipidoses

Gm_1 gangliosidosis with an onset from birth onwards shows an accumulation of Gm_1 ganglioside in the cells of the brain and viscera. In Gm_1 gangliosidosis there is also an accumulation of an abnormal acid mucopolysaccharide, resembling keratin sulphate in the generalized form (type 1). A deficiency of β-galactosidase A, B and C has been demonstrated (O'Brien, 1969a). These children may be thought to have gargoylism or Hunter's syndrome, and a number of different terms has been used to describe them. These include pseudo-Hurler's disease, familial neurovisceral lipidosis, and Landing's disease. These children are usually retarded from birth and become increasingly weak and inco-ordinate. There is frontal bossing, a depressed nasal bridge, large low-set ears, hypertrophied gums, a large tongue and kyphosis may develop. The hands are broad and the fingers short and stubby. There may be a cherry red spot at the macula, and the liver and spleen become palpable. Deterioration is rapid, with increasingly frequent epileptic seizures, and death usually occurs before the age of 2 years. The X-ray findings include beaking of the lumbar vertebrae at the site of the kyphosis, widening of the long-bones, elongation of the sella turcica, and flaring of the ilia. The urine shows a normal excretion of acid mucopolysaccharides. The findings on light

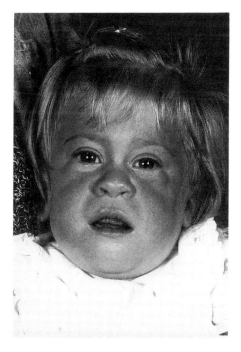

Figure 11.2   Child with I-cell disease.

and electron microscopy are similar to those in Gm_2 gangliosidosis. There is also at least one other form of Gm_1 gangliosidosis or type II, in which only cerebral symptoms occur (Klint, Dacremont and Vlientinck, 1968), and in this disease there is an absence of β-galactosidase B and C (O'Brien, 1969b). Early development is normal, but progressive deterioration starts in the second year of life. Death has been recorded between the ages of 3 and 10 years. There are usually no visceral and skeletal abnormalities, but if they do occur they are mild.

Type I Gm_1 gangliosidosis is an example of a group of conditions sometimes referred to as the 'mucolipidoses', as they exhibit symptoms and signs of both the sphingolipidoses and the mucopolysaccharidoses (Spranger and Wiedemann, 1970). Other examples include fucosidosis, mannosidosis and the four types of muco-lipidosis; known as ML I neuraminidase deficiency, divided into sialidosis I, II and III (the first is also known as the cherry red spot myoclonus syndrome), ML II lipo-mucopolysaccharidosis or I-cell disease (Fig. 11.2) (Gordon, 1973), and ML III pseudopolydystrophy or pseudo-Hurler's disease and ML IV. All these conditions are associated with varying degrees of psychomotor retardation, gargoyle-like appearance and dysostosis. They are probably all genetically determined, and most of them are associated with an inborn error of metabolism. I-cell disease due to a deficit of neuraminidase (Strecker *et al.*, 1976) must be suspected if there is strong evidence of gargoylism in the first 6 months of life. Gum hyperplasia is a very typical feature. Prenatal diagnosis of I-cell disease is possible by measuring altered alpha mannosidase activity in the amniotic fluid (Owada *et al.*, 1980). The main link between these various syndromes does seem to be the appearance of the children, and the term *pseudo-Hurler's syndrome* is often used (Gordon, 1978a). Mucosulphatidosis, referred to later, is another condition presenting in this way, and so are children with Hurler-like disorders; Winchester's syndrome, and Kniest's syndrome (Kelly, 1976). Also, it should not be forgotten that children on long-term treatment with phenytoin and those born of mothers taking phenytoin during pregnancy develop coarse facies.

Neuronal ceroid lipofuscinosis (Batten's disease)

There is increasing evidence that most of the children classified as having late infantile amaurotic idiocy (Janski-Bielschowski) have a disorder at present classified under the term 'neuronal ceroid lipofuscinosis', which is not a lipid storage disease. Batten (1903) may have been the first to describe this condition. The clinical picture and the routine histological findings are somewhat similar, but the main point of distinction from the diseases so far considered is the normal sphingolipid profile on thin layer chromatography of brain extracts. The age of onset may vary from infancy to adult life, but seems to remain constant within a single family, the mode of inheritance being autosomal recessive. So far three main types can be recognized; the infantile, late infantile and juvenile. The gene for the infantile form has been mapped to chromosome 1 and for the juvenile form to chromosome 16. The course of the disease varies considerably from a few months to many years; in fact the lack of change in the patient's condition suggests occasionally that the disease process has been arrested (Zeman and Dyken, 1969). The initial symptoms in the late infantile type (Janski-Bielschowski), which is the most common form in most countries, can be visual, epileptic, mental, behavioural or motor, with an onset from 18 months to 3 years, or even later. The clinical and histological spectrum of this disease can be wide (Santavuori *et al.*, 1991).

Visual signs are not always present, but typically consist of optic atrophy,

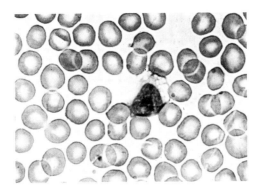

Figure 11.3   Neuronal ceroid lipofuscinosis (Batten's disease). Vacuolated lymphocyte in the peripheral blood—a non-specific finding although a common one in this disease.

attenuated retinal vessels, macular degeneration of the granular type, and pigmentation in the peripheral parts of the retina. Epileptic seizures are an integral part of the condition, often starting as generalized convulsions to be superseded by myoclonus, which becomes generalized and can develop into myoclonic status lasting for days on end. The frequency of the fits may be related to the severity of the cerebral degeneration. The dementia is usually but not always progressive, and in some patients personality changes predominate. Motor disturbances include dystonia, involuntary movements, ataxia and spastic quadraplegia.

The infantile type of neuronal ceroid lipofuscinosis has been described most frequently in Finland. Its onset is between the ages of 8 and 18 months, with rapid psychomotor deterioration, ataxia and hypotonia. Myoclonus is a particular feature, but convulsions are rare. Blindness is usual by the age of 2 years, with optic atrophy and retinal dystrophy (Santavuori *et al.*, 1973). The infantile type appears to be due to a disorder of fatty acid (linoleic acid) metabolism, and it has been suggested that it be called *polyunsaturated fatty acid lipidosis* (Svennerholm *et al.*, 1975). The diagnosis can be made by finding a raised level of arachidonic acid in the serum (Hagberg *et al.*, 1974).

The juvenile type (Spielmeyer-Vogt) usually starts with failing vision, optic atrophy and retinal pigmentation. It may be a number of years before neurological abnormalities appear with a typical Parkinsonian picture, and progression is usually slow. The metabolic defect in this type may involve the linolenic family of fatty acids, with a reduction of docosahexaemic acid in the leucocytes of affected patients (Pullarkat, Patel and Brockerhoff, 1978).

On the examination of a blood film the lymphocytes often show vacuoles (Fig. 11.3), and the neutrophils show azurophilic hypergranulation, but these are non-specific changes (Strouth, Zeman and Meritt, 1966). The EEG can show a number of interesting features: in most cases there are bursts of slow waves and irregular spike and wave complexes. At times the diffuse epileptic activity may be almost continuously present throughout the record and can be asymmetrical. An abnormal sensitivity to photic stimulation at a flash frequency of 2–5 per second is found in the late infantile type (Fig. 11.4). In the infantile type, the EEG rapidly becomes isoelectric, and there is an absence of sleep spindles.

Macroscopically there is cerebral atrophy with thinning of the cortex, as opposed to the megalencephaly characteristic of Gm_1 gangliosidosis. Microscopically there is a

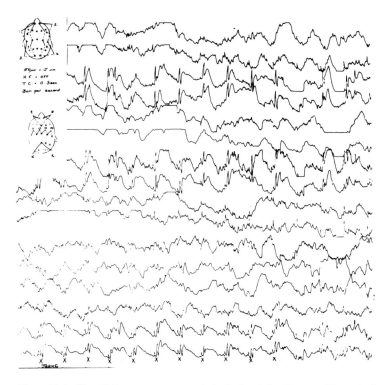

Figure 11.4   Slow flicker response seen only in the late infantile type of Batten's disease.

severe loss of neurons, and the surviving ones are swollen by granules which stain with Sudan Black B and periodic acid-Schiff (PAS) (Fig. 11.5), and give positive reactions with all stains for ceroid or lipofuscin. The findings on electron microscopy differ from those in Gm_1 and Gm_2 gangliosidosis. In the infantile type there is usually a homogeneous, finely granular appearance; in the late infantile type there is most often

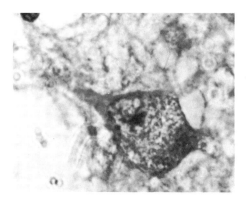

Figure 11.5   Neuronal ceroid lipofuscinosis (Batten's disease). Neuron showing swollen vacuolated cytoplasm.

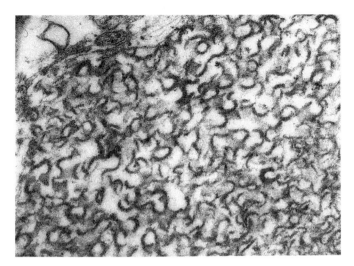

Figure 11.6   Neuron from patient with late infantile type of neuronal ceroid lipofuscinosis showing curvilinear pattern. Electron microscopy × 40 000.

a curvilinear pattern (Fig. 11.6); and in the juvenile type it is often finger-print like (Fig. 11.7). These varied pictures strongly suggest that this is indeed a syndrome of varying aetiology (Gonatas, Cambetti and Baird, 1968; Gordon, Marsden and Noronha, 1972). There is widespread degeneration of the rod and cone cells and the

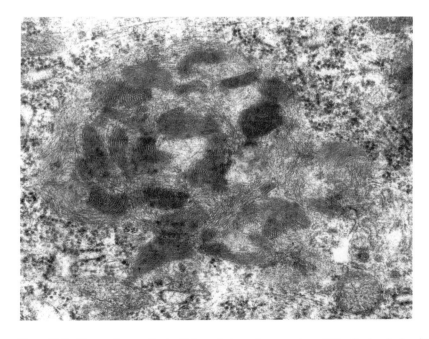

Figure 11.7   Neuron from patient with juvenile type of neuronal ceroid lipofuscinosis showing finger-print pattern. Electron microscopy × 40 000. Photograph courtesy of Professor B. D. Lake

pigment epithelial layer of the retina, whilst the ganglionic cell layer remains relatively preserved.

It is instructive that neuronal ceroid lipofuscinosis with its normal ganglioside pattern has remained hidden so long among conditions which are undoubtedly disorders of lipid metabolism. As Zeman and Dyken (1969) suggest, an unknown, genetically-determined defect may damage the neurons, and in those that survive there may be an accumulation of lipopigments (ageing pigments), the quantity of which is known to bear a relationship to the age of the individual. This may be a secondary phenomenon and possibly related to an inability to get rid of waste products or to an increased rate of production, although no doubt the accumulation of these pigments will eventually damage the cell. In the case of the late infantile and juvenile types a deficiency of peroxidase has been suggested (Armstrong, Dimmitt and van Wornier, 1974), but seems unlikely. Recent studies have shown an accumulation of dolichols and retinoid compounds which are involved in the synthesis of glycoproteins. An inability to recycle neuronal and retinal membrane glycoproteins could be the underlying metabolic defect (Santavuori, 1988). In the juvenile type there may be a failure to synthesize 'very low density lipoprotein', leading to a failure of membrane repair. A marked reduction in the fatty acid content of circulating blood cell membranes has been found, and giving dietary supplements of certain fatty acids may be of benefit.

Until the cause of neuronal ceroid lipofuscinosis has been identified with more certainty it may be worth trying to influence the accumulation of the 'ageing pigments' by large doses of vitamin E (Abrahams et al., 1964), or by giving drugs such as meclofenoxate hydrochloride. It has been claimed that if the condition is caused by a disorder of peroxidation its course can be favourably influenced by treatment, but no long-term follow-up study is available and personal experience has not been encouraging. Treatment consists of a daily dose of 2 g vitamin E and 200 mg butylated hydroxytoluene as antioxidants, 1 g DL methione as a radical scavenger, and 0.5 g vitamin C as a hydrogen donor (Zeman, 1974). Antioxidant treatment with vitamins E and C and selenium has also been proposed (Santavuori et al., 1985).

Metachromatic leucodystrophy (sulphatide lipidosis)

There are a number of other disorders of sphingolipid metabolism which present a somewhat different clinical picture. The first of these, metachromatic leucodystrophy, can start at almost any age, but most frequently starts in infancy, and different forms have been distinguished according to the age of onset. The course of the disease may be prolonged, especially in the juvenile and adult varieties, when the initial symptoms can be of a psychogenic type. In the late infantile type the clinical picture is sufficiently typical to at least suggest the diagnosis. Hagberg (1963) has divided the course of this illness into four stages. In stage 1 there are signs of a polyradiculitis and of an upper motor neuron lesion. In stage 2 there is progressive dementia and the paralysis increases, often with a change from hypotonia to hypertonia. The tendon reflexes can be increased or decreased and the plantar response is extensor. Pain in the limbs, ataxia, ocular palsies, and speech disorders may occur. In stage 3 (Fig. 11.8) myoclonus is frequent, as is hyperpyrexia. The physical and mental deterioration becomes profound and impaired vision is obvious. In Stage 4 the child is completely disabled, and bulbar symptoms are marked. The onset can be from birth to adult life, and the illness may last from weeks to years. There is evidence of a recessive mode of inheritance. There is another variety of metachromatic leucodystrophy first described

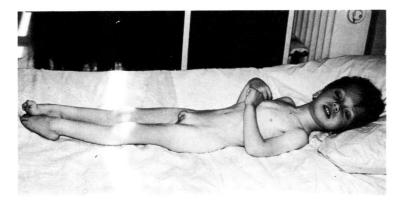

Figure 11.8   Child in stage 3 of metachromatic leudocystrophy (decorticate posture).

in 1965 (Austin, Armstrong and Shearer, 1965) and now referred to as *mucosulphatidosis* or *multiple sulphatase deficiency*. The child's facial appearance is suggestive of gargoylism. Development is slow and soon starts to regress with myoclonic seizures. The muscles become spastic, but with diminished reflexes due to a peripheral neuropathy. On X-ray examination there are globoid vertebral bodies and shortening, swelling and proximal pointing of the metacarpals. Increased amounts of sulphatides are found in the urine, as well as an excess of dermatan sulphate. There is raised cerebrospinal fluid protein and delayed conduction in the peripheral nerves. There is lack of arylsulphatase A, B and C in the liver, kidney and brain, and the multiple deficiency leads to an accumulation of many types of sulphate ester, including cerebroside sulphate and polysaccharides resembling dermatan and heparan sulphate (Ray, 1977).

The evidence of peripheral nerve involvement in metachromatic leucodystrophy can be confirmed by nerve conduction studies and nerve biopsy (Yudell *et al.*, 1967). The other suggestive finding is a pronounced increase in the protein level of the cerebrospinal fluid which also occurs in Krabbe's globoid cell leucodystrophy. Metachromatic granules can be found in the cells of the urinary deposit, but this is non-specific; although it may be possible to identify the sulphatide in the urine by chromatographic techniques (Hagberg, 1963). A deficiency of arylsulphatase A activity can be demonstrated in the leucocytes, but it is difficult to be sure if this is always diagnostic (Raine, 1970). It has become evident that there can be a wide variation in the clinical manifestations of this disease, and some affected children with a lowered serum level of the enzyme and a positive nerve biopsy may only be disabled by a very slowly progressive dementia and epilepsy. In these instances the lowered enzyme level may be due to a phenotype different from the one for the late infantile form of metachromatic leucodystrophy, or to coding for an enzyme with reduced activity, a pseudodeficiency (Kihara *et al.*, 1980).

Histological examination at autopsy will show marked demyelination in the cerebrum and cerebellum. Metachromatic material is often found in the neurons, especially in the basal ganglion and brain-stem and in the glial cells; as well as in the cells of the liver, kidney, lymph nodes and other organs (Hagberg, Somrander and Svennerholm, 1962). Loss of oligodendroglia is particularly marked in the late infantile type. There may be a failure in the anabolism of myelin in this disease, which results in intracellular storage of sulphatides (cerebroside sulphate) (Norman, 1962). Impaired metabolism within the oligodendrocytes, the cells responsible for the nutrition of the myelinated axons, could well be due to a deficiency of the enzyme complex cerebroside sulphatase, including arylsulphatase A (Pilz, 1970).

Gaucher's disease

Certain other diseases, more notable for their visceral manifestations, may also show cerebral involvement. The *cerebral form of Gaucher's disease* can present in the early years of life, or later, with hepatosplenomegaly, bone marrow depression, and mental and physical deterioration, associated with epilepsy. Cells in various parts of the body, including the brain, are distended by glucocerebroside, there being a deficiency of glucocerebrosidase which splits it into its component parts. The course of the disease is more often acute than chronic. The diagnosis may be suggested by an increased level of acid phosphatase in the serum, and by the appearance of distended cells obtained by bone marrow puncture. It will be confirmed by biochemical tests on biopsy specimens (Pilz, 1970); and a deficiency of glucocerebrosidase has been demonstrated in peripheral leucocytes (Sengers *et al.*, 1975).

Niemann-Pick disease

The cerebral form of Niemann-Pick's disease can present a similar clinical picture. A number of different types of this disease have been described, starting at any age up to adult life. Crocker (1961) suggested four groups, based on clinical and biochemical findings. In the most common—*type A*— the onset is early in life, with enlargement of the liver and spleen, physical and mental deterioration, and epileptic seizures. Spasticity, inco-ordination and dyskinesias may occur, and there is sometimes a cherry red spot at the macula. In *type B*, or the chronic form, the nervous system is not involved. In *type C*, or the juvenile form, the manifestations are similar to those in group A, but of later onset and slower course. Prenatal diagnosis is a possibility in this group by demonstrating abnormalities in intracellular processing of exogenous cholesterol in chorionic villus cells (Vanier *et al.*, 1989). In the fourth— *type D*—or the *Nova Scotian variety*, there are neurological symptoms of fairly late onset, but the biochemical disorder is different from the other groups. Circulating lymphocytes are vacuolated, and large 'foam cells' are found in the bone-marrow, liver and spleen. There is no storage of sphingomyelin in the brain or liver in types C or D.

There appears to be a deficiency of sphingomyelinase in groups A and B, and an intracellular accumulation of sphingomyelin and cholesterol in the brain and viscera. In group C, only the cholesterol may be increased in the cells of the brain (Crocker and Farber, 1958). There seems to be no doubt about the intracellular translocation of exogenous cholesterol, but the exact role of the cholesterol transport defect in the pathogenesis of Niemann-Pick type C is uncertain (Vanier *et al.*, 1991). The findings in the Nova Scotian group have not yet been definitely established (Pilz, 1970).

Doubts are now cast on this classification which appears over-simplified. Group C appears to include a number of conditions, some of which are characterized by foam cells in the bone marrow which stain blue with haematein, the so-called 'sea-blue histiocytes'.

Neurovisceral storage disease with vertical supranuclear ophthalmoplegia is a distinctive feature of one group showing these cells in the bone marrow (Neville *et al.*, 1973). In another there is a progressive encephalopathy with accumulation of lactose in an enlarged spleen. The activity of β-galactosidase is reduced (Hagberg *et al.*, 1978). In some other children in this group there is a reduction of both β-galactosidase and sphingomyelinase, or the properties of sphingomyelinase may be slightly altered. Recently it has been suggested that some of the conditions included in group C, such as the ophthalmoplegic type, are due to disturbed transport of several lysosomal enzymes from the ribosome to the lysosome, leading to lysosomal storage (Frank and Lasson, 1985).

Disorders of mucopolysaccharide (proteoglycan) metabolism— mucopolysaccharidoses

These disorders present in a variety of ways (Table 11.3), and some are undoubtedly progressive with involvement of the CNS. All have an autosomal recessive mode of inheritance, except Hunter's syndrome which is sex-linked recessive. Reference to these disorders has been made in Chapter 5.

The diagnosis is first suggested by the appearance of the patient. In Hurler's syndrome or *gargoylism* (Fig. 11.9) there is an excess of dermatan and heparan sulphate in the urine. The head is large, the bridge of the nose flattened, the tip broad with wide nostrils, and the lips and tongue are large with the mouth often held open. Growth is stunted and there is a marked kyphosis. There is shortening of the neck, deformity of the thorax, and protuberance of the abdomen. The hands are broad and the fingers shortened. Coxa valga, talipes and genu valgum are commonly seen, and

Table 11.3 Mucopolysaccharidoses

Syndromes	Inheritance	Excess urinary MPS	Enzyme deficiency
Hurler's syndrome MPS IH	Recessive	Dermatan sulphate Heparan sulphate	α-L-iduronidase
Scheie's syndrome MPS IS	Recessive	Dermatan sulphate	α-L-iduronidase
Hunter's syndrome MPS II	Sex-linked	Dermatan sulphate Heparan sulphate	Sulpho-iduronate-sulphatase
Sanfilippo syndrome MPS III	A Recessive	Heparan sulphate	Heparan sulphate N-sulphatase
	B Recessive	Heparan sulphate	N-acetyl-α-D-glucosaminidase
	C Recessive	Heparan sulphate	Acetyl CoA-α-glucosaminide-N-acetyl transferase
	D Recessive	Heparan sulphate	N-acetylglucosamine-6-sulphate sulphatase
Morquio syndrome MPS IV	Recessive	Keratan sulphate	Chondroitin-sulphate-N-acetyl-hexosamine-sulphate-6-sulphatase
Maroteaux-Lamy syndrome MPS VI	Recessive	Dermatan sulphate	Arylsulphatase-B
Sly's syndrome MPS VII	Recessive	Dermatan sulphate	β-glucuronidase

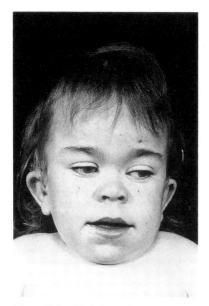

Figure 11.9   Hurler's syndrome.

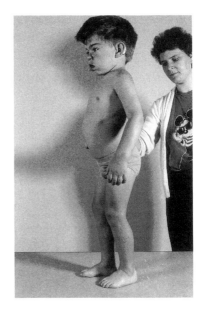

Figure 11.10   Hunter's syndrome.

there may be marked stiffness of the joints. Mental retardation becomes increasingly manifest, and the liver and spleen gradually enlarge. In Hunter's syndrome, deterioration tends to be slower but there is both a severe and mild form (Fig. 11.10). The clouding of the cornea, the lumbar gibbus, and the cardiovascular complications so typical of Hurler's syndrome do not occur. Also, deafness is more common in

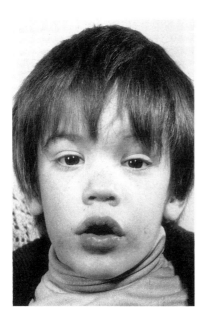

Figure 11.11   Sanfilippo syndrome.

Hunter's syndrome, and nodular skin lesions may be present (McCusick, 1972). Abnormalities on X-ray examination include a long and shallow sella turcica, wedge-shaped deformities of the bodies of vertebrae with anterior beaking, and shortening and deformity of the phalangeal bones. Hurler's syndrome (MPS IH) is due to diminished activity of α-L-iduronidase (Dorfman, 1972), and Hunter's syndrome (MPS II) to a deficiency of sulpho-iduronate-sulphatase (Eto *et al.*, 1974).

In the *Sanfilippo syndrome* (Sanfilippo *et al.*, 1963) (Fig. 11.11) the intellect deteriorates fairly rapidly and deafness is common, but the patient's height is usually normal and there is no clouding of the cornea, although retinitis pigmentosa may lead to blindness. The liver and spleen are only slightly enlarged, and there are few X-ray changes except for thickening of the vault of the skull. Also cardiovascular complications are unlikely to occur. There is an excess of heparan sulphate only in the urine. On the basis of enzyme studies this syndrome can be divided into types MPS III, A, B, C and D. The first results from impaired activity of heparan sulphate N-sulphatase, and the second of N-acetyl-α-D-glucosaminidase. A type C has been identified, due to a deficiency of acetyl CoA-α-glucosaminide-N-acetyl transferase, and a type D to lack of N-acetylglucosamine-6-sulphate sulphatase. Other syndromes; *Morquio, Scheie's* and *Maroteaux-Lamy*: show little if any impairment of intellectual functions. It is possible that some examples of Sly's syndrome (MPS VII) may be severely retarded (Sly *et al.*, 1973).

Mental deterioration is particularly marked in some cases of the Sanfilippo syndrome. As in other neuronal storage diseases, the cause of this is related to the distension of nerve cells which is usually conspicuous. There is evidence that the material stored by the neurons differs from the substance present in the liver and other organs. Mucopolysaccharides are found in the liver, but the substance stored in the neurons is partly a soluble lipid compound, probably ganglioside (Gordon and Thursby-Pelham, 1969). In Hurler's syndrome, extensive deposits can occur in the intima of the coronary arteries; these can lead to thrombosis and the sudden death that sometimes occurs among these patients. The carpal tunnel syndrome is a common complication of the mucopolysaccharidoses, and of the mucolipidoses (Wraith and Alani, 1990). The diagnosis of these syndromes is confirmed by the pattern of excess mucopolysaccharide excretion in the urine and the demonstration of enzyme deficiencies in cultured fibroblasts. Prenatal diagnosis may be possible, and in Hunter's syndrome it has been reported that this can be made as early as the ninth week of pregnancy by biochemical analysis of the chorionic villi cells, and termination of pregnancy offered (Kleijer *et al.*, 1984). A variety of therapies have been attempted. The possibility of replacing the missing enzyme in some of these disorders by transfusions of leucocytes is one, but it seems that this can have only a transient effect (Knudson, Ferrante and Curtis, 1971). Organ transplants are a way of ensuring a supply of a missing enzyme (Raine, 1975). Bone marrow transplantations are already giving encouraging results in children with Hurler's syndrome (Hugh-Jones, 1986).

Disorders of myelin

Myelin may suffer from a variety of noxious agents: toxic, infective and metabolic. As the aetiology of an increasing number of these diseases is discovered, they will be classified accordingly, but until then it seems convenient to describe certain conditions under this heading. Myelin may be destroyed by disease processes (myelinoclasis), or it may fail to form because of some defect of metabolism (dysmyelination). The latter is seen in a number of well-recognized metabolic disorders as a result of the chemical changes that occur. There is evidence of a lack of myelin in the brains of children with phenylketonuria, and it may be that this metabolic disorder interferes with the laying down of myelin. The autopsy findings in patients dying with maple-syrup-urine disease have been found to be consistent with oedema of the brain and a deficiency of myelin. The latter varied, but the axons were normal and there was no evidence of myelin breakdown (Woolf, 1962). A disturbance of myelination will also occur in the lipidoses, even though the enzyme defect in these conditions leads to an abnormal accumulation of substances in the neurons as the principle finding (Poser, 1968).

It seems likely that many, if not all, of the conditions classified as dysmyelinating with a failure of myelin formation, as opposed to myelinoclasis with myelin destruction, will be found to result from enzyme deficiencies. These enzymatic disturbances may be of a different type to those which result in a cell's inability to rid itself of metabolites which accumulate and prevent its normal function. The theory of 'glial insufficiency', a failure of the glial cells to maintain the nutrition of myelin, has been considered for a long time (Norman, 1962). In the leucodystrophies the abnormal lipids found contain breakdown products of myelin when metabolism has been arrested at a certain stage by enzymatic defects.

Myelinoclastic diseases

In these conditions the evidence favours a breakdown of previously normal myelin.

Schilder's disease, or diffuse cerebral sclerosis (encephalitis periaxialis diffusa)

The term 'Schilder's disease' is used for a variety of demyelinating disorders, and the question of its identity is still being discussed. For instance, it has been suggested that there is a close relationship with multiple sclerosis, the widespread nature of the lesions being related to the age of the patient and a possible hypersensitivity of the developing brain to noxious agents. Sporadic and familial instances of the disease have been recorded. Also, instances of adrenoleucodystrophy were included under this heading before the metabolic abnormalities of this disorder were clarified.

It usually starts in early childhood and is characterized by a downhill course over a period of several years. The onset tends to be insidious, with symptoms suggestive of a psychiatric disorder. Apathy, disorientation, hallucinations and intellectual deterioration occur. Seizures can sometimes accompany these changes. The progress of the disease is usually by stages, the patient becoming increasingly disabled, with loss of speech and impairment of vision and hearing. Occasionally, loss of sight or of hearing can be the presenting symptom. Examination will confirm that this is almost always of central origin due to lesions in the occipital or temporal lobes. Abnormal reactions of the pupils, and changes in the optic fundi have been reported, suggesting that the blindness is sometimes due to optic nerve lesions; but these patients may be examples of the transitional type of subacute cerebral sclerosis, transitional between myelinoclastic Schilder's disease and multiple sclerosis (Poser, 1968). There can also be evidence of hemiplegia and quadriplegia, and sometimes of ataxia. Occasionally, there are signs of raised intracranial pressure, including papilloedema. The cerebrospinal fluid may be under increased pressure, presumably the result of swelling of the brain. The level of protein in the fluid can be raised, and there is sometimes an increase in the number of cells. Immuno-electrophoresis of the cerebrospinal fluid may be a useful test (Tourtellotte, 1968), as may evidence of immunoglobulin production within the nervous system (Cohen and Bannister, 1967). The EEG is characterized by a non-specific excess of generalized slow-wave activity. After CT scanning and MRI a cortical biopsy is not likely to be needed in order to make a definite diagnosis, although the findings of large amounts of cholesterol esters will favour the diagnosis of myelinoclastic disease.

The pathological findings are characterized by a bilateral area of demyelination in the centrum ovale, often involving the occipital lobes, with scattered collections of perivascular and intercellular sudanophilic material. The cortical U-fibres are often spared. Severe perivascular cuffing with lymphocytes and phagocytes occurs in the acute stages. Scattered, small plaques of demyelination may be seen in the cerebral and cerebellar white matter and in the spinal cord, a finding which supports the possibility of a transitional type of sclerosis, that is between the diffuse and disseminated (Poser, 1968). Improvement may occur on treatment with immunosuppressants such as ACTH combined with cyclophosphamide (Konkal, Bonsounis and Kirban, 1987).

Balo's disease and Devic's disease

In some cases the demyelination may present a concentric appearance, as originally described by Balo. There is still disagreement on the classification of neuromyelitis optica or Devic's disease. The clinical picture of optic neuritis and spinal cord involvement can certainly complicate the infectious diseases of childhood and it seems reasonable to include this syndrome among the myelinoclastic diseases, and perhaps as an example of transitional sclerosis.

Among these conditions being considered there are grounds for treatment with steroids, as such myelin destruction occurs in experimentally induced allergic encephalomyelitis in animals. The steroids may have a significant effect on an allergic type of inflammatory reaction; and there are possibly other associations between cerebral sclerosis and adrenal insufficiency, as in adrenoleucodystrophy (or Addison-Schilder's disease) (Moser et al., 1984a). A humoral factor may be necessary for the development and maintenance of normal myelin (Gordon and Marsden, 1966). This condition will be considered among other peroxisomal disorders later in this chapter.

The leucodystrophies

Although there is a profound disorder of myelin metabolism in metachromatic leucodystrophy or sulphatide lipidosis, this condition has been included in the neuronal storage diseases. In some instances the accumulation of sulphatides in the cells is so marked that the findings are similar to those in the gangliosidoses, although the neuronal involvement is mainly in the brain-stem, dentate nuclei and the basal ganglia.

Globoid cell leucodystrophy or Krabbe's disease

No neuronal storage has been found in this condition, but there is an accumulation of cerebrosides in phagocytes which distend to form the globoid cells. Any division between the neuronal storage diseases and the leucodystrophies is a somewhat

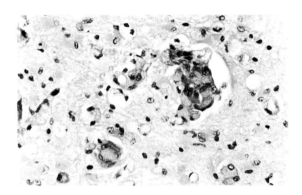

Figure 11.12   Krabbe's disease, showing collection of globoid cells.

artificial one, as both groups are genetically determined enzymatic defects affecting neurolipid metabolism.

The onset of the illness is within the first few months of life. Development ceases and the baby becomes increasingly irritable, and there may be episodes of fever. Then there is a rapid physical deterioration, with the development of an opisthotonic posture with flexion of the arms and extension of the legs. In spite of this, the tendon reflexes are often lost. The bouts of fever continue and seizures occur, particularly myoclonic twitching of the limbs. There are also episodes of screaming accompanied by hyperextension, usually a manifestation of excess muscle tone. Dribbling of saliva is common, and optic atrophy has been noted. Finally, the child is totally disabled, limp and wasted, often with evidence of bulbar palsy, before death during the first three years (Hagberg *et al.*, 1969).

There is a marked elevation of the protein level in the cerebrospinal fluid, often to more than 100 mg%. The EEG shows a progressive deterioration, with irregular slow-wave activity of moderate voltage. Spikes and sharp waves are infrequent, and a response to photic stimulation may disappear as the disease progresses (Kliemann, Harden and Pampiglione, 1969). The conduction velocity in peripheral nerves is reduced, which correlates with the degeneration of the myelin sheaths found on nerve biopsy (Gamstorp, 1968). The CT scan shows attenuation of the central white matter and dilatation of the ventricles. The histology of cerebral biopsies or of the brain at autopsy confirms the presence of the globoid cells in the white matter, but there is considerable variation in their distribution and amount (Fig. 11.12). The U fibres are spared, but secondary atrophy of the white matter occurs. The globoid bodies are PAS-positive and contain galacto-cerebroside. Similar material accumulates in the Schwann cells and endoneural phagocytes (Hagberg *et al.*, 1969). A deficiency of galactocerebroside β-galactosidase has been found in this condition and can be demonstrated in the peripheral leucocytes (Suzuki and Suzuki, 1971). It is suggested that this disease may be due to the death of the oligodendroglial cells, and that the primary lesion is an accumulation of highly cytotoxic galactosyl-sphingosine (psychosine) (Vanier and Svennerholm, 1975). This may be formed from galacto-cerebroside as a biochemical aberration, and if it is not degraded it is highly cytotoxic. Death of the oligodendroglial cells leads to a cessation of myelination, and may explain why the galactocerebroside does not accumulate outside the globoid cells. A variety of globoid cell leucodystrophy of late onset has been reported, with a normal cerebrospinal fluid protein level and no peripheral neuropathy (Crome *et al.*, 1973).

Spongy sclerosis of the van Bogaert/Bertrand type (Canavan's disease)

Reports have been published under a number of titles, including 'Schilder's disease' (Canavan, 1931). One of the characteristics of this condition is a progressive enlargement of the head. This is associated with increasing spasticity and dementia. It can be a familial disease, and then the mode of inheritance appears to be autosomal recessive. Its onset is within the first 9 months of life, and death usually occurs within 3 years. Episodes of sweating, vomiting and collapse can occur, and there may be a lack of tone rather than spasticity.

At *post mortem* examination the brain is large, heavy, soft and gelatinous. Status spongiosus is found in the subcortical white matter, in the lower layers of the cerebral cortex, and in the Purkinje cell layer in the cerebellum. There is a severe reduction in the number of myelinated axons in the white matter, and large glial nuclei occur throughout the grey and white matter. The appearances are consistent with an accumulation of water within the brain, and the myelin changes may be secondary to this. The oedema may be related to a disorder of the oligodendroglia (Zu Rhein, Eichmann and Puletti, 1960). It has been found that this condition may be due to a deficiency of aspartoacylase, causing elevated plasma levels and increased excretion of *N*-acetylaspartic acid (Matalon *et al.*, 1988). The CT scan and ultrasonography can be helpful in diagnosis by showing the cystic appearance of the white matter.

Somewhat similar, if less marked, spongiform changes have been noted in known metabolic disturbances such as maple-syrup-urine disease (Crome, Dutton and Ross, 1961), and in some toxic encephalopathies, for example from hexachlorophene when this is absorbed through the skin in neonates.

Fibrinoid leucodystrophy (Alexander type)

Enlargement of the head has also been described in fibrinoid leucodystrophy. Its onset is early in life, and its course is progressive, with death within a few years. Development remains grossly retarded, and convulsions are associated with increasing rigidity and opisthotonus (Crome, 1953). Signs of brain-stem involvement can occur (Russo, Aron and Anderson, 1976), and persistent hiccup can be a presenting feature (Wilson *et al.*, 1981). The brain is enlarged with status spongiosus of the white matter. There is a loss of nerve and glial cells, and numerous hyaline bodies are present throughout the nervous system. These are extracellular and similar to the so-called 'Rosenthal' fibres. They are most numerous on the pial surface and around the blood vessels. There is an extensive lack of myelin, but little in the way of sudanophil breakdown products. So far, no known cause has been found for the condition. CT scans and MRI may show attenuation of the white matter and ventricular enlargement, and brain biopsy can confirm the diagnosis.

Sudanophilic leucodystrophy (Pelizaeus-Merzbacher's disease)

This group contains a number of conditions included in the past as examples of diffuse sclerosis, and the term Pelizaeus-Merzbacher's disease has also been used to describe a collection of different diseases, many of them genetically determined (Norman, 1962). The classical Pelizaeus-Merzbacher type affects boys, starts in infancy, or early childhood, and runs a prolonged course. Another or connatal type starts very soon after birth, and there is a transitional type. There seems to be no doubt that in the classical type inheritance is sex-linked, while in the connatal type it may be sex-linked or autosomal recessive. Nystagmus is an early sign, as is a tremor of the head. The infant becomes progressively more spastic and ataxic, and extrapyramidal features may develop. In the first few years the progress of the disease is often rapid; then it can halt or even remit. Although the child is retarded, speech can develop but may be dysarthric.

Demyelination is diffuse in the centrum ovale and in the cerebellum, and the brainstem may be particularly affected. Scattered among the large areas of demyelination are small islands of intact nerve fibres and myelin sheaths. The U fibres are spared. The CT scan may show evidence of cerebral atrophy.

Norman (1962) also recognizes the *Seitelberger type* with an absence of stainable myelin in the brain and spinal cord, although the axis cylinders are well preserved; and the adult type of *Lowenberg and Hill*. Some cases have been classified under the term *Neutral fat leucodystrophy*, depending on how specific the category of Pelizaeus-Merzbacher's disease is considered to be. Occasionally there may be difficulties in distinguishing sudanophil leucodystrophies from diffuse cerebral sclerosis. A positive family history will be suggestive, as will biochemical findings, such as an increase of hexosamine in the white matter on histo-chemical examination of brain tissue (Edgar, 1961). However, increased hexosamine is found in other conditions such as globoid-cell dystrophy. There will still be reports of pathological findings which are difficult to fit into this type of classification; a more satisfactory classification will have to await the identification of the underlying biochemical defects.

Peroxisomal disorders

There are a number of conditions, mainly affecting children, which are characterized by increased levels of very-long-chain fatty acids because of impaired capacity to degrade these acids. This normally takes place in a subcellular organelle called the peroxisome so that they can now be classified in a new group of peroxisomal disorders (Gordon, 1987).

These conditions include the various types of adrenoleukodystrophy (Moser *et al.*, 1984b), the Zellweger cerebrohepatorenal syndrome (Moser *et al.*, 1984a) and infantile Refsum's disease (Budden *et al.*, 1986) The mode of inheritance of adrenoleukodystrophy is sex-linked recessive, and of the others autosomal recessive. The finding of high levels of very-long-chain fatty acids in the serum is useful in the diagnosis of these disorders. Treatment with various diets has been tried to influence the course of the illness, but more research is needed on these. Replacement of adrenal steroids can correct the adrenal insufficiency.

In the *childhood variety of adrenoleukodystrophy* (Addison-Schilder's disease) symptoms usually start between the ages of 4 and 8 years. The neurological symptoms can begin in an insidious manner and the course of the illness can vary greatly. Learning and behaviour difficulties may be noted and the child's behaviour can deteriorate. Then dementia becomes more obvious with motor disorders, visual failure with optic atrophy but sometimes of cortical origin, deafness and convulsions. Symptoms and signs of adrenal insufficiency, such as vomiting, hypotension and pigmentation may develop at any time; and sometimes not at all. The CT scan often shows areas of low attenuation, especially adjacent to the ventricular trigone, and there may be enhancement at the periphery of these zones in the area of the internal capsule. Nuclear magnetic resonance imaging may be even more effective in demonstrating the cerebral lesions (Nishio *et al.*, 1986). Tests of adrenocortical dysfunction are helpful, particularly raised levels of plasma ACTH (Rees, Grant and Wilson, 1975).

A first trimester prenatal diagnosis of adrenoleucodystrophy can be made on chorionic villi biopsy in the pregnancy of a carrier; and affected boys identified. This has been done with linkage analysis of DNA from the villi using the highly polymorphic probe St14, and by the determination of very-long-chain fatty acid levels in cultured chorionic villi (Boué *et al.*, 1985).

In *neonatal* or *connatal adrenoleucodystrophy* the onset is during the first year of life with severe seizures, retarded development, progressive auditory and visual dysfunction and profound hypotonia. There is usually retinal degeneration and the liver may be enlarged (Mobley *et al.*, 1983). The EEG shows the picture of hypsarrythmia. Death usually occurs before the age of 3 years, but life can be prolonged for several more years. At *post mortem* examination adrenal cortical atrophy and polymicrogyria has been described (Ulrich *et al.*, 1978). The level of very-long-chain fatty acids has been found to be raised in plasma and cultured skin fibroblasts. There is no evidence of overt adrenal insufficiency, but biochemical evidence of adrenocortical hypofunction has been reported, and at autopsy marked abnormalities of the adrenal cortices have been found (Jaffe *et al.*, 1982).

Zellweger's cerebrohepatorenal syndrome also presents with seizures, retardation and hypotonia. There are retinopathies; dysmorphic features such as high prominent forehead, widened sutures, puffy eyelids, hypertelorism, cataracts, abnormal ears and micrognathia; renal cortical cysts; hepatomegaly; and skeletal abnormalities, including camptodactyly, limited joint movement and chondrodysplasia punctata (Fig. 11.13). No adrenal abnormalities have been reported. Death usually occurs

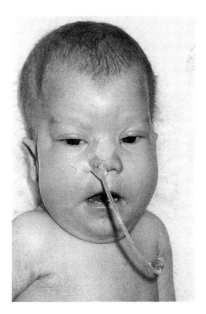

Figure 11.13   Child with Zellweger's syndrome.

within the first few month of life. Very-long-chain fatty acids are found to be increased in the plasma and in cultured fibroblasts. They are also found in cultured amniocytes in some women in whom the fetus was at risk of the Zellweger syndrome (Moser *et al.*, 1984b). Very-long-chain fatty acid analysis is a convenient method for the early diagnosis of the syndrome, and for prenatal diagnosis.

Other peroxisomal disorders include *hyperpipecolic acidaemia* (Anneson, Tipton and Ward, 1982) and *infantile Refsum's disease*. The latter shows evidence of retinitis pigmentosa, sensori-neural deafness, generalized developmental delay and hepatomegaly. In certain patients there may be evidence of a peripheral neuropathy (Poulas *et al.*, 1985).

Peroxisomes are subcellular organelles which contain enzymes for the β-oxidation of fatty acids, particularly of the long chain fatty acids. Peroxisomes in the sex-linked adrenoleucodystrophy appear normal but as the peroxisome has a β-oxidation system active towards very-long-chain fatty acids it is likely that this condition is associated with a specific peroxisomal enzyme defect confined to the pathway for the oxidation of very-long-chain fatty acids. The single peroxysomal enzyme defect in adrenoleuco-dystrophy may affect lignoceryl CoA synthetase (Wanders, Van Roermund and Van Wijland, 1987).

Conversely, in neonatal adrenoleucodystrophy and Zellweger's syndrome, and possibly infantile Refsum's disease, in which there are wide-ranging abnormalities more than one enzyme may be affected, the findings being secondary to a primary disturbance in the structure and/or function of the peroxisome (Poulas *et al.*, 1985). In the latter condition there is certainly an impaired capacity to degrade very-long-chain fatty acids in the peroxisomes, and these organelles are found to be absent in the livers in both neonatal adrenoleucodystrophy and Zellweger's syndrome (Farrell, Dimmick and Applegarth, 1983). These disorders are distinguishable on the basis of histology and peroxisomal biochemistry; with the former showing adrenal atrophy, systemic infiltration by abnormal lipid-laden macrophages and elevation of saturated very-long-chain fatty acids, while in the latter condition there is chondrodysplasia, glomerulocystic disease of the kidneys, demyelination of the cerebral white matter and elevation of unsaturated and saturated very-long-chain fatty acids, but no adrenal atrophy (Kelly *et al.*, 1986).

Various 'encephalopathies'

There are some diseases which cause widespread cerebral damage, but for which no definite cause has so far been found. Some may be due to metabolic disturbances, some may result from slow virus infections, and some may be found to lack a nosological entity.

Progressive neuronal degeneration of childhood (PNDC) (Alpers' disease) (poliodystrophia cerebri progressiva)

There are still doubts about the status of this condition, but there does seem to be a clinical entity consisting of an illness with intractable fits, progressive dementia and other neurological features coming on in early childhood. Liver function is abnormal due to hepatic cirrhosis, although there may be no symptoms of this. It is probably inherited in an autosomal recessive manner (Huttenlocher, Solitare and Adams, 1976). There may be a connection with some disorder of pyruvate oxidation (Harding *et al.*, 1986), and it may be a type of mitochondrial encephalopathy. It has been asked if in some patients the pathological changes follow a series of convulsions or if they cause them. Degenerative changes are found in the grey matter. In the cortex there is status spongiosus affecting the 3rd, and often the 5th layers. The striatum, thalamus, and cerebellum are also commonly affected. In the past the findings may well have been due to a number of different aetiological factors (Blackwood *et al.*, 1963).

Hereditary myoclonus epilepsy (progressive myoclonus epilepsy)

Myoclonus is often associated with degenerative changes, particularly affecting the extrapyramidal and cerebellar systems, and presumably due to a variety of causes, including anoxia, infections and metabolic disturbances. It may be also a symptom of a cerebral disease of known aetiology, for example Gm_2 gangliosidosis or subacute sclerosing panencephalitis. Finally, there is a group in which myoclonus is the presenting symptom of a very slowly progressive condition. There may be evidence of a genetic factor, but the cause is unknown.

This last category includes: *Unverricht-Lundborg disease*, or *hereditary myoclonus epilepsy*, and the *Ramsay Hunt syndrome* or *dyssynergia cerebellaris myoclonica*. The former disease usually begins around the age of 5 years, but sometimes later. Generalized seizures may be the first manifestation of epilepsy, to be followed by myoclonic twitching; although sometimes the myoclonus precedes the grand mal. There is a gradual physical and mental deterioration, extrapyramidal signs such as rigidity and tremor being a prominent feature. Amaurosis with normal ocular fundi has been reported (Schwarz and Yanoff, 1965). The course of the illness is prolonged over a period of 10 or more years. A positive family history suggesting a recessive mode of inheritance will support the diagnosis, as may abnormalities on electrophoresis of the serum mucoproteins (Miller and Neill, 1959). Close linkage has been noted with markers on the distal portion of the long arm of chromosome 21 (Lehesjoki *et al.*, 1991). At autopsy, or on examination of brain biopsy specimens, there are degenerative changes; and in some instances myoclonus or Lafora bodies are found in the cytoplasm of the neurons, with dislocation of the nucleus. These occur throughout the grey matter of the brain; in the cerebral cortex, basal ganglia, brain-stem and cerebellum, and sometimes in the retina. Deposits are also found in the cytoplasm of the liver cells and in the fibres of the cardiac muscle. The bodies have a basophil centre consisting of a polysaccharide, and the shell appears to be a weakly acid mucoprotein. It is suggested that the disease may be a generalized disturbance of intracellular polysaccharide metabolism, related to glycogen turnover. It is possible that those who have myoclonus epilepsy and are not of the Lafora body group are not so intellectually handicapped (Koskiniemi *et al.*, 1974).

The Ramsay Hunt syndrome is often classified among the hereditary ataxias; the cerebellar ataxia being associated with myoclonus, although the latter is not usually a pervading symptom.

Encephalopathy and fatty degeneration of the viscera (Reye's syndrome)

This syndrome, which affects glucose, amino acid and fatty acid metabolism, has been reported in a number of countries since it was originally reported by Reye, Morgan and Baral (1963). The aetiology has been the subject of much speculation, but no definite toxic or viral agent has been identified to account for all instances of the disease. The influenza virus has been implicated in some cases (Partin *et al.*, 1976). In the original report the main clinical features were an upper respiratory tract infection at the start of the illness, impairment of consciousness, fever, convulsions, vomiting and disturbed respiratory rhythm, but no jaundice although this may develop later. On examination there may be enlargement of the liver and abnormalities of tone and tendon reflexes. There is sometimes a characteristic posture, with flexion of the elbows, clenching of the hands, and extension of the legs. During the illness the transaminase levels are raised, and there may be hypoglycaemia although normal and raised blood sugar levels have also been recorded, metabolic acidosis, raised and sometimes fluctuating blood ammonia levels, lowered prothrombin levels, and uraemia and hypernatraemia. A blood ammonia level of over 300 mg/100 ml is rarely compatible with survival (Lovejoy *et al.*, 1974). The cerebrospinal fluid can also show a low sugar level, but lumbar puncture is to be avoided if there is a possibility of raised intracranial pressure. The EEG is often diffusely abnormal. Injections of glucose may have little effect, although a better response is obtained from continuous infusions, especially if combined with hydrocortisone. Oral neomycin, enemas, exchange transfusions and peritoneal dialysis have also been tried, as well as steroids and intravenous mannitol if the intracranial pressure is raised. Artificial ventilation may be required. L-citrulline has been given (De Long, Glick and Shannon, 1974), and large doses of ornithine and arginine have been suggested (Thaler, Hoogenraad and Boswell, 1974). The three lines of treatment under particular scrutiny are conservative management with vigorous anti-cerebral oedema therapy, exchange transfusion, and peritoneal dialysis (Lovejoy *et al.*, 1975). The first of these is of particular importance in a life-threatening situation, and such treatment is likely to be much more effective if it is controlled by intracranial pressure monitoring in this and other diseases complicated by cerebral oedema (Minns, 1977).

Death is frequent, often with evidence of brain-stem dysfunction, and the brain is swollen at autopsy. The cortical neurons may be swollen or shrunken, and there is swelling of the astrocytes and the oligodendroglia. The liver is enlarged and firm. Liver biopsy carried out early in the illness can be highly suggestive of the diagnosis, but may not be without risk in the presence of a coagulation defect. The characteristic findings are swelling of the parenchyma with neutral lipid, which is more evident in the periphery of the lobule around the portal vein than around the central vein. Evidence of inflammation is usually absent until necrosis occurs. Electron microscopy shows abnormalities of the mitochondria (Partin, 1974). The pathological findings do not suggest an infection, but are more in favour of a toxic cause (Becroft, 1966). As many of the children suffering from this condition are less than 6 months old, the risks of exposure to toxic agents are limited. Aspirin poisoning has been suggested, with an enzyme system involved in carbohydrate metabolism being hypersensitive to salicylates (Giles, 1965), and paracetamol is a known cause of fatty degeneration of the liver. The hypoglycaemia is most probably related to the liver damage, as may be the encephalopathy. Ammonia intoxication, perhaps associated with hypoglycaemia and anoxia, has also been considered as a possible cause (Huttenlocher, Schwartz and Klatzlin, 1969). One patient with Reye's syndrome has been shown to have a low activity of ornithine transcarbamylase, which suggests that the hyperammonaemia may be due to anorexia and vomiting causing a reduction of ornithine intake, rather than to a high protein load (Thaler, Hoogenraad and Boswell, 1974). It is this possibility which has led to the suggested treatment with L-citrulline or with ornithine and arginine. In spite of the absence of pathological findings of infections, the upper respiratory and gastrointestinal symptoms at the onset of the illness suggest that a viral aetiology cannot be excluded, at least as a precipitating cause (Randolph and

Gelfman, 1968). Cullity and Kakulas (1970) consider that the syndrome is most probably due to hypoxia following convulsions associated with non-specific infection, possibly complicated by disturbances of water and electrolyte balance. There seems to be no reason why such a syndrome should not have a varied aetiology, the possible causes mentioned being precipitating factors depending on an underlying mitochondrial dysfunction (Brown and Imam, 1991). Also, in this context it should be remembered that metabolic disorders can cause Reye-like syndromes, notably medium-chain acyl-CoA dehydrogenase deficiency. Sufferers must be given a high carbohydrate intake during any metabolic stress or acute infection (Roe and Coates, 1989).

Subacute necrotizing encephalomyelopathy of Leigh

The syndrome of an infantile encephalopathy, possibly a mitochondrial encephalo-pathy, with pathological findings suggestive of Wernicke's encephalopathy was first described by Leigh (1951). It may be inherited through an autosomal recessive gene, although spontaneous cases do occur. The illness usually starts during the first decade but there is no doubt that the age of onset can be later. Survival is rarely for more than 4 years. The symptomatology is variable, and it can be difficult to make a firm diagnosis during life (Montpetit *et al.*, 1971). The disease may present with feeding difficulties, vomiting and difficulty with swallowing or sucking. There is sometimes a rapid deterioration at the start of the illness, followed by a more gradual course characterized by recurring episodes. These may take the form of ataxia, chorea, athetosis, hypotonia and weakness, respiratory abnormalities, or vomiting. There is a suggestion that these can be precipitated by such factors as fever, excitement, or a high carbohydrate meal, possibly due to overloading of enzyme systems. Other signs include seizures, nystagmus, bizarre eye movements, ocular palsies and optic atrophy. As the condition progresses, dementia becomes more evident, and the pyramidal, extrapyramidal and cerebellar signs more obvious. Hyperventilation, dehydration and acidosis can occur (Clayton, Dobbs and Patrick, 1967). Death may be from respiratory paralysis.

The pathological findings are similar to those of Wernicke's encephalopathy. The damage is most marked in the caudate nucleus, putamen, peri-aqueductal tissues,

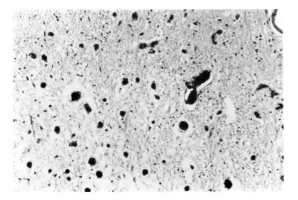

Figure 11.14 Leigh's encephalopathy. Proliferation of capillaries with rarefaction of tissue in the brain-stem.

tegmentum, and in the floor of the fourth ventricle. The mamillary bodies are not so often involved as in Wernicke's encephalopathy. Areas of softening of spongiform type occur. The dendrites and myelin are more damaged than the axons or neurons, with reactive gliosis and foci of round cell infiltration. There is a proliferation of the capillaries (Fig. 11.14) (Dayan, Ockenden and Crome, 1970). The posterior nerve roots and peripheral nerves can also be involved.

Raised levels of pyruvate and lactate have been reported, but these may be secondary to causes such as dehydration, hypoxia and hyperventilation. Hyperalaninaemia and hyperalaninuria have also been found (Lonsdale et al., 1969). The excess of alanine is presumably formed from pyruvate, and it appears in the urine when the plasma concentration overwhelms the renal clearance mechanism. It is possible that in some instances the condition may be related to a partial inability to oxidize pyruvate. A multienzyme complex is involved, and a deficiency or abnormal function of any part of this system may give rise to features similar to those of thiamine deficiency. Another explanation that has been suggested for this syndrome is the presence of an inhibitory factor which interferes with a neurophysiologically active form of thiamine, thiamine triphosphate, different from its co-enzyme form. Also, transketolase activity has been found to be raised in patients with Leigh's disease, suggesting an increased effect of thiamine pyrophosphate (Reed, 1976). These theories have led to treatment with thiamine, in large doses of several grams a day. Thiamine propyl disulfide has also been tried in a dose of 300 mg daily, as it enters cells by passive diffusion, and is then converted to thiamine. It does cause an unpleasant smell (Pincus et al., 1971). Thiamine pyrophosphate, lipoic acid, biotin, D-penicillamine, and vitamin B_6 and B_{12} have also been given, and in cases of pyruvate dehydrogenase deficiency (which occurs in some instances) a ketogenic diet, as during ketosis the brain can utilize ketone bodies and bypass a deficiency of the pyruvate dehydrogenase complex (Falk et al., 1975). Until the aetiology has been elucidated it seems reasonable to try all these methods consecutively or in combination; as this may well be a group of diseases. Some may be related to a deficiency of pyruvate dehydrogenase, others to a deficiency of pyruvate carboxylase (Van Biervliet et al., 1977), others to an impaired function of thiamine triphosphate, and, in quite a few cases, to unknown causes. There is a hope that there will be a response when the body is swamped by one or other of these substances, if the combining power of the enzyme is affected or there is an inhibitory substance present (Gordon, Marsden and Lewis, 1974).

If apnea attacks are a particular problem, and β-endorphins are elevated in the cerebrospinal fluid, treatment with naltrexone may be tried (Myer et al., 1990).

Subacute sclerosing panencephalitis

Evidence now suggests that this condition, originally described by Dawson (1934) and van Bogaert (1945), is most often related to infection with the measles virus, but it is mentioned in this section to include it in the differential diagnosis of progressive cerebral degenerative disorders, and because it may be found that a number of such conditions are due to slow virus infections. The illness may have an insidious onset with symptoms suggestive of a behaviour disorder, but it can be acute, with papilloedema. The first symptoms are usually noted from 3–15 years of age with a history of measles earlier in life, usually before the age of 18 months, with occasional doubts if the child has been developing normally in the interval. A possible association with measles vaccination has also been noted (Bellman and Dick, 1978). There is a progressive deterioration of varying rate in the child's condition. Cranial nerve palsies have been noted, and extrapyramidal disorders, including involuntary movements, tend to be more evident than cortico-spinal signs. Convulsions occur, but the characteristic seizure is of myoclonic type.

Serological tests reveal high levels of measles specific antibodies in the serum and cerebrospinal fluid, and although the possibility of other viruses being involved cannot definitely be excluded, it seems reasonable to include this finding as an essential feature of this condition.

The cerebrospinal fluid shows a paretic colloidal gold curve with a high concentration of gamma globulin, which has been shown to be immunoglobulin-G (IgG) (Tourtellotte *et al.*, 1968). Antibody may be synthesized by cells within the CNS as a result of a viral infection restricted to the brain which stimulates the emigration of plasma cells into the brain and the production of antibody; or by the virus incorporating brain protein into its structure, and locally synthesized antibody being directed against the brain itself (Cutler, Merler and Hammerstrad, 1968). If the presence of virus in the brain activates measles specific IgG and IgM synthesis within the CNS space, this will lead to large quantities of measles virus specific antibodies in the cerebrospinal fluid. In other types of measles infection this is largely prevented by the blood-brain barrier, however high the serum level may be, unless the barrier has been breached. There are methods which can check that this is intact, such as looking for haemaglutinating inhibiting antibodies against rubella virus in the serum and cerebrospinal fluid and seeing that the ratio is normal (Longson and Bailey, 1978).

In normal individuals the ratio of measles specific antibody titres between serum and cerebrospinal fluid is greater than 300 to 1, but in subacute sclerosing panencephalitis the ratio may fall to as low as 20 to 1 or even 5 to 1. The ratio can also fall in convalescence from acute measles encephalitis and in multiple sclerosis but these conditions will not cause diagnostic difficulties.

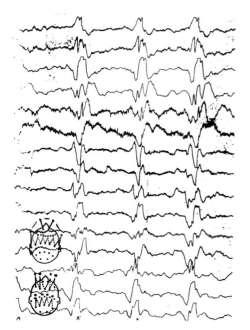

Figure 11.15   EEG in subacute sclerosing panencephalitis showing the periodic complexes so typical of this disease.

The EEG (Fig. 11.15) frequently reveals very suggestive findings, although they may be transient. The background activity consists of low-voltage, irregular, slow-wave activity, while every few seconds there are brief generalized outbursts of high voltage slow and sharp waves. These periodic complexes are sometimes associated with myoclonic jerks. They can be asynchronous, and can vary considerably in duration and timing (Ibrahim and Jeavons, 1974). The most sensitive diagnostic test is MRI (Miller *et al.*, 1990). On examination of cerebral biopsy specimens there may be immunofluorescent staining of measles antigen and identification of measles-virus-like tubules in glial cells. Measles virus, or a very similar agent, has been cultured from cerebral tissue taken from an affected child (Horta-Barbosa *et al.*, 1969).

Histological examination will show inflammatory exudate and gliosis in the white matter. The more acute the course of the disease the more prominent will be the inclusion bodies in the nuclei and cytoplasm of the cortical neurons and of the glial cells. In subacute sclerosing panencephalitis there is a slow infection of the brain with the virus spreading from cell to cell, both neurons and glial cells being affected. Burnett (1968) suggests that there may be a failure of the thymus-dependent immunocytes to attack the cells infected with the measles virus. He postulates that this may be due to an acquired anomaly preventing the recruitment of these immunocytes reactive against measles antigen, although the antibody response is normal. A possible explanation for this is the presence of antigen in the thymus where the stem cells differentiate to immunocytes, as this can result in the destruction of these cells. If this is so, there will be no recruitment of thymus-dependent immunocytes, so the harmful effects of the virus in the brain will only be prevented for as long as those immunocytes which are present in the brain at the time of the acute attack of measles survive. This theory has been questioned, for lymphocyte transformation has been found, which indicates an unimpaired T cell response. Perhaps brain damage is caused by an interaction between immunocompetent lymphocytes and cells containing virus.

The production of low-affinity antibody is another possibility, as such an abnormal pattern of immunological reactivity will result in immune complexes of measles antigen and IgG which cause tissue damage (Dayan and Stokes, 1972). Others (Valdimarsson, Agnaasdotir and Lachmann, 1974) have carried out experiments which seem to demonstrate the existence of a blocking factor in subacute sclerosing panencephalitis sera which prevents the elimination of measles-infected cells. Measles antibodies, together with complement, have been shown to be cytotoxic to measles infected cells. But when these grow in the presence of antibody, but without complement, the antigenic virus determinants are lost to the cells. Then, although harbouring virus internally, they cannot be identified and eliminated by the immune system. The effect of the serum in blocking the cytotoxic action of subacute sclerosing panencephalitis lymphocytes on the measles-infected cells is believed to be due to an immune complex which may have occurred in this way. The reasons for the absence of adequate amounts of complement *in vivo* may be explained by the way that measles infected cells are lysed (Agnarsdottir, 1977). As the main immunological abnormality in this disease is an unduly high antibody titre associated with the possible blocking of the cellular immune response to measles, transfer factor has been used to try to stimulate a supposed suppressor T cell function. It is such considerations that cause concern over a possible relationship between measles vaccination and subsequent encephalitis (Schneck, 1968).

It has been suggested that the measles or similar RNA paramyxovirus may be activated by a papova-like DNA virus, or, that the paramyxovirus, having caused fusion of brain cells, enables the papova-like DNA virus to spread throughout the brain and cause pathological changes (Koprowski, Barbanti-Brodano and Katz, 1970).

Prolonged treatment with corticosteroids, immunosuppressive therapy, and treatment with transfer factor have all been tried, but the results are difficult to assess in a disease subject to spontaneous remissions. Antiviral agents have also been given, for instance 5-bromo-2-desoxyuridine and cytosine arabinoside, but it is difficult to understand why substances which interfere with DNA synthesis should affect the RNA measles virus (Freeman, 1968). Perhaps the most encouraging agent so far has been isoprinosine, active against RNA viruses, which may at least delay the progress of the disease (Huttenlocher and Mattson, 1979). A combination of intrathecal interferon and isoprinosine may be the best treatment (Yoshioka et al.,1989). Because of the possibility of auto-immunity in this disease, and the role of the thymus in this type of reaction, thymectomy has been suggested and favourably reported on (Kolar et al., 1967). However, so far there is no absolutely reliable treatment. The condition usually progresses through stages of increasing disability to total incapacity or death within 6–12 months (Jabbour et al., 1969), but remissions can occur and the disease process appear to halt.

A similar condition related to rubella, congenital or acquired, *progressive rubella panencephalitis*, may be underdiagnosed.

Localized virus encephalitis (Rasmussen's syndrome) (chronic progressive epilepsia partialis continua of childhood)

There is some evidence that certain viruses can cause localized infection of the brain, resulting in focal seizures, which are often difficult to control, and focal signs such as hemianopia and hemiplegia. The diagnosis is difficult to make, except possibly by electron microscopy of biopsy material from the brain (Friedman, Ch'ien and Parham, 1977). The syndrome may well be due to infection with viruses, such as the Epstein-Barr virus or the cytomegalovirus (Power et al., 1990), which offers a chance of antiviral treatment with agents such as acyclovir. It is also possible that a virus triggers an autoimmune mechanism of cortical and white matter destruction. Surgical removal of an accessible part of the brain can be considered (Chapter 10).

Progressive multifocal leucoencephalopathy

This condition can also be included among the 'slow virus diseases' with long incubation periods. It complicates severe wasting diseases, such as cancer, notably the reticuloses. Histological examination shows demyelination and loss of oligodendroglia. It is suggested that a papova virus, the JC virus, invades the glial cells, causes nuclear abnormalities, and, indirectly, demyelination (Zu Rhein and Chou, 1965) (Chapter 10).

Other degenerative diseases of the nervous system of doubtful aetiology

There are a number of rare disorders of unknown aetiology which present with evidence of a slow degeneration of the nervous system.

Infantile neuroaxonal dystrophy (Seitelberger's disease)

The onset of infantile neuroaxonal dystrophy is usually in late infancy and there is a gradual physical and mental deterioration. There may be evidence of spasticity with appropriate reflex changes, or the increased tone may be the result of an extra-pyramidal rigidity. Conversely, the findings can be those of lower motor neuron lesion with hypotonia, muscle wasting and diminished reflexes. Evidence of both upper and lower neuron lesions may co-exist. Incontinence, optic atrophy and deafness can occur. Convulsions are uncommon, and their absence is suggestive diagnostically. The disease is inherited in many instances, probably autosomal recessive in type, but causation is unknown. The diagnosis is supported by EEG changes found after the age of 2 years. These consist of high amplitude, non-reactive, fast rhythms both in the waking and sleep records. Another helpful finding is EMG evidence of denervation of the anterior horn cell type with normal nerve conduction velocities (Aicardi and Castelein, 1979). Metachromatic leucodystrophy is the disease most likely to show clinical similarities but it can be diagnosed by enzyme tests and a high cerebrospinal fluid protein. Histological studies of biopsy material are characterized by spheroids. These occur in peripheral tissues, including skin and the conjunctivae, and in various parts of the CNS. They contain tubulovesicular structures, and these possibly represent a malformation of the synaptic vesicles (Ametani, 1974).

Hallervorden-Spatz disease

This is a familial disorder with an onset towards the second half of the first decade. Inheritance is almost certainly autosomal recessive (Dooling, Schoene and Richardson, 1974). There is a period of normal development and then a fairly rapid degeneration. Usually, rigidity first affects the legs, and an equinovarus deformity in the feet may be the presenting sign. Choreoathetosis involves the muscles of the face, tongue and palate, as well as the limbs, and causes difficulties of articulation and swallowing. Dementia accompanies the physical deterioration, but death may not occur for many years. The differential diagnosis is from conditions such as hepato-lenticular degeneration, dystonia musculorum deformans, and non-progressive disorders, caused, for instance, by jaundice and anoxia. The findings at autopsy are characterized by the deposition of brown or greyish-blue iron-containing pigment in the globus pallidus and substantia nigra, and the occurrence of spheroids mainly confined to the basal ganglia and thalamus. There is also diffuse neuronal loss and demyelination (Meyer, 1958). Although suggested, it has never been proven that there is any disorder of iron metabolism, but the increased iron uptake can be confirmed by scintillation counters on probes over the temples, and thus aid in diagnosis (Vakili *et al.*, 1977).

A number of syndromes somewhat similar both clinically and pathologically have been described, but it seems unlikely that they represent an entity (De Myer, Harter and Zeman, 1964). In some instances the onset can occur soon after birth. Histological examination may show only a moderate increase of pigment, with severe neuronal loss, demyelination and gliosis in the globus pallidus, zona reticularis, subthalamic bodies, dentate nucleus and inferior olives; all findings similar to those in kernicterus (Meyer and Earl, 1936). The common pathological finding in infantile neuroaxonal dystrophy and Hallervorden-Spatz disease is the presence of spheroids. Such axonal dystrophy can occur in other conditions such as ageing and injury to the neuron. Therefore, although it has been suggested that the two conditions may be variants of the same disease it seems best at this stage to regard them as separate entities (Gordon, 1978b). The concept of peroxidation as a common mechanism of pigment and spheroid formation can provide a possible link between them (Park,

Netsky and Betsill, 1975). Treatment with benztropine may be beneficial (Torch and Humphries, 1986).

Dystonia musculorum deformans (Torsion spasm)

This disease also has a gradual onset in middle childhood. It has a dominant mode of inheritance (Larsson and Sjogren, 1966), but can occur in the absence of a family history. There are abnormalities of gait, and bizarre movements develop. These are of a slow, writhing, twisting type, affecting mainly the trunk but also the facial and limb muscles. Dysarthria, torticollis and muscle wasting are other features, as well as a progressive dementia. The involuntary movements can cause considerable pain, especially if an injury occurs. Degenerative changes predominate in the putamen and caudate nuclei, but there does not appear to be anything specific about these findings. Muscle relaxants, such as mephenesin, can be given, and occasionally there is an unexpected response to L-dopa. Orphenadrine is a drug which is particularly worth trying. Stereotactic surgery may have a part to play, for the condition is only very slowly progressive.

Occasionally children may show fluctuating dystonia and sometimes they respond to very small doses of L-dopa.

Segawa's syndrome (dopa-responsive hereditary progressive dystonia)

Occasionally children show a fluctuating dystonia. The clinical picture of this syndrome can vary (Gordon, 1982), but the history is usually suggestive and should always indicate a trial of L-dopa treatment. The response can be dramatic and can change a severely disabled child to normality. The disorder may be due to defective storage of dopamine, or to impaired dopamine metabolism (de Jong *et al.*, 1989).

Huntington's chorea

The onset of Huntington's chorea is usually between 30 and 45 years of age, but it can start in childhood. The choreiform movements are of a coarse type and are associated with facial grimacing and dysarthria. Emotional tension aggravates the movements and they are absent during sleep. Dementia occurs, and can be the presenting symptom. There is a gradual deterioration of the patient's condition and, in the juvenile form, convulsions and rigidity are characteristic features (Byers and Dodge, 1967). The diagnosis depends on the positive family history, the inheritance of the condition being strongly dominant. The genetic defect is on the short arm of chromosome 4. Late-onset cases are most often associated with maternal transmission, while juvenile ones usually have affected fathers (Mann *et al.*, 1990). In older patients atrophy of the caudate nucleus on the CT scan may be helpful diagnostically.

There are widespread degenerative changes in the brain, particularly affecting the basal nuclei. The main finding in these areas is a very marked glial reaction and loss of neurons. There may also be a reduction of neurons in the cerebral cortex. As with other forms of chorea the mechanism may prove to be a relative or absolute excess of activity in dopamine systems of the corpus striatum. At autopsy there is a deficiency of GABA in the basal ganglia (Perry, Hansen and Kloster, 1973). The abnormal movements may be lessened by treatment with reserpine and tetrabenazine, combined if necessary with other drugs, such as haloperidol, chlorpromazine and pimozide (Dalby, 1969; Godwin Austin, 1979).

Sydenham's chorea

There can be no doubt that the introduction of antibiotics in the treatment of upper respiratory tract infections has dramatically reduced the incidence of acute rheumatism in childhood. This, in its turn, must have had an effect on the occurrence of Sydenham's chorea, which is now rare; although the exact association between the two conditions has never been elucidated. There is a possibility of antistreptococcal antibodies reacting with a chorea-producing system of neurons. Chorea was always an uncommon complication of acute rheumatism, and can occur with no evidence of the latter condition. Also, the abnormal movements may complicate other conditions, such as Henoch-Schonlein purpura, encephalopathies following infectious fevers, and systemic lupus erythematosis (Aron, Freeman and Carter, 1965).

The movements consist of sudden jerks of the limbs, which can be confused with tics and with myoclonus. These are sometimes so marked that the child cannot walk and may have to be fed. Writing can be severely affected (Fig. 11.16). Also, if the bulbar muscles are involved, speech may become impossible. If the chorea is unilateral, and is associated with anarthria, a mistaken diagnosis of a cortical lesion may be made. Typical postural findings are pronation of the arms when they are held above the head, and flexion of the wrists with extension of the fingers when they are outstretched. There is difficulty in protruding the tongue, and it may be held between the teeth to keep it from being retracted into the mouth. There is likely to be generalized hypotonia, and complaints of fatigue and muscle weakness are common. The tendon reflexes are sometimes diminished, and the knee jerk can show a characteristic slow or jerky relaxation, or may be pendular. The child is often emotionally labile and occasionally the disturbed mental state may dominate the clinical picture.

The diagnosis is from tics, other extrapyramidal disorders with involuntary movements, and from myoclonus; although it may be better to regard choreiform movements and myoclonus as being involuntary movements resulting from impaired

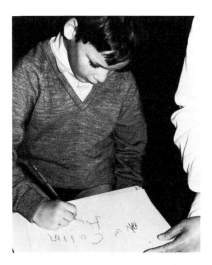

Figure 11.16 Abnormal writing of a 9-year-old with Sydenham's chorea, showing the distortion caused by the involuntary movements.

function at different levels of the nervous system rather than entities to be rigidly differentiated. Huntington's chorea is unlikely to cause diagnostic difficulties when the onset is later in life and there is a strong family history. Evidence of associated acute rheumatism, especially carditis, will support the diagnosis of Sydenham's chorea, and then there will be a raised erythrocyte sedimentation rate, and sometimes a raised antistreptolysin titre. Relapses are not uncommon, particularly in pregnancy, but carry no increased risk of carditis. If unnecessary investigations and treatment are to be avoided the possibility of benign familial chorea sometimes has to be considered. Evidence suggests that this condition is inherited as an autosomal dominant trait, so a careful family history will help (Sleigh and Lindenbaum, 1981). It is also an occasional cause of 'clumsiness' among young children and, apart from such disabilities, the prognosis is usually quite good (Burns, Neuhäuser and Tomasi, 1976).

The association with emotional disturbances is intriguing, as it is with a number of other extrapyramidal disorders (Matthews *et al.*, 1961). No definite reason has been established for this link, although various suggestions have been made, such as vascular lesions resulting from an abnormal response to stress. It is possible that the disease may be related to cross-reacting antigens, between an antigen on the surface of the streptococcal membrane and the caudate nucleus (Weiner and Hauser, 1982).

Apart from the management of an associated acute rheumatism and possibly carditis, Sydenham's chorea needs little treatment beyond rest and quiet. A sedative, such as phenobarbitone, can be given to ensure this, and diazepam and thioridazine may be helpful. Haloperidol has been used with particular benefit (Shenker, Grossman and Klawans 1973). If the involuntary movements are very severe or the condition shows a relapsing course, treatment with steroids can be tried.

References

Abrahams, C., Wheatley, A., Rubenstein, A.H. and Stables, D. (1964). Hepatocellular lipofuscin after excessive ingestion of analgesics. *Lancet*, **ii**, 621

Aicardi, J. and Castelein, P. (1979) Infantile neuroaxonal dystrophy. *Brain*, **102**, 727

Agnarsdottir, G. (1977) Subacute sclerosing panencephalitis. *Hospital Update*, **3**, 517

Ametani, T. (1974) Infantile neuroaxonal dystrophy (INAD). *Neuropädiatrie*, **5**, 63

Anneson, D.W., Tipton, R.E. and Ward, J.C. (1982) Hyperpipecolic acidemia. *Archives of Neurology*, **39**, 713

Armstrong, D., Dimmitt, S. and van Wornier, D.E. (1974) Studies in Batten disease. Peroxidase deficiency in granulocytes. *Archives of Neurology*, **30**, 144

Aron, A.M., Freeman, J.M. and Carter, S. (1965) The natural history of Sydenham's Chorea. *American Journal of Medicine*, **38**, 83

Austin, J.H., Armstrong, D. and Shearer, L. (1965) Metachromatic form of diffuse cerebral sclerosis V: the nature and significance of low sulphatase activity. *Archives of Neurology*, **13**, 593

Batten, F.E. (1903) Cerebral degeneration with symmetrical changes in the maculae in two members of a family. *Transactions of the Ophthalmological Society of the United Kingdom*, **23**, 386

Becroft, D.M.O. (1966) Syndrome of encephalopathy and fatty degeneration of viscera in New Zealand children. *British Medical Journal*, **ii**, 135

Bellman, M.H. and Dick, G.W.A. (1978) Surveillance of subacute sclerosing panencephalitis. *Journal of the Royal College of Physicians*, **12**, 256

Blackwood, W., Buxton, P.H., Cumings, J.N. *et al.* (1963) Diffuse cerebral degeneration in infancy. (Alpers' disease). *Archives of Disease in Childhood*, **38**, 193

Boué, J., Oberle, I., Heilig, R. *et al.* (1985) First trimester prenatal diagnosis of adrenoleucodystrophy by determination of very long chain fatty acid level and by linkage analysis to a DNA probe. *Human Genetics*, **69**, 272

Brett, E.M. and Lake, B.D. (1975) Reassessment of rectal approach to neuropathy in childhood. *Archives of Disease in Childhood*, **50**, 753

Brown, J.K. and Imam, H. (1991) Interrelationships of liver and brain with special reference to Reye syndrome. *Journal of Inherited Metabolic Disease*, **14**, 486

Budden, S.S., Kennaway, N.G., Buist, N.R.M. *et al.* (1986) Dysmorphic syndrome with phytanic acid oxidase deficiency, abnormal very long chain fatty acids, and pipecolic acidemia: studies on four children. *Journal of Pediatrics*, **108**, 33

Burnett, F.M. (1968) Measles as an index of immunological function. *Lancet*, **ii**, 610

Burns, J., Neuhäuser, G. and Tomasi, L. (1976) Benign hereditary chorea of early onset. *Neuropädiatrie*, **7**, 431

Byers, R.K. and Dodge, J.A. (1967) Huntington's chorea in children. *Neurology*, **17**, 587

Canavan, M.N (1931) Schilder's encephalitis periaxialis diffusa. *Archives of Neurology and Psychiatry*, **25**, 299

Carpenter, S., Karpati, G., Andermann, F. *et al.* (1977) The ultrastructural characteristics of the abnormal cytosomes in Batten-Kufs' disease. *Brain*, **100**, 137

Clayton, B.E., Dobbs, R.H. and Patrick, A.D. (1967) Leigh's subacute necrotizing encephalopathy: clinical and biochemical study with special reference to therapy with lipoate. *Archives of Disease in Childhood*, **42**, 467

Cohen, S. and Bannister, R. (1967) Immunoglobulin synthesis within the central nervous system in disseminated sclerosis. *Lancet*, **i**, 366

Crocker, A.C. (1961) The cerebral defect in Tay-Sachs disease and Niemann-Pick disease. *Journal of Neurochemistry*, **7**, 69

Crocker, A.C. and Farber, S. (1958) Niemann-Pick disease: a review of eighteen patients. *Medicine*, **37**, 1

Crome, L. (1953) Megalencephaly associated with hyaline pan-neuropathy. *Brain*, **76**, 215

Crome, L., Dutton, C. and Ross, C.F. (1961) Maple sugar urine disease. *Journal of Pathology and Bacteriology*, **81**, 379

Crome, L., Hanefeld, F., Patrick, D. and Wilson, J. (1973). Late-onset globoid cell leucodystrophy. *Brain*, **96**, 841

Cullity, G.J. and Kakulas, B.A. (1970) Encephalopathy and fatty degeneration of the viscera. *Brain*, **93**, 77

Cummings, J.N. (1960) *Modern Scientific Aspects of Neurology*, Cummings, J.N. (ed). Arnold, London

Cutler, R.W.P., Merler, E. and Hammerstad, J.P. (1968) Production of antibody by the central nervous system in subacute sclerosing pan-encephalitis. *Neurology*, **18**, 129

Dalby, M.A. (1969) Effect of tetrabenazine on extrapyramidal movement disorders. *British Medical Journal*, **ii**, 422

Dawson, J.R. (1934) Cellular inclusions in cerebral lesions of epidemic encephalitis. *Archives of Neurology and Psychiatry*, **31**, 685

Dayan, A.D. and Stokes. M.I. (1972) Immune complexes and visceral deposits of measles antigens in subacute sclerosing panencephalitis. *British Medical Journal*, **ii**, 374

Dayan, A.D., Ockenden, B.C. and Crome, L. (1970) Necrotizing encephalopathy of Leigh. *Archives of Disease in Childhood*, **45**, 39

de Jong, A.P.J.M., Haan, E.A., Mason, J.I. *et al.* (1989) Kinetic study of catecholamine metabolism in hereditary progressive dystonia. *Neuropediatrics*, **20**, 3

De Long, C.R., Glick, T.H. and Shannon, D.C. (1974) Citrulline for Reye's syndrome. *New England Journal of Medicine*, **290**, 1488

De Myer, W., Harter, D.H. and Zeman, W. (1964) Familial spasticity, hyperkinesia and dementia. Clinicopathological observations and comments on the nosology of Hallervorden-Spatz disease. *Acta Neuropathologica*, **4**, 28

Dooling, E.C., Schoene, W.C. and Richardson, E.P. (1974) Hallervorden-Spatz disease. *Archives of Neurology*, **30**, 70

Dorfman, A. (1972) The molecular basis of mucopolysaccharidoses: current status of knowledge. *Triangle*, **11**, 43

Edgar, C.W.F. (1961) Neurochemical aspects of leucodystrophy. *Psychiatria, Neurologia, Neurochirurgia*, **64**, 28

Eto, Y., Weismann, U.N., Carson, J.H. and Herschkowitz, N.N. (1974) Multiple sulfatase deficiencies in cultured skin fibroblasts. *Archives of Neurology*, **30**, 153

Falk, R.E., Cederbaum, S.D., Blass, J.P. *et al* (1975) Clinical and biochemical response to a ketogenic diet in two brothers with pyruvate dehydrogenase deficiency. *Paediatric Research*, **9**, 350

Farrell, K., Dimmick, J.E., Applegarth, D.A. *et al.* (1983) Peroxisomal abnormalities in neonatal adrenoleukodystrophy. *Annals of Neurology*, **14**, 379

Felding, I. and Hultberg, B. (1978) An atypical form of Sandhoff's disease. Case report and biochemical studies. *Neuropädiatrie*, **9**, 74

Frank, U. and Lasson, U. (1985) Ophthalmic neurolipidosis-storage cells in heterozygotes. *Neuropediatrics*, **16**, 3

Freeman, J.M. (1968) Treatment of subacute sclerosing panencephalitis with 5-bromo-2-deoxyuridine and pyran copolymer. *Neurology*, **18**, 176

Friedman, H., Ch'ien, L. and Parham, D. (1977) Virus in brain of child with hemiplegia, hemiconvulsions, and epilepsy. *Lancet*, **ii**, 666

Gamstorp, I. (1968) Polyneuropathy in childhood. *Acta Paediatrica Scandinavica*, **57**, 230

Giles, H. McC. (1965) Encephalopathy and fatty degeneration of the viscera. *Lancet*, **i**, 1075

Gloor, P., Kalabay, O. and Giard, N. (1968) The electroencephalogram in diffuse encephalopathies. Electroencephalographic correlates of grey and white matter lesions. *Brain*, **91**, 779

Godwin-Austin, R.B. (1979) The treatment of choreas and athetotic dystonias. *Journal of the Royal College of Physicians of London*, **13**, 35

Gonatas, N.K., Cambetti, P. and Baird, H. (1968) A second type of late infantile amaurotic idiocy with multilamellar cytosomes. *Journal of Neuropathology and Experimental Neurology*, **27**, 371

Gordon, N. (1973) I-cell disease-mucolipidosis II. *Postgraduate Medical Journal*, **49**, 359

Gordon, N. (1978a) The pseudo-Hurler syndrome. *Developmental Medicine and Child Neurology*, **20**, 383

Gordon, N. (1978b) Infantile neuroaxonal dystrophy and related disorders. *Developmental Medicine and Child Neurology*, **20**, 497

Gordon, N. (1982) Fluctuating dystonia and allied syndromes. *Neuropediatrics*, **13**, 162

Gordon, N. (1987) Peroxisomal disorders. *Brain and Development*, **9**, 571

Gordon, N. and Marsden, H.B. (1966) Diffuse cerebral sclerosis and adrenal atrophy. *Developmental Medicine and Child Neurology*, **8**, 719

Gordon, N. and Thursby-Pelham, D. (1969) The Sanfilippo syndrome: an unusual disorder of mucopolysaccharide metabolism. *Developmental Medicine and Child Neurology*, **11**, 485

Gordon, N., Marsden, H.B. and Noronha, M. (1972) Neuronal ceroid lipofuscinosis (Batten's disease). *Archives of Disease in Childhood*, **47**, 285

Gordon, N., Marsden, H.B. and Lewis, D. (1974) Subacute necrotising encephalomyelopathy in three siblings. *Developmental Medicine and Child Neurology*, **16**, 64

Hagberg, B., Sourander, P. and Svennerholm, L. (1962) Sulfatide lipidosis in childhood. *American Journal of Diseases of Children*, **104**, 644

Hagberg, B. (1963) Clinical symptoms, signs and tests in metachromatic leucodystrophy. In *Brain Lipids and Lipoproteins and the Leucodystrophies* (eds. J. Folch-Pi and H. Bauer), Elsevier, Amsterdam

Hagberg, B., Kollberg, H., Sourander, P. and Akesson, H.O. (1969) Infantile globoid cell leucodystrophy (Krabbe's disease). *Neuropädiatrie*, **1**, 74

Hagberg, B., Halta, M., Sourander, P. *et al.* (1974) Polyunsaturated fatty acid lipidosis. Infantile form of so-called neuronal ceroid lipofuscinosis. *Acta Paediatrica Scandinavica*, **63**, 753

Hagberg, B., Haltia, M., Sourander, P. *et al.* (1978) Neurovisceral storage disorder simulating Niemann-Pick disease. *Neuropädiatrie*, **9**, 59

Harding, B.N., Egger, J., Portmann, B. and Erdohazi, M. (1986) Progressive neuronal degeneration of childhood with liver disease. *Brain*, **109**, 181

Horta-Barbosa, L., Fuccilo, D.A., Sever, J.L. and Zeman, W. (1969) Subacute sclerosing pan-encephalitis: isolation of measles virus from a brain biopsy. *Nature*, **221**, 974

Hugh-Jones, K. (1986) Psychomotor development of children with mucopolysaccharidosis, type 1-H following bone marrow transplantation. *Birth Defects*, **22**, 25

Huttenlocher, P.R. and Mattson, R.H. (1979) Isoprenosine in subacute sclerosing pan-encephalitis. *Neurology*, **29**, 763

Huttenlocher, P.R., Schwartz, A.D. and Klatskin, G. (1969) Reye's syndrome: ammonia intoxication as a possible factor in the encephalopathy. *Pediatrics*, **43**, 443

Huttenlocher, P.R., Solitare, G.B. and Adams, G. (1976) Infantile diffuse cerebral degeneration with hepatic cirrhosis. *Archives of Neurology*, **33**, 186

Ibrahim, M.M. and Jeavons, P.M. (1974) The value of electroencephalography in the diagnosis of subacute sclerosing panencephalitis. *Developmental Medicine and Child Neurology*, **16**, 295

Jabbour, J.T., Garcia, J.H., Lemmi, H. *et al.* (1969) Subacute sclerosing pan-encephalitis: a multidisciplinary study of eight cases. *Journal of the American Medical Association*, **207**, 2248

Jaffe, R., Crumrine, P., Hashida, Y. and Moser, H.W. (1982) Neonatal adrenoleukodystrophy. Clinical, pathological and biochemical delineation of a syndrome affecting both males and females. **108**, 100

Kelly, T.E. (1976) Hurler-like disorders in infancy. *Clin. Perinatal*, **3**, 115

Kelly, R.I., Datta, N.S., Bobyns, W.B. *et al.* (1986) Neonatal adrenoleukodystrophy: new cases, biochemical studies, and the differentiation from Zellweger and related peroxisomal polydystrophy syndromes. *Journal of Medical Genetics*, **23**, 869

Kihara, H., Ho, C-K., Fluharty, A.L. *et al.* (1980) Prenatal diagnosis of metachromatic leukodystrophy in a family with pseudo arylsulphatase A deficiency by the cerebroside sulfate loading test. *Pediatric Research*, **14**, 224

Kingston, H.M. (1989) Prenatal diagnosis. *British Medical Journal*, **289**, 1868

Kleijer, W.J., van Diggelen, O.P., Jonse, H.C. *et al.* (1984) First trimester diagnosis of Hunter's syndrome on chorionic villi. *Lancet*, **ii**, 472

Kliemann, F.A.D., Harden, A. and Pampiglione, G. (1969) Some EEG observations in patients with Krabbe's disease. *Developmental Medicine and Child Neurology*, **11**, 475

Klint, J.S., Dacremont, C. and Vlientinck. R. (1968) Type II Gm₁, gangliosidosis. *Lancet*, **ii**, 1080

Knudson, A.C., Di Ferrante, N. and Curtis, J.E. (1971) Effect of leukocyte transfusion in a child with type II mucopolysaccharidosis. *Proceedings of the National Academy of Sciences of the United States of America*, **68**, 1738

Kolår, O., Obrucnik, M., Behounkova, L. *et al.* (1967) Thymectomy in subacute sclerosing leucoencephalitis. *British Medical Journal*, **iii**, 22

Konkal, R.J., Bonsounis, D. and Kirban, K.C. (1987) Schilder's disease: additional aspects and a therapeutic option. *Neuropediatrics*, **18**, 149

Koprowski, H., Barbanti-Brodano, G. and Katz, M. (1970) Interaction between Papova-like virus and paramixovirus in human brain cells: a hypothesis. *Nature*, **225**, 1045

Koskiniemi, K., Donner, M.. Majuri, H. *et al.* (1974) Progressive myoclonus epilepsy. *Acta Neurologica Scandinavica*, **50**, 307

Larsson, T. and Sjögren, T. (1966) Dystonia musculorum deformans. A genetic and clinical population study of 121 cases. *Acta Neurologica Scandinavica*, **42**, Suppl. 17, 1

Lehesjoki, A.E., Koskiniemi, M., Sistonen, P. *et al.* (1991) Localization of a gene for progressive myoclonus epilepsy to chromosome 21q22. *Proceedings of the National Academy of Sciences, USA*, **88**, 3696

Leigh, D. (1951) Subacute necrotizing encephalomyelopathy in an infant. *Journal of Neurology, Neurosurgery and Psychiatry*, **14**, 216

Libert, J., Martin, J.J., Evrard, P. *et al.* (1977) Les céroide-lipofuscinosis. Ultrastructure oculaire et diagnostic par biopsie conjunctivale. *Arch. Opht. (Paris)*, **37**, 613

Longson, M. and Bailey, A.S. (1978) Early diagnosis and treatment of virus infections of the central nervous system. *The Practitioner*, **221**, 47

Lonsdale, D., Faulkner, W.R., Price, J.W. and Smeby, R.R. (1969) Intermittent cerebellar ataxia associated with hyperpyruvic acidemia, hyperalaninemia and hyperalaninuria. *Pediatrics*, **43**, 1025

Lovejoy, F.H., Smith, A.L., Bresnan, M.J. *et al.* (1974) Clinical staging in Reye's syndrome. *American Journal of Diseases of Children*, **128**, 36

Lovejoy, F.H., Bresnan, M.J., Lombroso, C.T. and Smith, A.L. (1975) Anticerebral oedema therapy in Reye's syndrome. *Archives of Disease in Childhood*, **50**, 933

MacLeod, P.M., Wood, S., Jan, J.E. *et al.* (1977) Progressive cerebellar ataxia, spasticity, psychomotor retardation, and hexosaminidase deficiency in a 10 year-old child: Sandhoff disease. *Neurology*, **27**, 571

Mann, V.M., Cooper, J.M., Javoy-Agid, F. *et al.* (1990) Mitochondrial function and parental sex effect in Huntington's chorea. *The Lancet*, **336**, 749

Matalon, R., Michals, K., Sebasta, D. *et al.* (1988) Aspartoacylase deficiency and N-acetylaspartic aciduria in patients with Canavan's disease. *American Journal of Medical Genetics*, **29**, 463

Matthews, R., Williams, H., Rickards, W. *et al.* (1961) Sydenham's chorea: its relationship to rheumatic infection and psychological illness. *Medical Journal of Australia*, **47**, 771

Max, S.R., Maclaren, N.K., Brady, R.O. *et al.* (1974) Gm₃ (hematoside) sphingolipodystrophy. *New England Journal of Medicine*, **291**, 929

McCusick, V.A. (1972) *Heritable Disorders of Connective Tissue*. 4th edn, C.V. Mosby, St Louis

Meyer, A. (1958) The Hallervorden-Spatz syndrome. In *Neuropathology* (eds. J.G. Greenfield, W. Blackwood, W.H. McMenemey *et al.*), Arnold, London

Meyer, A. and Earl, C.J.C. (1936) Studies on lesions of the basal ganglia in defectives: a case of état dysmyélinisé (Hallervorden-Spatz disease). *Journal of Mental Science*, **82**, 798

Miller, D.H., Robb, S.A., Ormorod, E.C. and Pohl, K.R.E. (1990) Magnetic resonance imaging of inflammatory and demyelinating white matter diseases of childhood. *Developmental Medicine and Child Neurology*, **32**, 97

Miller, J.H.D. and Neil, D.W. (1959) Serum mucoproteins in progressive familial myoclonic epilepsy. *Epilepsia*, **1**, 115

Minns, R.A. (1977) Clinical application of ventricular pressure monitoring in children. *Z. Kinderchir.*, **22**, 430

Mobley, W.C., White, C.L., Tennekoon, G. *et al.* (1983) Neonatal adrenoleukodystrophy. *Annals of Neurology*, **12**, 204

Montpetit, V.J.A., Andermann, F., Carpenter, S. *et al.* (1971) Subacute necrotizing encephalomyelopathy. A review and a study of two families. *Brain*, **94**, 1

Moser, A.E., Inderjit Singh, A.B., Brown, F.R. *et al.* (1984a) The cerebrohepatorenal (Zellweger) syndrome. *New England Journal of Medicine*, **310**, 1141

Moser, H.W., Moser, A.E., Singh, I. and O'Neill, B.P. (1984b) Adrenoleukodystrophy: survey of 303 cases: biochemistry, diagnosis and therapy. *Annals of Neurology*, **16**, 628

Myer, E.C., Morris, D.L., Brase, D.A. *et al.* (1990) Naltrexone therapy of apnea in children with elevated cerebrospinal fluid β-endorphin. *Annals of Neurology*, **27**, 75

Neville, B.G.R., Lake, B.D., Stephens, R. and Sanders, M.D. (1973) A neurovisceral storage disease with vertical supranuclear ophthalmoplegia and its relationship to Niemann-Pick disease. *Brain*, **96**, 97

Nishio, T., Sia, H., Nohara, R. *et al.* (1986) A case of adrenoleukodystrophy. *Brain and Development*, **8**, 192

Norman, R.M. (1962) Lipid disease of the brain. In *Modern Trends in Neurology* (ed. D. Williams), Butterworths, London

O'Brien, J. (1969a) Generalized gangliosidosis. *Journal of Pediatrics*, **75**, 167

O'Brien, J. (1969b) Five gangliosidosis. *Lancet*, **ii**, 805

Okada, S. and O'Brien, J.S. (1969) Tay-Sachs' disease: generalized absence of a beta-D-N-acetyl-hexosaminidase component. *Science*, **165**, 698

Owada, M., Nishiya, O., Sakiyama, T. and Kitagawa, T. (1980) Prenatal diagnosis of I-cell disease by measuring altered alpha-mannosidase activity in amniotic fluid. *Journal of Inherited Metabolic Disease*, **3**, 117

Park, B.E., Netsky, M.G. and Betsill, W.L. (1975) Pathogenesis of pigment and spheroid formation in Hallervorden-Spatz syndrome and related disorders. *Neuropathogy*, **25**, 1172

Partin, J.C. (1974) Liver ultrastructure in Reye's syndrome. In *Raye's Syndrome* (ed. J.D. Pollock), Grune and Stratton, New York

Partin, J.C., Schubert, W.K., Partin, J.S. *et al.* (1976) Isolation of influenza virus from liver and muscle biopsy specimens from a surviving case of Reye's syndrome. *Lancet*, **ii**, 599

Perry, T.L., Hansen, S. and Kloster, M. (1973) Huntington's chorea: deficiency of gamma-amino-butyric acid in brain. *New England Journal of Medicine*, **288**, 337

Pilz, H. (1970) Clinical, morphological and biochemical aspects of sphingolipidoses. *Neuropädiatrie*, **1**, 383

Pincus, J.H., Cooper, J.R., Itokawa, Y. and Gumbinas, M. (1971) Subacute necrotizing encephalomyelopathy. Effects of thiamine and thiamine propyl disulphide. *Archives of Neurology*, **24**, 511

Poser, C.M. (1968) Disease of the myelin sheath. In *Pathology of the Nervous System* (ed. J. Minckler), McGraw-Hill, New York

Poulas, A., Sharp, P., Fellenberg, A.J. and Danks, D.M. (1985) Cerebro-hepato-renal (Zellweger) syndrome, adrenoleucodystrophy, and Refsum's disease: plasma changes and skin fibroblast phytanic acid oxidase. *Human Genetics*, **70**, 172

Power, C., Poland, S.D., Blume, W.T. *et al.* (1990) Cytomegalovirus and Rasmusson's encephalitis. *Lancet*, **336**, 1282

Pullarkat, R.K., Patel, V.K. and Brockerhoff, H. (1978) Leukocyte decosahexaenoic acid in juvenile form of ceroid lipofuscinosis. *Neuropädiatrie*, **9**, 127

Raine, D.N., (1970) Biochemical relationships in the neuronal sphingolipidoses. *Developmental Medicine and Child Neurology*, **12**, 348

Raine, D.N. (1975) *The Treatment of Inherited Metabolic Disease*, Medical and Technical Publishing, Lancaster

Randolph, M. and Gelfman, N.A. (1968) Acute encephalopathy in children associated with acute hepatocellular dysfunction. Reye's syndrome revisited. *American Journal of Diseases of Children*, **116**, 303

Ray, A.B. (1977) Sulphatase deficiencies. In *The Cultured Cell and Inherited Metabolic Disease* (eds. R.A. Harkness and F. Cockburn), MTP Press, Lancaster

Reed, M.A. (1976) Leigh's disease: a family study. *Lancet*, **i**, 1237

Rees, L.H., Grant, D.B. and Wilson, J. (1975) Plasma corticotrophin levels in Addison-Schilder's disease. *British Medical Journal*, **iii**, 201

Reye, R.D.C., Morgan, G. and Baral, J. (1963) Encephalopathy and fatty degeneration of the viscera. A disease entity in childhood. *Lancet*, **ii**, 749

Roe, C.R. and Coates, P.M. (1989) Acyl CoA dehydrogenase deficiencies. In *The Metabolic Basis of Inherited Disease*, 6th edn (eds. C.R. Scriver, A.L. Beaudet, W.S. Sly and D. Valle), McGraw Hill, New York

Russo, L.S., Aron, A. and Anderson, P.J. (1976) Alexander's disease: a report and reappraisal. *Neurology*, **26**, 607

Sandhoff, K.V., Andreae, U. and Jatzkewitz, H. (1968) Deficient hexosaminidase activity in an exceptional case of Tay Sachs disease with additional storage of kidney globoside in visceral organs. *Life Sciences*, **7**, 283

Sanfilippo, S.J., Podosin, R., Langer, L. and Good, R.A. (1963) Mental retardation associated with acid mucopolysacchariduria heparitin sulphate type. *Journal of Pediatrics*, **63**, 837

Santavuori, P. (1988) Neuronal ceroid-lipofuscinosis in childhood. *Brain and Development*, **10**, 80

Santavuori, P., Haltia, M., Rapola. J. and Raitta, C. (1973) Infantile type of so-called neuronal-ceroid lipofuscinosis. 1 A clinical study of 15 patients. *Journal of the Neurological Sciences*, **18**, 257

Santavuori, P., Westermarck, T., Rapola, J. *et al.* (1985) Antioxidant treatment in Spielmeyer-Sjögren's disease. *Acta Neurologica Scandinavica*, **21**, 136

Santavuori, P., Rapola, J. Nuutila, A. *et al.* (1991) The spectrum of Janski-Bielschowski disease. *Neuropediatrics*, **22**, 92

Schneck, L., Friedland, J., Valenti. L. *et al.* (1970) Prenatal diagnosis of Tay-Sachs' disease. *Lancet*, **i**, 582

Schneck, S.A. (1968) Vaccination with measles and central nervous system disease. *Neurology*, **18**, 78

Schwarz, C.A. and Yanoff, M. (1965) Lafora's disease. Distinct clinico-pathologic form of Unverricht's syndrome. *Archives of Neurology*, **12**, 172

Seitelberger, F. (1968) Myoclonus body disease. In *Pathology of the Nervous System* (ed. J. Minckler), McCraw-Hill, New York

Sengers, R.C.A., Lamers, K.J.B., Bakkeren, J.A.J.M. *et al.* (1975) Infantile Gaucher's disease: glucocerebrosidase deficiency in peripheral blood leukocytes and cultured fibroblasts. *Neuropädiatrie*, **6**, 377

Shenker, D.M., Grossman, H.J. and Klawans, H.L. (1973) Treatment of Sydenham's chorea with haloperidol. *Developmental Medicine and Child Neurology*, **15**, 19

Sleigh, G. and Lindenbaum, R.H. (1981) Benign (non-paroxysmal) familial chorea. Paediatric perspectives. *Archives of Disease in Childhood*, **56**, 616

Sly, W.S., Quinton, B.A., McAlister, W.H. and Rimoin, D.L. (1973) Beta glucoronidase deficiency: report of clinical, radiologic and biochemical features of a new mucopolysaccharidosis. *Journal of Pediatrics*, **82**, 249

Spranger, J.W. and Wiedemann, H.R. (1970) The genetic mucolipidoses. *Humangenetik*, **9**, 113

Strecker, G., Michalski, J.C., Montreil, J. and Farriaux, J.P. (1976) Deficit in neuraminidase associated with mucolipidosis II (I-cell disease). *Biomedicine*, **25**, 238

Strouth, J.C., Zeman, W. and Merritt, A.D. (1966) Leucocyte abnormalities in familial amaurotic idiocy. *New England Journal of Medicine*, **274**, 36

Suzuki, K., Suzuki, K., Rapin, I. *et al.* (1970) Juvenile Gm_2 gangliosidosis. Clinical variant of Tay-Sachs disease or a new disease. *Neurology*, **20**, 190

Suzuki, Y. and Suzuki, K. (1971) Krabbe's globoid cell leukodystrophy: deficiency of galactocerebrosidase in serum, leukocytes, and fibroblasts. *Science*, **171**, 73

Svennerholm, L., Hagberg, B., Haltia, M. *et al.* (1975) Polyunsaturated fatty acid lipidosis. *Acta Paediatrica Scandinavica*, **64**, 489

Thaler, M.M., Hoogenraad, N.J. and Boswell, M. (1974) Reye's syndrome due to a novel protein-tolerant variant of ornithine transcarbamylase deficiency. *Lancet*, **ii**, 438

Torch, W.C. and Humphreys, H.K. (1986) Pharmological therapy of Hallervorden-Spatz syndrome. Two cases responsive to benztropine. *Annals of Neurology*, **20**, 445

Tourtellotte, W.W. (1968) Cerebrospinal fluid and its reactions in diseases. In *Pathology of the Nervous System* (ed. J. Minckler), McCraw-Hill, New York

Tourtellotte, W.W., Parker, J.A., Herndon, R.M. and Cuardros, C.V. (1968) Subacute sclerosing panencephalitis: brain immunoglobulin-G, measles antibody and albumin. *Neurology*, **18**, 117

Ulrich, J., Herschkowitz, N., Heitz, Ph. *et al.* (1978) Adrenoleukodystrophy. Preliminary report of a connatal case. *Acta Neuropathologica*, **43**, 77

Vakili, S., Drew, A.L., Schuching, S. *et al.* (1977) Hallervorden-Spatz syndrome. *Archives of Neurology*, **34**, 729

Valdimarsson, H., Agnaasdotir, C. and Lachmann, P.J. (1974) Cellular immunity in subacute sclerosing panencephalitis. *Proceedings of the Royal Society of Medicine*, **67**, 1125

Van Biervliet, J.P.G.M., Bruinins, L., van der Herden, C. *et al.* (1977) Report of a patient with severe chronic lactic acidaemia and pyruvate carboxylase deficiency. *Developmental Medicine and Child Neurology*, **19**, 392

van Bogaert, L. (1945) Une leuco-encéphalite sclérosante subaigue. *Journal of Neurology, Neurosurgery and Psychiatry*, **8**, 101

Vanier, M.T. and Svennerholm, L. (1975) Chemical pathology of Krabbe's disease. *Acta Paediatrica Scandinavica*, **64**, 641

Vanier, M.T., Rousson, R.M., Mandon, G. *et al.* (1989) Diagnosis of Niemann-Pick disease Type C on chorionic villus cells. *Lancet*, **i**, 1014

Vanier, M.T., Pentchev, P., Roderiguez-Lafrasse, C. and Rousson, R. (1991) Niemann-Pick disease type C: an update. *Journal of Inherited Metabolic Disease*, **14**, 580

Wanders, R.T.A., Van Roermund, C.W.T. and Van Wijland, M.J.A. (1987) Peroxisomal fatty acid beta-oxidation in human skin fibroblasts: X-linked adrenoleucodystrophy, a peroxisomal very long chain acyl-coA synthetase deficiency. *Journal of Inherited Metabolic Disease*, **10**, 220

Weiner, H.L. and Hauser, S.L. (1982) Neuroimmunology II: antigenic specificity of the nervous system. *Annals of Neurology*, **12**, 499

Willner, J.E., Grabowski, G.A., Gordon, R.E. *et al.* (1981) Chronic Gm_2 gangliosidosis masquerading as atypical Friedreich's ataxia: clinical, morphological and biochemical studies in nine cases. *Neurology*, **31**, 787

Wilson, J. (1972) Investigation of degenerative disease of the central nervous system. *Archives of Disease in Childhood*, **47**, 163

Wilson, J., Manners, B.T.B., Robins, D.G. and Erdohazi, M. (1981) Persistent hiccups as a presenting feature of Alexander's leucodystrophy. *Developmental Medicine and Child Neurology*, **23**, 660

Woolf, L.I. (1962) Recent work on phenylketonuria and maple syrup urine disease (leucinosis). *Proceedings of the Royal Society of Medicine*, **55**, 824

Wraith, J.E. and Alani, S.M. (1990) Carpal tunnel syndrome in the mucopolysaccaridoses and related disorders. *Archives of Disease in Childhood*, **65**, 962

Yoshioka, H., Nishimura, O., Nakagawa, M. *et al.* (1989) Administration of human leukocyte interferon to patients with subacute sclerosing panencephalitis. *Brain and Development*, **11**, 302

Yudell, A., Gomez, M.R., Lambert, E.H. and Docherty, M.B. (1967) The neuropathy of sulfatide lipidosis (metachromatic leucodystrophy). *Neurology*, **17**, 103

Zeman, W. and Dyken, P. (1974) Neuronal ceroid lipofuscinosis (Batten's disease): relationship to amaurotic family idiocy. *Paediatrics*, **44**, 570

Zeman, W. (1974) Studies in the neuronal ceroid lipofuscinoses. *Journal of Neuropathology and Experimental Neurology*, **33**, 1

Zu Rhein, G.M. and Chou, S.M. (1965) Particles resembling papova viruses in human cerebral demyelinating disease. *Science*, **148**, 1477

Zu Rhein, G.M., Eichmann, P.L. and Puletti, F. (1960) Familial idiocy with spongy degeneration of the central nervous system of van Bogaert-Bertrand type. *Neurology*, **10**, 998

12 Neurological disorders complicating general medical conditions; and neurosurgical problems

Neurological disorders can complicate a large number of systemic diseases, diseases which do not primarily involve the nervous system but often affect it to a serious degree. Some examples of these will be discussed to illustrate the importance of a careful examination of all systems of the body. With the rapid increase of knowledge that has occurred in this century specialization has become a necessity, but the good specialist is likely to be the good physician with a widely based experience of medicine. Paediatric neurosurgery is a subject of its own, and only certain aspects can be considered which particularly involve the paediatric neurologist. Congenital anomalies, including spina bifida, diastematomyelia and hydrocephalus are discussed in Chapter 4.

System diseases

Affecting the central and peripheral systems and the muscles

Gastrointestinal diseases

The dangers of gastroenteritis in infancy are well recognized, and vascular complications of dehydration have already been mentioned. Hypernatraemia with a plasma sodium level greater than 150 mEq per litre is associated with a high incidence of neurological symptoms and signs. Those occurring at the time of the illness include irritability, increased muscle tone and convulsions, and may occur in more than a third of affected children (Morris-Jones, Houston and Evans, 1967). Persistent neurological disabilities are also common, particularly mental handicap, spasticity and epilepsy (Macaulay and Watson, 1967). The brain damage is thought to be due to vascular lesions, both thrombotic and haemorrhagic. Cerebral oedema also plays a part, particularly during rehydration with salt-poor solutions, and is related to the onset of convulsions. The blood pressure should be restored using plasma; and subsequent fluids must be given slowly, aiming to produce normal electrolytes in 36–48 hours. Half normal saline and dextrose may be the best therapy, with no more than the daily fluid requirements of 150 ml/kg body weight during the first 48 hours. Plasma osmolarity must be carefully monitored and hypocalcaemia corrected if necessary (Chambers, 1975). Cerebral oedema is more likely to arise when too rapid rehydration induces a significant discrepancy between serum and cerebrospinal fluid osmolarity (dysequilibrium syndrome).

Renal and hepatic diseases

Coma and convulsions can be due to the biochemical disorders which accompany renal failure, but these are unlikely to cause diagnostic difficulties. Occasionally a child is admitted to hospital with signs of raised intracranial pressure including papilloedema and retinal haemorrhages, and an intracranial space-occupying lesion may be suspected. If this is due to hypertension caused by renal disease, such as acute glomerulonephritis, then the correct diagnosis will be made as long as the blood pressure is recorded as a routine.

The coma resulting from hepatic failure may develop insidiously, and the patients seem to be asleep. A flapping tremor of the arms is a finding which is very suggestive of this diagnosis.

Respiratory diseases

Hypercapnia can result from chronic pulmonary disease, such as cystic fibrosis, and from hypoventilation resulting from severe chest deformities and disorders of the motor system like muscular dystrophy (McCormack and Spalter, 1966). It can be associated with papilloedema, but rarely with other signs of raised intracranial pressure. The primary clinical concern will focus on respiratory function, but the appearance of the optic fundi can be misleading. Pulmonary oedema associated with an intracranial lesion causing raised pressure is not likely to be confused with this state. Treatment to rectify the raised CO_2 tension has to be given with caution.

The association of a polio-like illness with asthma has been mentioned in Chapter 10.

Endocrine and metabolic disorders

Myopathies associated with hypo- and hyperthyroidism are excessively rare in childhood (Johnston, 1974). Hypokalaemic periodic paralysis and myasthenia gravis have been reported in thyrotoxicosis, and myotonia in hypothyroidism. These conditions have been considered in Chapter 7. Cretinism will have to be considered in the differential diagnosis of infants who fail to thrive, have prolonged jaundice in the newborn period, hypotonia or a hoarse cry. Hypokalaemia, which can cause transient muscle weakness, occurs in a variety of conditions, such as primary aldosteronism, adrenal hyperplasia, hypokalaemia associated with renal disease, gastroenteritis and an excessive intake of licorice.

Diabetes insipidus presenting with polydipsia and polyuria can result from lesions in the anterior hypothalamus or pituitary. These may be due to trauma, tumours, meningitis or encephalitis. Occasionally the diabetes insipidus is nephrogenic in origin due to a lack of response of the kidneys to endogenous or exogenous antidiuretic hormone (ADH). There is evidence that this is genetically determined, with a sex-linked recessive mode of inheritance. Dehydration can occur easily, and this may be related to the physical and mental retardation that occurs in the nephrogenic type unless it is diagnosed at an early stage and carefully treated.

The diagnosis can present certain difficulties. The 8-hour water deprivation test, which must be carried out under careful supervision, will show if the patient can excrete concentrated urine and prevent the plasma osmolarity rising. If there is a possibility of compulsive water drinking, a careful watch will have to be kept to prevent surreptitious drinking (Besser, 1972).

Occasionally the opposite may occur, with inappropriate secretion of ADH. This can complicate a number of conditions, including some causing brain damage, such as meningitis, raised intracranial pressure, subarachnoid haemorrhage and trauma. In view of the widely different causes, and the fact that treatment varies, so that in some cases giving hypertonic saline may be harmful, it may be best to restrict the use of the term inappropriate secretion of ADH. It has been suggested that it should only refer to tumour secretion of ADH (Thomas *et al.*, 1978). There is concentration of the urine and hypernatraemia. Mental confusion and seizures can result.

Pituitary diabetes insipidus is most effectively treated with I-desamino-8D-arginine vasopressin (DDAVP), a synthetic vasopressin which is given intranasally 5–10 mg twice daily (Kauli and Laran, 1974). ADH in the form of 'pitressin' tannate in oil can be given by intramuscular injection. Chlorpropamide can also be effective by increasing the renal response to the hormone. In the nephrogenic type there will be no response to pitressin analogues. An adequate water intake must be assured, and sodium and protein intake restricted. Paradoxically, a chlorothiazide diuretic causes salt depletion and increased proximal tubular reabsorption (Schotland, Grumbach and Strauss, 1963). Potassium supplements will be needed.

Diabetes mellitus can be complicated by a polyneuritis, especially if the condition is poorly controlled; in fact, the stricter the treatment of the diabetes the better the chance of improvement of the neurological signs. The most common form is a sensory neuropathy, and an autonomic neuropathy can occur with disturbances of bladder function and other symptoms. A predominantly motor neuropathy in a patient on dietary therapy may be reversed by giving insulin. The aetiology is partly metabolic and partly vascular. It is certainly rare in young children.

Hypoglycaemic attacks, sometimes producing convulsions, not infrequently complicate the course of diabetes mellitus in childhood, and, if prolonged, can cause brain damage. The hyperosmolar state of diabetic kctoacidosis can present problems similar to those of gastroenteritis, with the risk of cerebral oedema on rehydration. Hypertension and excessive blood viscosity, particularly when associated with hyperlipidaemia, can lead to cerebral infarction. Excessive use of bicarbonate can cause cardiorespiratory arrest.

Hypertension due to hormonal disorders can also cause diagnostic difficulties if it leads to symptoms and signs of raised intracranial pressure, and especially if it is intermittent as sometimes occurs in association with a pheochromocytoma. This is a rare tumour growing from chomaffin tissue, usually of the adrenal medulla. If the history is of headaches and convulsions a cerebral tumour can easily be falsely suspected. There is an abnormal production of adrenalin and noradrenalin, and the diagnosis is confirmed by finding an excess of these substances in the serum or of their metabolites in the urine. The site of the tumour is confirmed by special X-ray examination, selective aortography being the most helpful; and it is usually possible to remove it (Swenson, 1962). Pre-operative expansion of the total vascular space for two weeks using phenoxybenzamine, an alpha-blocker, with blood transfusion if anaemia results, and partial beta-blockade, for example with propranolol, have markedly reduced operative mortality.

Hypertension can complicate Cushing's syndrome, often due to a tumour or hypertrophy of the adrenal cortex with over-production of steroids, although occasionally it may result from a basophil adenoma of the pituitary. The appearance of the child is usually characteristic enough, with rounded facies, obesity, hirsutism and acne (Hayles *et al.*, 1966). An adrenal tumour can also cause an excessive production of aldosterone. This will cause hypertension, muscular weakness, polydipsia and polyuria. Serum bicarbonate and sodium is raised, and the potassium level is depressed, as has already been mentioned (Conn, 1955).

Deficiency diseases

Diseases such as rickets can occur in the presence of adverse social conditions, and, owing to difficulties of feeding, can affect any child who is severely mentally and physically handicapped. Rickets can also complicate anti-epileptic therapy. It can present as pain in the limbs, which may be thought to be of neurological origin. Malabsorption complicating conditions such as coeliac disease can result in failure to thrive and delayed motor development. Occasionally this can be so marked that neurological diseases, such as infantile spinal muscular atrophy, may be suggested.

Vitamin E deficiency linked to a number of diseases such as cholestatic liver disease and intestinal malabsorption can affect the nervous system, and in particular cause a spinocerebellar syndrome and a peripheral neuropathy (Gordon, 1987).

Encephalopathies

Terms such as 'encephalitis' and 'encephalopathy' are obviously dangerous if they delude anyone into thinking that a diagnosis has been made merely by using such names. This is well illustrated in the case of *acute lead encephalopathy*, a diagnosis which is easy to miss if it is not thought of. There is still plenty of lead in old paintwork and in the lead piping in old properties which can be ingested, by children, and even plastic toys can be a danger if made in lead moulds. An increase in atmospheric lead levels in areas of high traffic density, and parental involvement in lead-using industries may also increase the risk of poisoning, as may a history of pica.

The child becomes drowsy and irritable, and there may be abdominal pain and constipation. Epileptic seizures are an early symptom, and evidence of raised intracranial pressure is soon manifest, including papilloedema in many instances. Hemiplegia and cerebellar ataxia are not uncommon.

Findings such as punctate basophilia of red cells, raised erythrocyte protoporphyrin, excess secretion of coproporphyrin III in the urine, and the lead lines at the ends of the long bones (Fig. 12.1) are obviously suggestive, but a definite

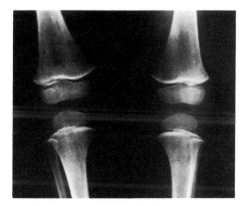

Figure 12.1   Lead lines at ends of long bones in lead poisoning.

diagnosis can only be made by finding a raised level of lead in the serum. If the serum lead level is borderline it may be justifiable to carry out an edathomil calcium disodium diagnostic test (Whitaker, Austin and Nelson, 1962). This consists of an intramuscular dose of edathomil calcium disodium (75 mg/kg body weight in a 20% solution, with 15% procaine divided into three doses at 8-hourly intervals), and a subsequent collection of urine over 24 hours. If the excretion of lead in the urine is more than 500 mg per litre there has been an excessive ingestion of lead-containing substances, and the child must be removed from the source of exposure and treatment considered.

In classical lead poisoning, or if the serum level of lead is persistently about 50 µg per 100 ml, treatment can be given with a combination of 2,3-dimercapto-1-propanol (BAL) and edathamil calcium disodium (calcium EDTA). The dose of the former is 500 mg/m² per 24 hours, and of the later 1500 mg/m² per 24 hours, with procaine added to the 20% calcium EDTA concentrate in a final concentration of 0.5% to lessen pain. Each is given by deep intramuscular injection at separate sites in divided doses 4-hourly for 5 days. This is a maximum dosage and can be modified for the treatment of the more chronic syndromes, for example by giving calcium EDTA alone in a dose of 500 mg/m² 12-hourly intramuscularly for 3–5 days (Chisolm and Barltrop, 1979). Such treatment should not be given if lead, which can still be absorbed, is demonstrated in the alimentary canal by X-ray examination; until this has been removed. D-penicillamine is given when the condition is mild, or to prevent the rebound in blood lead after treatment with BAL and calcium EDTA, in two oral doses a day of 10 mg/kg body weight for a week at a time. Intravenous diazepam or paraldehyde must be given if convulsions occur, and mannitol may be necessary to re-establish adequate urine flow before calcium EDTA is given (Chisolm and Barltrop, 1979). A course of dexamethazone may be required if there is cerebral oedema.

Burns encephalopathy can lead to unexpected death, as it can occur with relatively small burns or scalds (sometimes as little as 5% of the body surface). It usually occurs during the first 48 hours after the burn. It may be mild, but the symptoms include vomiting, impairment of consciousness and twitching. The blood pressure and temperature are usually raised. Sometimes increasing coma ensues, and death may be associated with status epilepticus or respiratory arrest. The condition is related to cerebral oedema, and therefore treatment is directed towards reducing this. A dose of 7 ml/kg body weight of 20% mannitol, followed by 4 mg dexamethazone intravenously 4-hourly for 36–48 hours is usually an effective regime. Anticonvulsants are also indicated, and intravenous diazepam or other emergency treatment, may be needed initially, if fits occur. The exact cause of the encephalopathy is unknown (Warlow and Hinton, 1969).

Other instances of 'encephalopathies' may be due to such causes as uraemia, glycine, anoxia, hypertension or poisoning; and the post-ictal state which can lead to permanent brain damage may result not only from anoxia but also from metabolic disturbances. An addition to the differential diagnosis is toluene intoxication due to glue sniffing. This can result in an encephalopathy with coma, hallucinations, ataxia, convulsions and behaviour disturbances (King et al., 1981). Every effort must be made to find a cause for the symptoms and to exclude conditions requiring specific therapy, but symptomatic treatment (e.g. to reduce cerebral oedema) can often prevent subsequent disability and death.

These are only a few reminders that the body functions as a whole, and that disorders of one system will affect others to a greater or lesser degree, just as there is no line of division between disorders of function and those of structure.

Iatrogenic disease

It is well recognized that some diseases may be iatrogenic or self-induced: one obvious example is the long-term effects of anti-epileptic treatment and the possibility that this may seriously affect the child's development. Not enough consideration has been given to these problems in the past, and criticism (Illich, 1974) can only be refuted if a child's progress is assessed more carefully than it has sometimes been, and this applies to both surgical and medical treatment.

Sarcoidosis

The cause of this condition is unknown, but the three most favoured theories are: (1) a form of tuberculosis; (2) some other type of infection; and (3) a tissue hypersensitivity.

Patients with sarcoidosis fail to react to inoculation with tuberculin, although this is not a specific feature of the disease. There is always the possibility of a virus infection, but this has not yet been proven. The third possibility puts sarcoidosis in the same category as collagen diseases (Jefferson, 1957).

The sarcoid granuloma or follicle may occur in a variety of organs, and may coalesce to form tumour-like masses. It consists of a variety of cells, including giant cells and large polyhedral epithelioid cells.

The condition is rare in childhood, and damage to the nervous system is rare at any age. There may be involvement of the cranial nerves, particularly the optic nerve and both facial nerves. Peripheral neuropathies, meningitis and focal cerebral lesions can occur alone or in combination.

If there are no conveniently enlarged lymph nodes to biopsy, or suggestive involvement of the skin or lungs, diagnosis can be very difficult. The Mantoux reaction may be negative, the blood calcium increased, and the erythrocyte sedimentation rate raised. The Kveim test is not absolutely reliable.

Treatment is with ACTH or adrenocortical steroids, and with cyclosporin. Intracranial space-occupying lesions may need surgical intervention.

Cardiovascular diseases

Although cardiovascular diseases do not present so many problems in childhood as in later life, they are, when they occur, just as serious, and can be considered under the same headings. There are those intracerebral cardiovascular disorders complicating generalized diseases, and primary intracerebral vascular lesions.

Cerebral haemorrhage

Intracerebral haemorrhage in the newborn will not be considered in this chapter. In older children, apart from trauma and bleeding from vascular anomalies, intracranial haemorrhage occurs in blood disorders such as aplastic anaemia, idiopathic thrombocytopaenic purpura, clotting factor deficiencies and acute leukaemia, as well as in very severe infections with septicaemia, and associated with hypertension. Haemorrhage can also result from consumption coagulopathy (the defibrination syndrome) following endothelial damage after anoxia, severe infections or some other cause. The platelet count will drop, as will the levels of clotting factors V and VIII and fibrinogen (de Gruchy, 1970). Haemorrhages may occur into the brain and into other tissues.

There will be a sudden onset of focal neurological signs and the cerebrospinal fluid will be blood-stained. Such episodes can also result from haemorrhage into a tumour. If the bleeding spreads to the subarachnoid space an aseptic meningitis will result, and vasospasm and raised intracranial pressure are likely to occur. The former may cause focal symptoms and signs, and the latter can demand medical treatment. Giving calcitonin-gene-related peptide by infusion may reverse the cerebral ischaemia (Johnston *et al.*, 1990).

Cerebral thrombosis

Arterial and venous thrombosis can complicate severe dehydration and infections, particularly meningitis. It also occurs in the presence of polycythaemia resulting from certain types of congenital heart disease, and in 'collagen' diseases of various types, and in moyamoya disease and fibromuscular hypoplasia. The neurological defect may be of sudden or gradual onset, sometimes preceded by episodes of transient symptoms or signs. These will depend on the part of the brain deprived of a normal blood supply.

Venous sinus thrombosis has been considered in Chapter 10.

Thrombosis affecting major vessels

Thrombosis of the carotid arteries in the neck is unlikely to be due to atheroma in childhood and adolescence. However, it does occur in response to external injury to the artery. This can result from trauma to the neck or tonsillar fossa, or from inflammation spreading from infected cervical glands (Edwards, Gordon and Rob, 1960). In childhood there is a greater tendency for the thrombosis to spread to the intracranial arteries, which at first sight is surprising. This is possibly the result of external injuries involving the cervical sympathetic plexus on the surface of the carotid artery leading to spasm of the whole of the carotid artery, rather than atheromatous plaques affecting the intima. If this does happen, impairment of intellectual function and hemiplegia will be inevitable.

Thrombosis can also involve the vertebro-basilar system (Ouvrier and Hopkins, 1970). Recurrent attacks of dizziness, ataxia and vomiting occur, and lead to varying degrees of paralysis and sometimes coma. Horner's syndrome, ocular palsies, dysarthria and ataxia are other possible findings on examination. The aetiology is frequently obscure, although some form of arteritis is often suspected. This may be secondary to meningitis, septicaemia or infected emboli. Treatment with anti-coagulants can be considered if the condition is progressive and there is no definite evidence of infection or haemorrhage.

In moyamoya disease (so called because of the net-like collaterals seen on the carotid arteriogram looking like 'a puff of smoke drifting in the air') there is occlusion of a number of the main intracranial arteries. A total of 50% of affected patients present before the age of 10 years. Sometimes there is one episode only with partial or full recovery, but in others there is rapid deterioration with recurrent acute attacks and death. The hemiplegia can alternate between right and left sides, and there can be sensory disturbances and mental disorders. Headaches and seizures induced by crying and hyperventilation often occur between and during ischaemic episodes. On histological examination eccentric and laminated hypertrophy of the intima has been noted, with abnormal tortuosity and duplication of the internal elastic lamina and thinning of the media. Similar but unilateral appearances (moyamoya phenomenon) can occur in other conditions such as neurofibromatosis, tuberous sclerosis, encephalo-trigeminal-angiomatosis, tuberculous meningitis, periarteritis nodosa, Down's syndrome and previous radiation therapy. A possible cause may be a generalized immunological arteritis, especially affecting arteries which receive their innervation from the superior cervical sympathetic ganglia. The prognosis is poor, as dementia and progressive neurological deterioration can occur. Surgical treatment is sometimes possible, with the best operation likely to be a combination of perivascular sympathectomy and superior cervical ganglionectomy, with an interval of several weeks between sides, and some form of arterial bypass. If haematomas collect they must be removed (Gordon and Isler, 1989). In fibromuscular hypoplasia there are defects in the walls of medium-sized vessels which results in the 'string of beads' appearance revealed by arteriography. The aetiology of both conditions is unknown (Isler, 1971).

Cerebral embolism

Cerebral embolism is a relatively common cause of neurological lesions of vascular aetiology in childhood. The embolus can occur in the context of cyanotic congenital heart disease, rheumatic heart disease and bacterial endocarditis, including infection of the valves used in the treatment of hydrocephalus. The onset of the symptoms will be sudden and, with septic emboli, the problems of infection are added to those of brain damage. Fat emboli can occur after fractures, and air emboli during open heart surgery. Loss of consciousness is common, as well as seizures, dysphasias, hemianopia and hemiplegia.

Hypertension

As will be seen, hypertension in childhood can complicate a variety of conditions from endocrine disturbances to renal and respiratory diseases, to encephalopathies and cerebral tumours, particularly of posterior fossa location. The hypertension is sometimes paroxysmal and blood pressure should therefore be monitored at frequent intervals in acute neurological diseases. The most satisfactory treatment for sudden rises of blood pressure is diazoxide in a dose of 5 mg/kg body weight intravenously. Alternatives are diazepam if convulsions are also occurring, and frusomide (0.5–1.5 mg/kg body weight parenterally) in milder cases. A possible mechanism for acute hypertension may be a loss of integration between the control of blood volume and the capacity of the vascular bed (Eden, Sills and Brown, 1977).

'Collagen diseases'

Collagen diseases can be both acute and chronic, but they are rare in childhood. An example of the chronic type is polymyositis, which has been considered with other muscle disorders (Chapter 7). The acute diseases, such as periarteritis nodosa and disseminated lupus erythematosis, can present with evidence of damage to the central and peripheral nervous systems. Lesions will result if small vessels are involved in the inflammatory process, and thrombose. The peripheral neuropathy may be of gradual onset, but other lesions occur suddenly. Rare as these diseases may be, when such an unusual episode occurs in childhood it is worthwhile keeping them in mind. The diagnosis is supported by the presence of anaemia, eosinophilia and a raised erythrocyte sedimentation rate. To make a definite diagnosis of lupus erythematosis (LE), LE cells must be identified. The typical vascular abnormalities found in a skin or muscle biopsy will confirm the diagnosis of polyarteritis nodosa. As there is a good chance of a favourable response to treatment with steroids, early diagnosis is essential.

Heart disease

The risk of emboli in rheumatic heart disease has already been mentioned. If an intracranial arterio-venous anomaly shunts enough blood through large vessels congestive heart failure can occur. This may present before the vascular lesion has been recognized, although neurological signs will usually be present.

A cardiomyopathy occurs in Friedreich's ataxia and may be a cause of death among these patients. An abnormal ECG with conduction defects, inversion of the T wave and other evidence of left ventricular hypertrophy can be present before there is any clinical evidence of cardiac involvement. There is a similar association in Refsum's syndrome (Gordon and Hudson, 1959). The heart muscle can also be involved in a variety of myopathies, from glycogen storage diseases to Duchenne muscular dystrophy, and it is as well to examine the ECG in all cases of muscle disease.

If the conducting tissues of the heart are involved, for example in rheumatic or congenital heart disease, the child may present with attacks of unconsciousness, and epilepsy can be suspected (Stephenson, 1990). A careful history can reveal an absence of a tonic or clonic phase in the attack, although the latter can certainly occur during syncope. The child is more likely to be limp, pale or cyanotic. Such attacks may be caused by paroxysmal atrial tachycardia, and sometimes by heart block. Particularly when they start during exercise the possibility of the sick sinus syndrome should be considered, as it occasionally occurs during childhood (Scott, McCartney and Deverall, 1976). The evidence of sinus bradycardia may be hard to find, even with provocative tests, and repeated examination may be needed. Techniques of prolonged ECG recording over 24 hours can reveal transient abnormalities in this and other arythmias and establish the diagnosis. If sinus arrest occurs and is not replaced by other rhythms there are obvious dangers to life. Occasionally it is necessary to insert an artificial demand pacemaker (Ferrer, 1973).

Cardiomyopathy can complicate a number of infections which also involve the nervous system, such as Coxsackie virus infections and toxoplasmosis.

Aneurysms and angiomas of the brain

The so-called 'berry' or 'congenital aneurysms' can occur at any age, and may cause subarachnoid haemorrhage in childhood. They are due to a weakness in the wall of the cerebral arteries at their bifurcations, resulting from a deficiency of the muscle layer. These malformations will have been present from birth, but the prolapse of the intima through the gap will take time to enlarge, and, although it may rupture when very small, it will rarely cause focal signs until adult life. If subarachnoid haemorrhage does occur xanthochromia has been detected within a few hours and may persist for several weeks. Lumbar puncture is contra-indicated if there are gross neurological signs, evidence of increased intracranial pressure, or a deteriorating level of consciousness.

Angiomas are quite likely to cause trouble in childhood. These consist of collections of vessels over the surface of the brain and within the cerebral hemispheres. They may cause focal symptoms and signs, or may result in a gradual dementia due to their

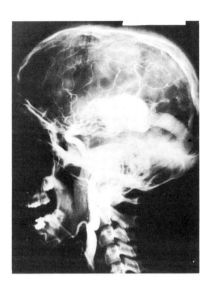

Figure 12.2   Arteriovenous malformation draining into the vein of Galen. The course of the anterior cerebral artery indicates hydrocephalus.

action as a vascular shunt depriving the brain of an adequate blood supply. Subarachnoid haemorrhage in childhood is more likely to arise from an angioma than an aneurysm.

The focal features of an aneurysm prior to rupture most often result from pressure on the cranial nerves, particularly the optic and oculomotor nerves. Occasional confusion can be caused by the Tolasa-Hunt syndrome, with ophthalmoplegia being caused by inflammatory changes within the cavernous sinus. This can respond to treatment with steroids (Terrence and Samaha, 1973). The focal symptoms of angioma more frequently involve the cerebrum. Repeated focal seizures without evidence of raised intracranial pressure may be suggestive, and evidence of more permanent damage such as hemianopia or hemiplegia can occur. Presumably these signs arise either as a result of impaired local blood supply or destruction of tissue from compression, thrombosis, or haemorrhage. If the vascular malformation affects the posterior cerebral artery and the vein of Galen there can be obstruction of the aqueduct resulting in internal hydrocephalus (Fig. 12.2), and, as in the case of any arterio-venous shunt, congestive heart failure may occur (Gomez *et al.*, 1963).

An intracranial bruit can sometimes be heard, especially over the orbits, but bruits are not uncommon during childhood due to no discoverable cause, and are probably related to haemodynamic effects of increased blood flow, or changes in the composition of the blood such as anaemia (Dodge, 1956). They are often transmitted from the chest. Even unilateral bruits do not necessarily indicate the presence of a vascular lesion. The EEG may show focal abnormalities, but, if such a lesion is suspected, scans and arteriography are the investigations of choice to try to confirm the diagnosis.

It is sometimes possible to remove these vascular lesions at operation, but if not, the main feeding artery may be ligated. Carotid ligation is not likely to affect an angioma, as they are located well beyond the major arterial bifurcations at the base of the brain, but it can be helpful in cases of certain aneurysms which are not amenable to more direct attack.

Angiomas of the spinal cord

Such vascular anomalies sometimes cover large areas of the spinal cord. Signs of damage to the cord can appear suddenly or gradually, depending on whether there is sudden bleeding into the tissues or an interference with the blood supply. Pain may be a predominant symptom, and signs of spastic paraplegia are the most common finding on examination. Occasionally, a bruit is heard on auscultation over the spinal column. Bleeding into the cerebrospinal fluid can occur, but usually there is only an elevation of the protein level. A myelogram is likely to show a pattern compatible with the tortuous vessels over the surface of the cord, and, although it is a highly specialized technique, spinal arteriography can be helpful in showing the vascular supply. Removal of these vessels at operation is occasionally possible (Shepherd, 1963).

Head injuries

The complications of head injuries are many and varied. The skull may be fractured, and, if the fracture is depressed, operative treatment may be needed to re-elevate the bone. Haemorrhage can occur inside and outside the brain. Extradural haematomas due to arterial bleeding are likely to lead to deepening unconsciousness soon after the injury. Such a change in the level of consciousness may obviously be due to laceration of the brain, but, particularly when this is sudden, the possibility of an extradural haematoma should be considered. Computerized axial tomography (CT scan) can resolve this dilemma.

Subdural haematomas

Subdural haematomas are one of those conditions in medicine which have to be constantly kept in mind as a possible diagnosis, even when the symptoms and signs are not particularly suggestive, and this is especially true in infancy. They can occur after relatively trivial head injuries, including trauma at birth, and after severe dehydration; and they may cause misleading symptoms, e.g. failure to thrive and vomiting in infancy. When diagnosed in the early stages the condition is particularly amenable to treatment. The presence of retinal haemorrhages, especially subhyaloid ones, is a very suggestive finding.

Classically, but by no means always, there is a stage in which the patient's condition improves and is then followed by gradual deterioration; and unless a careful watch is kept on such parameters as pulse rate, respiration rate, blood pressure, and size and reactions of the pupils, the patient may be thought to be sleeping rather than suffering from a dangerous degree of cerebral compression. In the case of subdural haematomas the bleeding is venous, due to tearing of the diploic veins which cross the subdural space from the scalp veins to those in the subarachnoid space. The force in most head injuries is a shearing one, and it is not surprising that these delicate veins are torn.

Sometimes the blood accumulates so slowly that there is nothing to suggest a complication, apart from perhaps a failure to improve as rapidly as might be expected. The bleeding may stop and the haematoma cease to enlarge. Although the causal mechanism is uncertain, the encysted fluid can occasionally increase again in volume with a resulting rise in the intracranial pressure. As the haematomas are frequently bilateral, they can in early life mimic the appearances of hydrocephalus, and, if undiagnosed, may calcify, thus preventing the expansion of the developing brain and causing mental retardation.

A normal cerebrospinal fluid pressure and protein level do not exclude the presence of a subdural haematoma, and once the suspicion has been raised investigations must be done to prove or disprove this diagnosis. When the fontanelles are still open, subdural taps can be carried out, otherwise brain scans are the most useful tests. Very occasionally subdural haematomas may not be defined by computerized axial tomography, as their density gradually decreases and for a time is the same as that of the brain. Repeated taps and drainage, but not aspiration, of the subdural space until there is no evidence of further accumulation of fluid may be all that is required. Care must be taken not to remove too much fluid at one time. Sometimes burr-holes accompanied by washing through the cavity with saline will be needed, or continuous drainage in the hope that the inner wall of the cavity will become adherent; and if a more rigid capsule has formed it may have to be removed at craniotomy to enable the underlying brain to expand. A shunt into the peritoneal space may occasionally be necessary. Blood transfusions are often needed in infancy to counteract the shock resulting from the large loss of blood into the haematoma (Sparacio, Khatib and Cook, 1971).

Some other complications

Among the other short-term complications of head injury, intracerebral haematomas have to be considered. If their presence is confirmed, by isotope or CAT scan, they should be evacuated immediately. In fact the use of computerized axial tomography has greatly simplified the management of head injuries. The high density haematomas can be identified even in unusual sites, and they can be differentiated from the low density cerebral contusions or chronic subdural haematomas. Also, serial scans can monitor the response to therapy (Ambrose *et al.*, 1975a). Raised intracranial pressure from cerebral oedema in the absence of haematoma can be life-threatening unless treated urgently, and the use of intracranial pressure monitoring helps to rationalize treatment (Lewin, 1976). Infections such as meningitis and cerebral abscess may occur. Air may be found to have collected within the cranium, and cerebrospinal fluid otorrhoea and rhinorrhoea, and carotico-cavernous fistulae are other rare findings. Almost any of the cranial nerves can be damaged, particularly if a fracture line cuts across their exit foramina. The oculomotor nerves, the facial nerve and the auditory nerve are the ones most often affected.

In the period immediately following a head injury, apart from treatment of such complications, the nursing care of the patient will be of fundamental importance. If unconscious, the patient will be nursed best lying on one side, and every care will have to be taken to ensure an adequate airway. Sometimes it is necessary for a tracheostomy with controlled ventilation to be considered. If there is a drop in blood pressure it is advisable to raise the patient's legs to encourage venous return to the heart, but not the foot of the bed which may increase intracranial venous pressure. A particular watch must be kept for hyperpyrexia and electrolyte disturbances. Dexamethazone may be given to counteract the possibility of cerebral oedema, although there is no positive proof of its effectiveness, and if raised intracranial pressure does occur urgent treatment must be started with drugs such as urea or mannitol.

In the case of any unconscious patient it is important to chart the pulse rate, respiration rate and blood pressure at frequent intervals, as any change may herald the onset of complications. X-ray of the skull can warn of some of these; for example, if there is a fracture line suggesting the possibility of infection spreading from a sinus, damage to the middle meningeal artery, or the development of cerebrospinal fluid rhinorrhoea. External hydrocephalus necessitating ventriculoatrial shunting can occur after severe head injury.

Post-traumatic epilepsy

Among the long-term effects of a head injury, post-traumatic epilepsy is one of the most worrying, especially as its onset may be delayed for a number of years. Jennett (1975) has estimated that the risk of late post-traumatic epilepsy is only about 1% for all injuries uncomplicated by early epilepsy within the first week after the accident, acute haematoma and depressed fracture; even when the post-traumatic amnesia is of more than 24 hours duration. The overall risk of one or more seizures occurring after the first week following a blunt head injury is about 3–5% if the period of observation is 4 years or more, although it varies widely. A quarter of those with fits occurring within the first week after the accident, 31% of those with acute haematoma and 15% of those with depressed fracture develop post-traumatic epilepsy. The incidence of late epilepsy after depressed fracture can be estimated if three of the following four factors are known: post-traumatic amnesia of over 24 hours, dural tear, focal signs and the occurrence of early epilepsy during the first week. The risk varies from 70% to 2% and from this the need for prophylactic treatment can be gauged. In Jennett's series, just over half the patients who developed post-traumatic epilepsy had their first fit within a year of the injury, but in more than a quarter it was delayed beyond the fourth year. He found that the EEG did not help in predicting the occurrence of post-traumatic epilepsy. Although these figures are not applicable to all ages, the differences between the age groups are slight. The incidence of early epilepsy was twice as high among the under fives but the same among older children. The incidence of late epilepsy was much the same at all ages, but mild injuries were more often followed by epilepsy in children than in adults (Jennett, 1973).

Vertigo

This is a relatively common symptom after head injuries. It can result from damage to the brain-stem, the vestibular nerve, or labyrinth, but one variety which is easily overlooked is benign positional vertigo. This seems to result from damage to the utricle and can follow trauma. The patient complains of sudden, intense vertigo lasting only a few seconds when the head is placed in a certain position (Gordon, 1954). Routine examination is usually negative, but if the head is placed backwards and to one side so that the affected labyrinth is underneath there is a sudden onset of vertigo accompanied by a rotary nystagmus lasting about 20 seconds. This may recur on assuming the erect posture again. If the patient realizes that the vertigo is precipitated by certain positions of the head, efforts can be made to avoid them. Otherwise, treatment is symptomatic, with drugs such as dimenhydrinate. After varying periods of time the symptoms usually disappear.

Post-traumatic syndrome

All kinds of disorders, many of them uncommon (e.g. diabetes insipidus), can follow head injury, but one of the main problems is the so-called 'post-traumatic syndrome'. This may be of more significance among adults than children, especially when there is impending litigation. The symptoms of anxiety may not be so troublesome, but many children will be worried about their condition. Headaches, giddiness, difficulty with sleeping. and 'nervousness' may occur. The child's personality changes, and the happy, carefree child becomes anxious and depressed. Also there can be evidence of an impairment of intellect with consequent failure at school. This will be particularly evident if language function is affected, as has been discussed under acquired speech disorders (Chapter 6).

Assessment by appropriate psychological tests will obviously be of importance so that advice can be given to the teacher on the best means of helping the child, and it will be essential to see that undue academic pressures are avoided. If there is a severe emotional disturbance a psychiatric opinion may be needed, but improvement can usually be obtained by reassurance and advice to both the parents and the child. These various problems emphasize that the paediatrician must be involved in the rehabilitation of children who have suffered head injuries.

Non-accidental injury

Child abuse syndrome (battered baby syndrome)

Whenever a child is seen to be suffering from the effects of trauma it is necessary to consider whether this really has resulted from an accident. Babies may be battered as a result of a sudden loss of temper, for example after persistent crying which has kept parents awake for nights on end, or the cruelty may be more premeditated and persist over long periods of time. There can be contributing factors, such as ignorance, single parents, the low intelligence of parents, and poverty, but sometimes a child is singled out for repeated injury for reasons that are hard to understand. The parents rarely suffer from psychoses, but often from neuroses. Emotional immaturity is one of the reasons why they are unable to cope. The fact that battering is particularly common among babies who have been in special care baby units emphasizes the importance of the emotional ties between mother and baby which will be disturbed by separation at this time. This is supported by the increased incidence among victims of child abuse, not only of neonatal separation, but of difficult pregnancies and early ill-health of the baby and parents (Lynch, 1975). The child is usually under the age at which the ability to run is firmly established when the cruelty begins, so that he or she cannot get out of the way quickly, but this is not always so. A child brought for treatment after an unduly long interval after injury, and with a history of repeated admissions to hospital for somewhat trivial reasons is suggestive, and discrepancies in the parents' stories must always be questioned (Jackson, 1972). Also multiple injuries of a mixed type and of different vintages are suspicious. Failure to thrive and slow development are definite features.

The key to diagnosis is often the level of suspicion and recognition of the evidence, which is well-illustrated in the book by O'Doherty (1982). The signs include bruising, fractures, burns and scalds. Once suspicions of this kind are aroused, the child must be admitted to a place of safety (usually the hospital ward), and a skeletal survey is mandatory to discover X-ray evidence of fractures or previous trauma. Suspicious X-ray findings are metaphysial fractures, fractured ribs, a thick involucrum from periosteal haemorrhages, and epiphyseal dislocations. Skull fractures are usually multiple and complex, and may be depressed (Fig. 12.3). They are often associated with complications such as subdural haematoma and intracranial haemorrhage (Hobbs, 1989). The injuries can often be only too evident, but sometimes bruising can

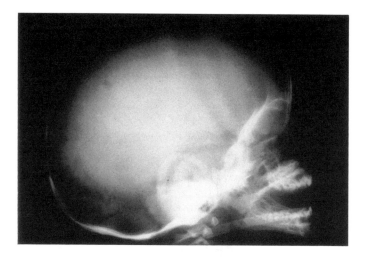

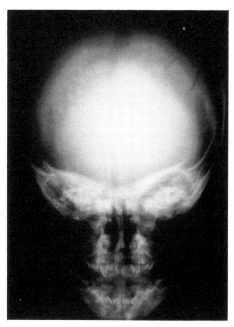

Figure 12.3   X-rays of skull, fracture due to
non-accidental injury.

be very slight, even in the presence of multiple fractures. Also, bilateral subdural
haematoma can occur without evidence of external injury. Guthkelch (1971) suggests
that this is due to violent shaking. In these instances retinal haemorrhages are a very
suggestive finding (Fig, 12.4). In some cases scalds and burns are inflicted by cigarette
ends or by placing the child on a hot stove. Characteristic bite marks and finger-grasp
marks must also be looked for. The child may show a fear of all adults. Very
occasionally, parents may deliberately poison their child, particularly with drugs,
which are so readily available these days (Munchausen by proxy). Bizarre symptoms

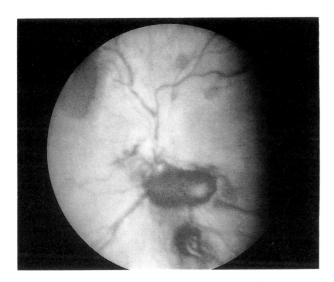

Figure 12.4   Retinal haemorrhages due to shaking a child (non-accidental injury).

and signs should raise the possibility and blood and urine collected for toxicological analysis (Rogers *et al.*, 1976; Meadow, 1982).

The differential diagnosis is from conditions such as fragilitas ossium (osteogenesis imperfecta), and certain skin conditions including erythema nodosum and focal epidermal necrosis, and the mongolian blue spot, a common birthmark in the lumbar region. The management of the problem involves the whole family, and will necessitate help from a number of specialties: doctors (including the family doctor), health visitors, the social services and voluntary societies such as the National Society for the Prevention of Cruelty to Children (NSPCC). The advice of experienced members of the police force can also be helpful. An urgent case conference should be arranged as soon as possible after the child has been admitted to hospital. It has been estimated that the incidence of cases of non-accidental injury in the UK is 3000 a year; of these about 100 die, and 400 suffer permanent physical and mental handicap (MacKeith, 1974). These figures are obviously hard to come by and larger numbers have been suggested by the Royal College of Psychiatrists; in England and Wales some 3000 children are injured each year of whom 6 will die each week and 1 in 4 become brain damaged or mentally retarded (report from the Select Committee on Violence in the Family, 1977). This is a rapidly expanding subject, which has been reviewed in many excellent books.

Abnormalities of the skull

Craniostenosis

Fibrous union between the bones of the skull usually occurs towards the end of the first 6 months of life, but solid bony union not until the sixth to eighth decade. More than 50% of all postnatal increase in the skull circumference occurs during the first year, and normal growth of the brain is only possible when the skull bones remain un-united. Therefore, premature closure of the sutures is bound to interfere with the

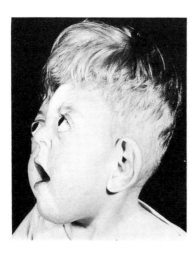

Figure 12.5   Child with Crouzon's disease.

development of the brain. This has to be differentiated from the closure of the sutures which occurs in microcephaly and happens because the brain is small and there is no impetus for the skull to expand. Although the cause of craniosynostosis is unknown there may be a familial incidence, and it is sometimes associated with other anomalies such as hypophosphatasia.

The final shape of the head will depend on the particular sutures which close. The earlier in life the sutures close the more likely it is that raised intracranial pressure will occur, and this increased pressure is most common when the coronal suture is affected. Closure of this suture is sometimes associated with fusion of the sutures of the facial bones, with beaked nose, prognathism, small maxilla and exophthalmos (Crouzon's disease) (Fig. 12.5), which is inherited as a dominant trait. Cardiac complications can occur in this condition. The narrowing of the oral and nasal airways can give rise to carbon dioxide retention and hypoxia resulting in the development of pulmonary hypertension and severe cor pulmonale, as can occur in the Pierre Robin syndrome and in Down's syndrome (Gordon, 1988). Adenotonsillectomy does result in improvement. If the orbit is involved there will be an increased risk of damage to the eyes and optic nerves from compression. Epileptic seizures and mental handicap may result from the raised intracranial pressure, although the possibility always has to be considered that they are due to an associated deformity of the brain. X-rays of the skull will confirm the presence of fused sutures and the premature closure of the anterior fontanelle. There may be increased density, and sometimes raising up of the bone adjacent to the fused sutures. Increased digital markings and erosion of the posterior clinoid processes can also be seen.

In order to be successful surgical treatment when indicated must be carried out in the first few months of life to allow the brain to grow normally. One possibility is a linear craniectomy along the line of the affected suture and a polyethylene film placed over the edges of the bone on each side. If there is marked exophthalmos, an orbital decompression may be necessary in addition to a coronal craniectomy.

Platybasia (basilar impression)

This deformity is caused by the upward displacement of the cervical spine. It may be associated with other anomalies, such as the Arnold-Chiari malformation, syringobulbia, and the Klippel-Feil syndrome. There is a familial occurrence in some instances, particularly in association with the last of these syndromes (Bull, Nixon and Pratt, 1955). The condition may be asymptomatic, but there is a risk of complications arising at any time, although rarely before adolescence. The neck is short and tends to be hyperextended. If there is compression of the cerebellum or cervical cord there will be ataxia, nystagmus, spastic weakness of the limbs and sometimes sensory loss. The lower cranial nerves can be damaged, and if the distortion of the structures in the posterior fossa blocks the flow of cerebrospinal fluid there will be symptoms and signs of raised intracranial pressure.

An X-ray examination will confirm the diagnosis. It will show the widening of the angle between the basisphenoid and the basilar portion of the occipital bone, normally between 110 and 140 degrees; and the deformity of the foramen magnum. In the lateral view of the skull the odontoid process will be seen above a line joining the posterior end of the hard palate to the posterior lip of the foramen magnum, but the plane of the axis relative to that of the hard palate is a more reliable guide. With basilar impression they form an acute angle instead of being parallel (Bull, Nixon and Pratt, 1955). X-ray examination will also show fusion of the cervical vertebrae if this is present. The differential diagnosis is from tumours of the posterior fossa and upper cervical cord, multiple sclerosis and hydrocephalus. If it is not congenital, the condition may be caused by bone diseases, such as osteogenesis imperfecta and rickets. When complications arise, treatment is by surgical decompression of the posterior fossa and upper cervical cord, and, if necessary, appropriate management of the hydrocephalus.

Benign intracranial hypertension

Raised intracranial pressure can occur in the absence of any intracranial space-occupying lesion or obstruction to the flow of cerebrospinal fluid, except possibly at the point of absorption. There are likely to be symptoms such as headache, vomiting and sometimes double vision. The presence of marked papilloedema in a patient who is alert and well is a suggestive finding, but papilloedema does not always occur. In addition to papilloedema the signs will include ataxia, inferior nasal quadrantic visual field defect and bilateral external rectus palsies. The excess of affected females found among adults does not occur during childhood, when there is no sex difference (Grant, 1971).

The condition is often related to infections of the middle ear, presumably resulting in thrombosis of the lateral venous sinus (Symonds, 1931). When it occurs after head injuries, which may be quite trivial, sinus thrombosis may be a factor. Bilateral external rectus palsy seems to be a frequent sign in that event. A number of drugs, such as nalidixic acid, tetracyclines, steroids, and vitamin A, have been implicated. Accidental intoxication with hexochlorophane has been reported with resulting raised intracranial pressure and spinal cord damage, most probably due to massive intramyelinic oedema. The hexachlorophane was contained in talcum powder used on intact skin (Goutières and Aicardi, 1977). It may also be associated with severe anaemia, hypocalcaemia and Addison's disease. The respiratory distress of cystic fibrosis can cause a rise of venous pressure and, subsequently, of intracranial pressure (Katznelson, 1978).

In these latter instances it is suggested that the raised pressure is related to cerebral oedema, although why this should occur has not been elucidated, and the general well-being of these patients makes it an unlikely cause. Steroids are often given to reduce cerebral oedema, which seems paradoxical. However, benign intracranial hypertension occurs most often when steroids are being withdrawn; and it is always important to watch for this possibility, and, if it occurs, to consider increasing the dose again. Perhaps the most plausible theory on the aetiology of benign intracranial hypertension is reduced cerebrospinal fluid absorption, due either to a reduced pressure gradient between the subarachnoid space and the superior sagittal sinus or to an increased resistance to flow across the absorptive channels (Johnson, 1973). Excessive production of fluid is also a possibility, and occasionally interference with lymphatic drainage from the intracranial structures due to inflammatory changes may result in raised intracranial pressure.

Usually full neuroradiological investigations will be needed to exclude tumours or hydrocephalus, but sometimes if the intracranial hypertension is found in association with a well-recognized cause (such as one of the drugs mentioned) it may be justifiable to withdraw it and see if there is rapid improvement (Grant, 1971).

If symptoms persist, treatment with diuretics, such as chlorthalidone, or with steroids is justifiable. Repeated lumbar punctures can be tried, although care will have to be taken that this does not cause brain-stem compression. A watch will also have to be kept on the patient's visual acuity when the papilloedema is long-standing, and if there is any evidence of failing vision, such treatment must be given as a matter of urgency. Subtemporal decompression is no longer used because of the resulting deformity and high incidence of post-operative epilepsy (Jefferson and Clark, 1976). The prognosis is almost always good, with rapid recovery and no sequelae, except for occasional visual impairment.

Intracranial and spinal tumours

Tumours of the brain may be rare in childhood. but their presence has to be constantly considered in the differential diagnosis of progressive cerebral disorders. They are much more likely to occur subtentorially than supratentorially. The most common types are malignant glioma, astrocytoma, medulloblastoma and ependymoma. Craniopharyngioma is the most frequent supratentorial tumour in childhood. Different tumour types cannot be considered in detail, but a few comments will be made on the more common ones.

The symptoms and signs of raised intracranial pressure headache, vomiting and papilloedema may not be present in early childhood when the skull is able to expand with spreading of the suture lines. Expansion of the head circumference at too rapid a rate will raise the question of hydrocephalus, and a cerebral tumour will always have to be considered as a possible cause of this. Additional symptoms and signs related to the raised pressure can occur, e.g. convulsions and false localizing signs like double vision.

Posterior fossa tumours

Tumours of the posterior fossa in childhood will include brain-stem gliomas, astrocytomas and medulloblastomas of the cerebellum, hemanglioblastoma and ependymomas. The symptoms and signs of these tumours can be very similar, although their rate of progress may vary considerably. Due to the confined space within the posterior fossa, the signs of raised intracranial pressure will quickly develop, except in an infiltrating tumour such as a glioma of the brain-stem.

One of the first symptoms will be unsteadiness of gait. The child will start falling more often than is usual for his or her age, and will be seen to stagger and walk on a wide base. A lack of interest and a tendency to tire very easily will develop. Headache and vomiting due to raised intracranial pressure may proceed or follow these symptoms, depending on the rate of growth of the tumour in terms of volume, and the extent to which the flow of cerebrospinal fluid is obstructed. A persistent head tilt is a suggestive finding, usually with flexion and rotation to the side of the lesion. The occiput is directed to the shoulder towards which the head is flexed.

Brain-stem glioma

This tumour infiltrates the pons and medulla; it may enlarge in size, but rarely blocks the flow of cerebrospinal fluid. CAT scans and contrast radiological studies are therefore likely to show distortion of the fourth ventricle and aqueduct, but not necessarily in the very early stages, so that they may need to be repeated. The clinical picture will be dominated by lesions of the cranial nerves, and various combinations of cranial nerve palsies may ensue with certain of the nerves escaping damage, so that exact localization of the lesion proves difficult. The 5th to 12th nerves are the ones usually affected. Long tract signs and truncal ataxia will appear, and if vomiting and drowsiness occur it is likely to be due to the brain-stem lesion rather than the result of raised intracranial pressure.

Virus encephalitis and demyelinating diseases affecting the brain stem can cause diagnostic difficulties, although in these conditions improvement should start after a few weeks.

Astrocytomas and medulloblastomas of the cerebellum

Astrocytomas and medulloblastomas affect the mid-line structures of the cerebellum: the former is one of the most benign of cerebral tumours; the latter one of the most malignant. The main characteristic of the cerebellar astrocytoma is its cystic structure containing a mural nodule. Signs of cerebellar dysfunction will gradually appear, sometimes localized to one side of the body to begin with, and then the nystagmus (quick phase) will be to the side of the lesion. Unsteadiness in walking may be the only sign of a cerebellar disorder. Central hypertension and a labile heart rate can be features. The course of the illness often lasts for many years, and sometimes a second operation is needed. Medulloblastomas are fortunately rarer than astrocytomas of the cerebellum. They grow rapidly, and symptoms and signs of raised intracranial pressure are often the first evidence of such a lesion. There may also be ataxia and cranial nerve palsies, and the tumour can seed down the spinal canal and cause additional lesions at this level. Death usually occurs within 6 months of diagnosis, but the prognosis has considerably improved. This appears to be due to a combination of surgical advances and improved radiation techniques (McIntosh, 1979).

Ependymomas

These tumours invade the floor of the fourth ventricle. They may not be rapidly growing or particularly invasive growths, but their situation makes complete removal impossible. The clinical picture is sometimes dominated by the symptoms and signs of raised intracranial pressure. The extension or seeding of the tumour down into the upper cervical spinal canal can cause stiffness and tenderness of the neck and shoulder muscles, and the head may be tilted to one side. As in the other cerebellar tumours described, truncal ataxia may occur with difficulty in walking, but little if any inco-ordination of limb movements.

Supratentorial tumours

Supratentorial tumours are less common in childhood than those of the posterior fossa. The most frequent are craniopharyngiomas, followed by astrocytomas (Fig. 12.6) and ependymomas of the cerebral hemispheres. Focal symptoms do occur with these latter tumours, but the younger the child the harder they will be to elicit. Focal epileptic seizures and signs of hemiparesis will help in localization. Gliomas of the optic nerve are sometimes a manifestation of Von Recklinghausen's disease, as may be neurofibroma on the auditory and other cranial nerves.

Craniopharyngiomas

These tumours are also referred to as 'Rathke's pouch cysts', 'adamantinomas', 'suprasellar cysts', and 'hypophyseal duct tumours'. They arise from squamous cell rests in the region of the pars tuberalis or infundibulum of the hypophysis, and they can cause symptoms at any age.

The onset of symptoms and signs can be insidious, with a gradual enlargement of the head if the patient is a young child, and perhaps a few other signs such as severe lack of appetite and retarded growth, the significance of which can easily be missed. However, there is more often unequivocal evidence of raised intracranial pressure due to internal hydrocephalus (Fig. 12.7). The site of the tumour in the suprasellar region means that the visual pathways are likely to suffer at an early stage, and the most

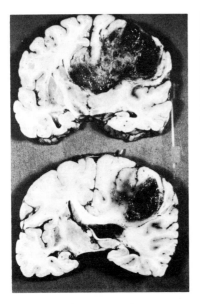

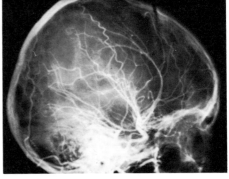

Figure 12.7 Craniopharyngioma. Lateral view of carotid arteriogram showing gross raised intracranial pressure, with elevation and stretching of the peri-callosal artery, and slight depression of the posterior cerebrals. (There is reflux into the basilar system.)

Figure 12.6 Supratentorial astrocytoma.

frequent defect is in the temporal fields. Apart from stunted growth, severe pituitary dysfunction can occur, with a low basal metabolic rate, low blood pressure, and sometimes even severe cachexia simulating anorexia nervosa. If the hypothalamus is involved there can be drowsiness (unrelated to raised intracranial pressure), polydipsia and polyuria, failure of the onset of puberty and precocious puberty. Cranial nerve palsies also occur, particularly of the oculomotor nerves.

Spinal tumours

The rarity of spinal tumours in childhood is an adequate reason for constantly bearing in mind the possibility of this diagnosis, so that a chance of successful removal of the tumour is not missed.

The onset of symptoms is often insidious, but can be sudden if the blood supply to the cord is disturbed. Pain, paraesthesiae and sensory impairment may not dominate the early stages of the condition as they are apt to do among adults. Sphincter disturbances, although more easily attributed to other causes in infancy and early childhood, can be a sign of cord compression. If the first symptom is difficulty in walking and weakness of the legs, the rate of progress can be rapid. Meningiomas and neurofibromas are very rare in childhood. The common tumours are teratoma, dermoid cysts, intramedullary glioma and extradural sarcoma.

Neuroblastomas

This tumour arises from embryonic tissue of the adrenal medulla and sympathetic ganglia. It is a common intra-abdominal tumour arising in relation to the kidney, and also occurs within the thoracic cavity, especially just below the inlet and in the neck. It presents as a mass, and may show evidence of calcification on X-ray examination. Direct spread can occur to within the spinal canal and result in compression of the spinal cord. This may not cause any striking bony changes, so that myelography may be needed to localize the lesion. Metastases are common, particularly to the liver (Pepper type) and to the skeleton (Hutchinson type). In the Hutchinson type the bony lesions in the skull can usually be felt, and the peri-orbital metastases will displace the eye. Myoclonic encephalopathy occasionally occurs in association with this tumour.

As epinephrine metabolism disturbed, the diagnosis can often be confirmed by examination of the urine for an excess of 3-methyl, 4-hydroxymandelic acid (VMA) (Voorhess and Gardner, 1961). This is not present in every instance, possibly because the tumour is sometimes very anaplastic. Cystathioninuria may also be found (von Studnitz, 1970). The prognosis is better the younger the child, and spontaneous cures do occasionally occur, due, presumably, to maturation of the tumour cells. The tumour should be removed if possible, but the primary lesion and the metastases respond well to radiotherapy, and cytotoxic drugs can be used.

Ganglioneuromas are a more mature form of neuroblastoma, and are not progressive if they do not contain small areas of malignant cells.

Metastatic tumours

These tumours are rare in childhood, but there are a few important examples. Wilm's tumour or nephroblastoma may metastasize to the brain and other parts of the body. There will be raised intracranial pressure as well as neurological signs, depending on the site of the secondary tumour. Neuroblastomas with their frequent metastasis to the liver and skeleton have already been considered.

Leukaemia

This malignancy can result in invasion of the nervous system; the brain and the spinal cord and nerve roots. Leukaemic infiltration of the brain and cord can also occur, and this may involve the meninges as well; then the cerebrospinal fluid sometimes shows leukaemic cells and a low sugar content. Even if there is no direct involvement, the CNS may well be affected by the vascular complications of this condition. Symptoms and signs, in order of decreasing frequency, tend to be manifestations of raised intracranial pressure, ocular disturbances, cranial and peripheral nerve dysfunction, psychic disorders, Cushing's syndrome, auditory disturbances, evidence of autonomic nervous system dysfunction and speech disorders (Hyman *et al.*, 1965). Central nervous system leukaemia is compatible with prolonged survival, but once established it is increasingly difficult to eradicate (Gribben, Hardistry and Chessells, 1977). Among children under treatment for the disease, the greatest neurological hazards arise from viral infections and from the toxic effects of drugs such as methotrexate, and from radiation (Campbell, Marshall and Chessells, 1977). These can include convulsions, encephalopathy, myelopathy; and with some drugs a polyneuropathy (Hanefeld and Riehm, 1980). Studies have confirmed the particular vulnerability of younger children with leukaemia treated with cytotoxic drugs and cranial irradiation (Chessells *et al.*, 1990). Many of these children will have difficulties when they return to school, due to brain damage, often confirmed by CT scanning. Said *et al.* (1989) assessed 106 children with acute lymphoblastic leukaemia who had been treated with cranial irradiation for the prevention of CNS leukaemia some years previously. As controls 45 siblings of comparable age were used. The index group had a lower IQ, performance more than verbal and they were more distractable and less able to concentrate. The less aggressive treatment now used may do less damage, but it is still of the greatest importance to monitor the progress of these children in school.

Paraneoplastic syndromes

These syndromes are not as common in childhood as in later life. The best established paraneoplastic syndrome is the myoclonic encephalopathy associated with neuro-blastoma (Brandt *et al.*, 1974). A polyneuropathy syndrome has been reported in children with Hodgkin's disease (Kurczynski *et al.*, 1980), a myasthenic syndrome among children with leukaemia, and central pontine myelinolysis with both these diseases (Crosley *et al.*, 1978). Progressive multifocal encephalopathy has been reported in patients with acute leukaemia with areas of demyelination in the cerebral hemispheres. The clinical picture is due to progressive dementia and spasticity. A papova-like virus has been demonstrated in this condition. It may be that there are other such syndromes, which are so far unrecognized.

Diagnosis of neoplasia

The history and clinical examination will frequently raise the suspicion of a tumour. Headaches related to raised intracranial venous pressure tend to wake the child early in the morning and gradually ease off over the day. These are sometimes associated with vomiting. Swelling of the optic discs in the early stages is seen as a pinkish colour with obliteration of the physiological cup and then burying of the fine vessels at the edge of the disc and obvious engorgement of the veins. The appearances of early papilloedema can sometimes be mimicked by those seen in hypermetropia and in optic neuritis. If the latter condition is bilateral, is already causing defective vision and the child is too young to describe this, the impaired pupillary reaction to light will help in the differentiation. Pseudo-papilloedema is a congenital anomaly which can cause considerable worry until a firm diagnosis can be made, often by using fluorescein angiography (Dollery, 1967). The drusen, which are deposits of hyaline-like material, can very rarely be associated with retinal haemorrhages. There is often a familial incidence of drusen which may help in diagnosis (Hitchins *et al.*, 1976). In the young child, raised intracranial pressure will cause an abnormally rapid enlargement of the head, so that serial measurements are essential. Before this occurs there may be obvious separation of the sutures and, when the head is percussed, a 'cracked-pot' sound may be elicited. Head tilt with posterior fossa tumours has already been mentioned. It is not uncommon for symptoms of raised pressure due to a cerebral tumour to follow a relatively trivial head injury or infection, and their true implication may be missed if they subside quickly. Occasionally papilloedema occurs in chronic respiratory insufficiency, in polycythemia and in cystic fibrosis.

Electroencephalography

The electroencephalogram can be of help, but in posterior fossa tumours it may show only a generalized increase of slow wave activity, although this may be asymmetrical, and sometimes paroxysmal when there is dilatation of the third ventricle. Such abnormalities may be the one sign leading to the increasing suspicion of a space-occupying lesion. When the EEG shows only generalized abnormalities of a non-specific type the single recording is of limited value, but serial recordings showing a progressive deterioration can be highly significant. In supratentorial tumours, focal abnormalities are likely to occur. Sometimes the EEG will show changes suggestive of some other conditions, such as minor status epilepticus or certain types of degenerative cerebral disease.

X-ray examination

Plain X-ray examination can show a number of abnormalities. The 'beaten silver' (Fig. 12.8) appearance due to convolutional impression of the inner table of the skull vault is almost certain to occur with raised intracranial pressure of any duration, but it

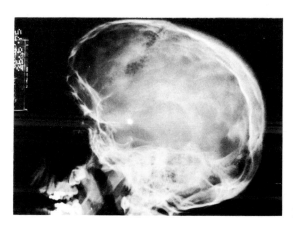

Figure 12.8   'Beaten-silver' appearance.

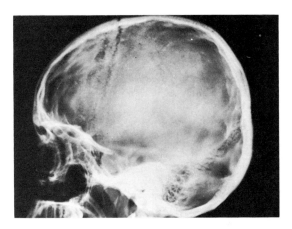

Figure 12.9   Plain lateral view of the skull showing excavation of the pituitary fossa and evidence of raised intracranial pressure (copper-beaten vault and diastasis of coronal suture).

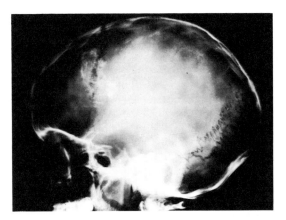

Figure 12.10   Calcified astrocytoma in the fronto-parietal region, with evidence of raised intracranial pressure.

is by no means always an indication of this. Separation of the sutures is a much more reliable sign (Fig. 12.9). Erosion of the posterior clinoid process is also highly suggestive, but it does not occur so often among children as adults. Thinning or sclerosis of the bone in relation to an underlying tumour can be an important localizing sign, as can the presence of intracranial calcification in, for example, a craniopharyngioma or astrocytoma (Fig. 12.10). If a glioma of the optic nerve is suspected, special views should be taken to show any enlargement of the optic foramen.

CT scan, MRI and other tests

There can be no doubt that the CT scan, which is only slightly more invasive than a plain X-ray of the skull, will be the investigation of choice in the majority of diagnostic problems affecting the nervous system (Fig. 12.11) (Ambrose, 1974; Ambrose, Gooding and Richardson, 1975a; Day, Thomson and Schutt, 1978). Its accuracy has been proven, and it reduces the need for other complex investigations, but the dose of radiation must always be considered. It will help in the diagnosis of cerebral and spinal lesions, and in the differentiation between benign and malignant tumours, haemorrhage and infarction, and post-traumatic cerebral oedema and haematoma. It is also particularly helpful in the case of a suspected cerebral abscess, and can sometimes be utilized to follow the progress of other inflammatory and degenerative conditions, particularly where there is demyelination. Intravenous

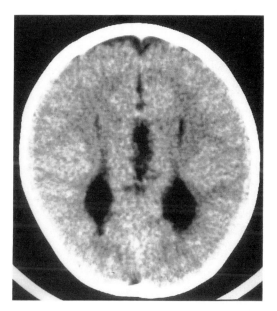

Figure 12.11   CAT scan in patient with absent corpus callosum.

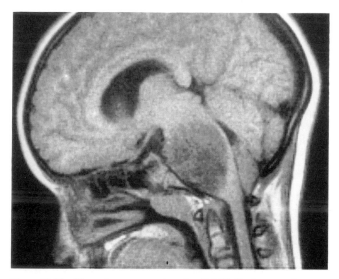

Figure 12.12   Magnetic resonance imaging (MRI). Brain stem glioma.

injection of sodium iothalamate improves accuracy by the enhancement of tissue density (Ambrose, Gooding and Richardson, 1975b). Occasionally the findings may be misleading if not interpreted with care; for example the appearance of cerebral atrophy when the patient is on treatment with steroids, presumably due to diminished brain volume from water loss (Bentson, Reza and Winter, 1978). Other techniques, such as magnetic resonance imaging (MRI) (Fig. 12.12), are going to open up even greater possibilities in the diagnosis of intracranial lesions of various kinds, including disorders of myelination (Levene *et al.*, 1982; Elias-Jones *et al.*, 1990); as well as enabling aspects of brain metabolism to be studied. It is now recognized as the investigation of choice in the diagnosis of suspected white matter abnormalities (Miller *et al.*, 1990).

Positron emission tomography (PET) and single photon emission computed tomography (SPECT) are proving of use in studying the activity of certain areas of the brain, for example if a particular function is impaired (Lou, Henriksen and Bruhn, 1984; Chugani, Phelps and Mazziotta, 1987). Other investigations, such as arteriography, are now rarely used in childhood except in special circumstances.

Myelography

Spinal tumours can be confirmed on plain X-ray films, but myelography is often needed. Air myelography, or the use of water-soluble contrast medium, is sometimes more helpful in infancy and childhood than using oily contrast media (Vogelsang and Busse, 1976). Now an increasing use will be made of MRI with enhancement, or CT scanning with intrathecal metrizamide (Hyman and Gorey, 1988).

Brain-stem death

Pallis (1983) has discussed the subject of brain-stem death in detail, and this book should be consulted by all those likely to be involved in withdrawing the use of life-support systems for patients in coma who require mechanical ventilation. This decision is based on the concept that brain-stem death is incompatible with recovery, and means that organs can be removed for transplantation.

O'Brien (1990) has set out a form which can be placed in the patient's records when the transplant of organs is being considered and the cause of the coma is known. The diagnosis should not be considered, if errors are to be avoided, until at least 6 hours after the onset of coma; or, if anoxia or cardiac arrest was the cause of the coma, until 24 hours after the circulation has been restored, and then only if preconditions have been satisfied. These include the exclusion of hypothermia, drugs, or metabolic-endocrine abnormalities contributing significantly to the apnoeic coma, the use of neuromuscular blocking drugs during the preceding 12 hours, and a rectal temperature below 35°C. The plasma and urine can be checked for drugs, plasma pH, glucose, sodium and calcium; and patients with a low temperature can be warmed and then reassessed.

When the preconditions have been met, the patient should be examined, to answer the following questions. When the head is fully rotated to either side is there contraversive conjugate deviation of the eyes (doll's eye movements)? Do the pupils react to light? Is there any response to corneal stimulation on either side? Do the eyes deviate when either ear is irrigated with 50 ml of ice-cold water for 30 seconds? (after ensuring the tympanic membranes are intact). Is there a gag reflex? Is there a cough reflex following bronchial stimulation with a suction catheter? Is there any motor response within the distribution of the cranial nerves following stimulation of any somatic area (supraorbital and nail-bed pressure)? The responses must be negative to confirm the diagnosis.

Are there any respiratory movements? If there are, record carbon dioxide and oxygen levels after preoxygenating the patient for 10 minutes with 100% oxygen (before disconnection the P_aCO_2 must exceed 5.3 kPa: if it is less, then slow ventilation must be carried out until it rises to this level). An alternative is ventilation with 95% O_2 and 5% CO_2. The patient is disconnected from the ventilator and given oxygen at 6 l/min via a suction catheter in the trachea. After 10 minutes the blood gases are measured (P_aCO_2 must exceed 6.65 kPa at the end of the disconnection period). The patient is then assessed for any spontaneous respiratory movement.

The assessment should be made by two experienced medical practitioners of senior status; and the respiratory disconnection should be performed by an anaesthetist and witnessed by one of the assessors. The British Paediatric Association have now published the report of a Working Party on the Diagnosis of Brain Death in Infants and Children. It is concluded that it is rarely possible to diagnose brain death between 37 weeks' gestation and 2 months of age, and that among infants below 37 weeks' gestation the concept of brain-stem death is inappropriate.

References

Ambrose, J. (1974) The EMI-scanner: clinical use. *British Journal of Hospital Medicine.* **11** (Equipment suppl.), 14

Ambrose, J., Gooding, M.R. and Richardson, M.E. (1975a) An assessment of the accuracy of computerized transverse axial scanning (EMI scanner) in the diagnosis of intracranial tumour. *Brain*, **98**, 569

Ambrose, J., Gooding, M.R. and Richardson, A.E. (1975b) Sodium iothalamate as an aid to diagnosis of intracranial lesions by computerized transverse axial scanning. *Lancet*, **ii**, 669

Bentson, J., Reza, M. and Winter, J.W.G. (1978) Steroids and apparent cerebral atrophy on computed tomography scans. *Journal of Computer Assisted Tomography*, **2**, 16

Besser, G.M. (1972) The hypothalamus and pituitary gland. *Medicine*, **2**, 97

Brandt, S., Carlsen, N., Glenting, P. and Helweg-Larsen, J. (1974) Encephalopathia myoclonica infantiles (Kinsbourne) and neuroblastoma in children. A report of three cases. *Developmental Medicine and Child Neurology*, **16**, 286

Bull, J.W.D., Nixon. W.L.B. and Pratt, R.T.C. (1955) The radiological criteria and familial occurrence of primary basilar impression. *Brain*, **78**, 229

Campbell, R.H.A., Marshall, W.C. and Chessells, J.M. (1977) Neurological complications of childhood leukaemia. *Archives of Disease in Childhood*, **52**, 850

Chambers, J.L. (1975) Hypernatraemia: a preventable cause of acquired brain damage? *Developmental Medicine and Child Neurology*, **17**, 91

Chessells, J.M., Cox, T.C.S., Kendall, B. *et al.* (1990) Neurotoxicity in lymphoblastic leukaemia: comparison of oral and intramuscular methotrexate and two doses of radiation. *Archives of Disease in Childhood*, **65**, 416–22

Chisolm, J.J. and Barltrop, D. (1979) Recognition and management of children with increased lead absorption. *Archives of Disease in Childhood*, **54**, 249

Chugani, H.T., Phelps, M.E. and Mazziotta, J.C. (1987) Positron emission tomography study of human brain functional development. *Annals of Neurology*, **22**, 487

Conn, J.W. (1955) Primary aldosteronism. *Journal of Laboratory and Clinical Medicine*, **45**, 661

Crosley, C.J., Rorke, I.B., Evans, A. and Nigro, M. (1978) Central nervous system lesions in childhood leukaemia. *Neurology*, **28**, 678

Day, R.E., Thomson, J.L.G. and Schutt, W.H. (1978) Computerized axial tomography and acute neurological problems of childhood. *Archives of Disease in Childhood*, **53**, 2

de Gruchy, G.C. (1970) *Clinical Haematology in Medical Practice*, Blackwell Scientific, Oxford

Dodge, H.W. (1956) Cephalic bruits in children. *Journal of Neurosurgery*, **13**, 527

Dodge, H.W., Wood, M.W. and Kennedy, K.L.J. (1959) Craniofacial dysostosis: Crouzon's disease. *Pediatrics*, **23**, 98

Dollery, C.T. (1967) Fluorescence retinal photography. In *Modern Trends in Ophthalmology* (ed. A. Sorsby), Butterworth, London

Eden, O.B., Sills, J.A. and Brown, J.K. (1977) Hypertension in acute neurological diseases of childhood. *Developmental Medicine and Child Neurology*, **19**, 437

Edwards, C.H., Gordon, N.S. and Rob, C. (1960) The surgical treatment of internal carotid artery occlusions. *Quarterly Journal of Medicine*, **29**, 67

Elias-Jones, A.C., Jaspan, T., Mellor, D.H. and Worthington, B.S. (1990) Magnetic resonance imaging in neurological disorders. *Archives of Disease in Childhood*, **65**, 922–9

Ferrer, M.I. (1973) The sick sinus syndrome. *Circulation*, **47**, 635

Goebel, H.H., (1992) Neuronal ceroid-lipofuscinosis: the current status. *Brain and Development*, **14**, 203

Gomez, M.R., Whitten, C.F., Nolke, A. *et al.* (1963) Aneurysmal malformation of the great vein of Galen causing heart failure in early infancy. *Pediatrics*, **31**, 400

Gooding, M.R. and Uttley, D. (1976) EMI scan in the management of head injuries. *Lancet*, **i**, 847

Gordon, N. (1954) Post-traumatic vertigo. with special reference to positional nystagmus. *Lancet*, **i**, 1216

Gordon, N. (1987) Vitamin E deficiency and illness in childhood. *Developmental Medicine and Child Neurology*, **29**, 646

Gordon, N. (1988) Nasal obstruction in childhood: the obstructive sleep apnea syndrome. *Developmental Medicine and Child Neurology*, **30**, 261

Gordon, N. and Hudson, R.E.B. (1959) Refsum's syndrome, heredopathia atactica polyneuritiformis. *Brain*, **82**, 41

Gordon, N. and Isler, W. (1989) Childhood moyamoya disease. *Developmental Medicine and Child Neurology*, **31**, 103

Goutières, F. and Aicardi, J. (1977) Accidental percutaneous hexachlorophane intoxication in children. *British Medical Journal*, **ii**, 663

Grant, D.N. (1971) Benign intracranial hypertension. A review of 79 cases in infancy and childhood. *Archives of Disease in Childhood*, **46**, 651

Gribben, M.A., Hardistry, R.M. and Chessells, J.M. (1977) Long-term control of central nervous system leukaemia. *Archives of Disease in Childhood*, **52**, 673

Guthkelch, A.N. (1971) Infantile subdural haematoma and its relationship to whiplash injuries. *British Medical Journal*, **ii**, 430

Hanefeld, F. and Riehm, H. (1980) Therapy of acute lymphoblastic leukaemia in childhood: effects on the nervous system. *Neuropädiatrie*, **11**, 3

Hayles, A.B., Hahn, H.B., Sprague, R.G. *et al.* (1966) Hormone-secreting tumours of the adrenal cortex in children. *Pediatrics*, **37**, 19

Hitchins, R.A., Corbett, J.J., Winkleman, J. and Schatz, N.J. (1976) Haemorrhages with optic nerve drusen. *Archives of Neurology*, **33**, 675

Hobbs, C.J. (1989) Head injuries. *British Medical Journal*, **296**, 1169

Hyman, C.B., Bogle, J.M., Brubaker, C.A. *et al.* (1965) Central nervous system involvement by leukaemia in children: 1. Relationship to systemic leukaemia and description of clinical and laboratory manifestations. *Blood*, **25**, 1

Hyman, R.A. and Gorey, M.T. (1988) Imaging strategies for MR of the spine. *Radiological Clinics of North America*, **26**, 505

Illich, I.D. (1974) *Medical Nemesis*, Calder and Boyars, London

Isler, W. (1971) *Acute Hemiplegias and Hemisyndromes in Childhood*, Clinics in Developmental Medicine, Nos. 41/42, SIMP, William Heinemann, London

Jackson, G. (1972) Child abuse syndrome: the cases we miss. *British Medical Journal*, **ii**, 756

Jefferson, M. (1957) Sarcoidosis of the nervous system. In *Modern Trends in Neurology* (ed. D. Williams), Butterworth, London

Jefferson, A. and Clark, J. (1976) Treatment of benign intracranial hypertension by dehydrating agents with particular reference to the measurement of the blind spot as a means of recording improvement. *Journal of Neurology, Neurosurgery and Psychiatry*, **39**, 627

Jennett, W.B. (1973) Trauma as a cause of epilepsy in childhood. *Developmental Medicine and Child Neurology*, **15**, 56

Jennett, W.B. (1975) *Epilepsy after Non-missile Head Injuries*, William Heinemann Medical Books, London

Johnson, I. (1973) Reduced CSF absorption syndrome. Reappraisal of benign intracranial hypertension, and related conditions. *Lancet*, **ii**, 418

Johnston, D.M. (1974) Thyrotoxic myopathy. *Archives of Disease in Childhood*, **49**, 968

Johnston, F.G., Bell, B.A., Robertson, I.J.A. *et al.* (1990) Effect of calcitonin-gene-related peptide on postoperative neurological deficits after subarachnoid haemorrhage. *Lancet*, **335**, 869–72

Katznelson, D. (1978) Increased intracranial pressure in cystic fibrosis. *Acta Paediatrica Scandinavica*, **67**, 607

Kauli, R., Laren, Z. (1974) A vasopressor analogue in treatment of diabetes insipidus. *Archives of Disease of Childhood*, **49**, 482

King, M.D., Day, R.E., Oliver, J.S. *et al.* (1981) Solvent enchephalopathy. *British Medical Journal*, **ii**, 663

Kurczynski, T.W., Choudhury, A.A., Horwitz, S.J. *et al.* (1980) Remote effects of malignancy on the nervous system in children. *Developmental Medicine and Child Neurology*, **22**, 205

Levene, M.I., Whitelaw, A., Dubowitz, V. *et al.* (1982) Nuclear magnetic resonance imaging of the brain in children. *British Medical Journal*, **ii**, 774

Lewin, W. (1976) Changing attitudes to the management of severe head injuries. *British Medical Journal*, **ii**, 1234

Lou, H.C., Henriksen, L. and Bruhn, P. (1984) Focal cerebral hypoperfusion in children with dysphasia and/or attention deficit disorders. *Archives of Neurology*, **41**, 825

Lynch, M.A. (1975) Ill-health and child abuse. *Lancet*, **ii**, 317

Macaulay, D. and Watson, M. (1967) Hypernatraemia in infants as a cause of brain damage. *Archives of Disease in Childhood*, **42**, 485

MacKeith, R. (1974) Speculations on non-accidental injury as a cause of chronic brain damage. *Developmental Medicine and Child Neurology*, **16**, 216

McCormack, W.M. and Spalter, H.F. (1966) Muscular dystrophy, aveolar hypoventilation and papilloedema. *Journal of the American Medical Association*, **197**, 957

McIntosh, N. (1979) Medulloblastoma-a changing prognosis? *Archives of Disease in Childhood*, **54**, 200

Meadow, R. (1982) Munchausen's syndrome by proxy. *Archives of Disease in Childhood*, **57**, 92

Miller, D.H., Robb, S.A., Ormorod, E.C. and Pohl, K.A.E. (1990) Magnetic resonance imaging of inflammatory and demyelinating white matter diseases of childhood. *Developmental Medicine and Child Neurology*, **32**, 97

Morris-Jones, P.H., Houston, I.B.and Evans, R.C. (1967) Prognosis of the neurological complications of acute hypernatraemia. *Lancet*, **ii**, 1385

O'Brien, M.D. (1990) Criteria for diagnosing brain stem death. *British Medical Journal*, **301**, 108–9

O'Doherty, N. (1982) *The Battered Child*, Baillière Tindall, London

Ouvrier, R.A. and Hopkins, I.J. (1970) Occlusive disease of the vertebro-basilar arterial system in childhood. *Developmental Medicine and Child Neurology*, **12**, 186

Pallis, C. (1983) *ABC of Brain Stem Death*, British Medical Journal, London

Rogers, D., Tripp, J., Bentovia, A. *et al.* (1976) Non-accidental poisoning: an extended syndrome of child abuse. *British Medical Journal*, **i**, 793

Said, J.A., Waters, B.G.H., Cousens, P. and Stevens, M.M. (1989) Neurophysiological sequelae of central nervous system prophylaxis in survivors of childhood acute lymphoblastic leukaemia. *Journal of Consulting and Clinical Psychology*, **57**, 251–6

Schotland, M.G., Grumbach, M.M. and Strauss, J. (1963) The effects of chlorothiazides in nephrogenic diabetes insipidus. *Pediatrics*, **31**, 741

Scott, O., McCartney, F.J. and Deverall, P.B. (1976) Sick sinus syndrome in childhood. *Archives of Disease in Childhood*, **51**, 100

Select Committee on Violence in the Family (1977) *Violence to Children, Vol. 1 HC 329*, HMSO, London

Shepherd, H.H. (1963) Observations on intradural angioma; treatment by excision. *Neurochirurgia*, **6**, 58

Sparacio, R.R., Khatib, R. and Cook, A.W. (1971) Acute subdural haematoma in infancy. *New York State Journal of Medicine*, **71**, 212

Stephenson, J.B.P. (1990) *Fits and Faints*, MacKeith Press, Oxford

Swenson, O. (1962) *Pediatric Surgery*, 2nd edn. Appleton-Century-Crofts, New York; Butterworth, London

Symonds, C.P. (1931) Otitic hydrocephalus. *Brain*, **54**, 55

Terrence, C.F. and Samaha, F.J. (1973) The Tolasa-Hunt syndrome (painful opthalmoplegia) in children. *Developmental Medicine and Child Neurology*, **15**, 506

Thomas, T.H., Moggan, D.B., Swarminathan, R. *et al.* (1978) Severe hyponatraemia. A study of 17 patients. *Lancet*, **i**, 621

Vogelsang, H. and Busse, O. (1976) Neuroradiological diagnosis of intraspinal tumours in childhood. *Neuropädiatrie*, **7**, 3

Voorhess, M.L. and Gardner, L.I. (1961) Urinary excretion of nor epinephrine, epinephrine, and 3-methoxy-4-hydroxymandelic acid by children with neuroblastoma. *Journal of Clinical Endocrinology and Metabolism*, **21**, 321

von Studnitz, W. (1970) Cystathioninuria in children with neuroblastoma with and without metastasis. *Acta Paediatrica Scandinavica*, **59**, 80

Warlow, C.P. and Hinton, P. (1969) Early neurological disturbances following relatively minor burns in children. *Lancet*, **ii**, 978

Whitaker, J.A., Austin, W. and Nelson, J.D. (1962) Edathamil calcium disodium (Versenate) diagnostic test for lead poisoning. *Pediatrics*, **29**, 384

13 Emotional and functional disorders

The chapters on psychogenic disorders in textbooks of neurology are of necessity brief, but none-the-less important. Apart from the inevitability of the emotional accompaniments of any illness or disability, there are a number of other conditions which overlap the two specialties. There is no sharp division between neurology and psychiatry, merely a difference of emphasis and, possibly, approach, resulting from a number of factors such as training and differences in the personalities of those trained. In discussing such subjects as epilepsy the role of stress in increasing the incidence of seizures has been indicated, and the same applies to a number of other symptoms. Whatever the illness, there will be an associated emotional problem, whether the condition is a progressive cerebral degeneration, such as one of the gangliosidoses, syncope in adolescence, or a specific learning disorder in the young school-child. Such problems affect not only the child but the whole family. It has also been shown that children with physical handicaps are more likely to suffer from psychiatric disorders than their normal peers. The incidence is highest among children with lesions above the brain-stem associated with epilepsy (Rutter, Graham and Yule, 1970). In this group, Rutter, Graham and Yule (1970) found that the incidence was 58.3%, a figure which should dispel forever the feeling that if there is a physical handicap all evidence of impaired function is due to this, and that such a person has no business to suffer from emotional disorders as well.

The psychiatric presentation of neurological diseases

In addition to the emotional disturbances frequently associated with progressive neurological diseases and chronic handicaps, there are a number of conditions which can present as a change of personality with disorders of behaviour. Minor epileptic status can occur in a child who has never had a fit, and the confusion can initially be mistaken for a psychosis. Among the degenerative diseases of the CNS which can begin with abnormal behaviour and with no abnormal physical signs on examination are: subacute sclerosing panencephalitis, late-onset metachromatic leucodystrophy and adrenoleucodystrophy. Under these circumstances an unexpectedly abnormal EEG can be a suggestive finding.

The overactive child

Many children are considered to be overactive, but few suffer from the hyperkinetic syndrome (see Chapter 6). The parents often base their judgement of the child on adult standards of behaviour, and their anecdotal evidence must therefore be accepted with caution. The doctor can also be misled if he or she bases the assessment of the child on his or her behaviour in the clinic. The clinic is bound to be an artificial setting and the child's fear can result in aggressive and destructive behaviour. The teacher, also, may blame the child for inattention and failure to concentrate, when in reality the fault is due to inappropriate teaching when specific learning disorders are present. It follows, therefore, that a careful analysis of each situation is required before prescribing tranquillizers or other treatment.

Functional symptoms and hysteria

It is obviously dangerous to diagnose a symptom or sign as hysterical just because a cause cannot be found. However, such functional disorders do occur in childhood, particularly among adolescent girls. There may well be suggestive features in the child's history and environment, e.g. personality traits, sleep-walking, family history.

Symptoms such as headache, dizziness and abdominal pain can present a difficult diagnostic problem. If they occur without associated symptoms or signs, certain investigations may be necessary to exclude organic causes, but these should be reduced to a minimum, and, if necessary, the patient should be kept under careful observation for a while. It seems reasonable in these circumstances to give symptomatic treatment while enquiring into the child's background at home and at school to discover if there are any stressful situations.

Hysterical symptoms can take a variety of forms. Seizures can occur which may closely mimic epilepsy, and this may be especially true of a child who does, or has, suffered from epilepsy, or who has seen another member of the family have a fit (pseudo seizures) (Taylor, 1982). The occasional difficulties of diagnosing syncope, particularly in adolescent girls, has been mentioned elsewhere. In this context, the role of hyperventilation may be important. In its chronic form there can be a lack of awareness of the disorder of respiration, and voluntary hyperventilation may not reproduce the symptoms unless the patient is rendered emotionally disturbed. Such a disorder is likely to occur among those who are tense, anxious or depressed (Gordon, 1970). In these situations, as Taylor (1986) has stressed, it may be better to concentrate on the patient's predicament rather than using a play-safe strategy for fear of missing an organic lesion.

Hysterical motor weakness and loss of sensation often does not fit the anatomical pattern or other neurological findings. Paralysis is not accompanied by the expected alterations in tone or reflex changes, and the numbness ends exactly at the mid-line or has a glove-and-stocking distribution. Abnormal movements of a functional nature can often be surprisingly complicated in their form, but conversely the fact that they seem only to occur when the patient is being observed can equally apply to involuntary movements resulting from disorders of the basal ganglia. Attention to a limb tends to make organically determined movements less obvious, and functional movements worse. The staggering gait is bizarre in its form, and is unassociated with falling and injury. Hysterical blindness often takes the form of tunnel vision and, even when apparently complete, the pupil reactions will be normal. Similar findings may be produced by damage to the occipital areas of the brain, following anoxia for instance, but the clinical picture is likely to be so different that there is seldom confusion. Deafness may also be an hysterical symptom on rare occasions, but it is not often necessary to go to the lengths of eliciting evoked potentials on the EEG to prove it. Aphonia caused by bilateral adductor paralysis of the vocal cords can be surprisingly resistant to treatment, even though it can be demonstrated that coughing is still present. All these various symptoms can cause considerable diagnostic difficulties, especially when it is remembered that the most florid hysteric is in no way immune to organic illness. A clear distinction between hysteria and malingering is not always possible.

A good example of how easy it is to attribute uncommon diseases to hysteria is the frequency with which the initial symptoms of myasthenia gravis are thought to be hysterical. Conversely, it is obviously important to avoid unnecessary investigations which may only aggravate the patient's anxieties, even if they help to reassure the doctor. Unless there is a rapid response to explanation and reassurance referral to a psychiatrist is likely to be needed. The situation involving the child and the family which has led to such symptoms is often complex and difficult to analyse.

Neuroses and psychoses

The frequent association of anxiety and depression with physical and mental handicap has already been emphasized. In an otherwise healthy child depression can cause symptoms such as headaches, pains in the limbs and deterioration in school performance, especially in a child with learning disorders; and the correct aetiology is often difficult to establish. Similar problems arise in the context of such illnesses as myalgic encephalomyelitis, and it should be remembered that depression is treatable while most viral infections are not. Suicide before puberty is very rare (Barker, 1971), but must always be considered a possibility during adolescence; it is often a greater risk during the period of recovery than when the child is in the depth of depression. The association of epilepsy and depression in adolescence is, understandably, not uncommon in view of all the problems involved. This may result in an increased frequency of fits, and it does add to the complexities of treatment. It must always be remembered that patients with epilepsy have a readily available source of dangerous drugs (Betts, 1982).

Other psychiatric disorders, such as anorexia nervosa, can sometimes be closely simulated by neurological diseases. The profound distaste for food, and resulting loss of weight, and the endocrine disturbances can result from a lesion such as a slowly growing craniopharyngioma. The problems of infantile autism are considered in Chapter 6. The condition does not appear to be related to schizophrenia but to result from a profound defect in perception and symbolisation. Disintegrative psychoses have been described (Heller's disease, dementia infantalis), but although there may be no evidence of a disorder of cerebral metabolism or of diseases such as tuberous sclerosis, even after a long period of observation, such possibilities cannot be excluded in the present state of knowledge (Evans-Jones and Rosenbloom, 1978).

The tradition in Britain has been to separate the training of neurologists and psychiatrists. There are merits in the difference of approach that result from this, apart from the fact that no-one can be an expert in fields as wide as those encompassed by the whole of neurology and psychiatry. The disadvantages result from the kind of attitude that regards diseases as either organic or functional. The borderland becomes particularly indistinct when studying higher cerebral functions. It may now be a cliché to say that the brain works as a whole and that localization, except in a very limited sense, is an out-moded concept. However, it is important to realize that this applies not only to sensorimotor functions, but to the integration of such functions with memory and, above all, with emotion. In fact it would seem that the latter is all-important in governing the efficacy of what we do.

Asperger's syndrome

In Chapter 6 on disorders of learning, the diagnosis of autism was mentioned, and the effect this condition has on a child's development, particularly of language. Asperger's syndrome can describe children who have a 'touch of autism'; that is to say they have many of the symptoms but are not so severely handicapped. Their intelligence can be average and language function may be unimpaired, although they may talk in a stilted way. However, they are often significantly clumsy. Their behaviour problems include poor eye contact, eccentric and all absorbing interests and a need for sameness and routine. There is also a lack of reciprocal social skills, such as poor turn-taking and an apparent lack of empathy for the feelings of others (Green, 1990). The treatment of these children requires intervention at many levels, but improvement can undoubtedly result. The sex ratio, family history and the presence of neurological disease in some cases suggests the aetiology of the disorder is similar to that of autism (Szatmari, Bremner and Nagy, 1989).

Narcolepsy and cataplexy

Narcolepsy can occur among adolescents. It may be symptomatic after head injuries, encephalitis or tumours involving the hypothalamus, but more often occurs for no discoverable reason; but even then can be associated with other evidence of a hypothalamic disorder, such as obesity or genital atrophy. The irresistible sleepiness tends to occur in situations when anyone might feel sleepy, as after a heavy meal, riding in a bus, or attending a dull lecture. Occasionally the narcolepsy only occurs under special circumstances, for example in relation to the menstrual periods (Parks, 1977). The sleep is usually brief, and if woken there is often no feeling of drowsiness.

Those with narcolepsy may be affected by cataplexy, falling to the ground because of a sudden loss of postural tone precipitated by emotions such as laughter or anger. The attack will not last for more than a few seconds, but during this time movement is impossible, although consciousness is not impaired. As with the sleepiness of narcolepsy, it seems to be an accentuation of what is usually regarded as a normal phenomenon like 'weak at the knees with laughter'.

Other phenomena can be associated with this syndrome, e.g. sleep paralysis, when movement is not possible for a short period on waking from sleep, or vivid and frightening visual hallucinations, usually on falling asleep. The latter are particularly evident in childhood.

These conditions appear to be a disturbance of sleep, particularly affecting REM sleep (Corfariu and Popoviciu, 1974). In true narcolepsy there is an initial REM period of sleep instead of the normal entry into sleep through a prolonged non-REM period. If the symptoms are disabling, the narcolepsy can be treated with methyl-phenidate or amphetamines, and the cataplexy by clomipramine (Guilleminault, Carskadon and Dement, 1974).

Tics or habit spasms

Tics are not associated with other abnormal physical signs, except in such rare cases as part of a post-encephalitic syndrome. The movements usually occur at irregular intervals and are abrupt and spasmodic; for instance, blinking of an eye, jerking of the head, sniffing, facial grimacing, clearing the throat, and shrugging of the shoulders. They can be controlled, but feelings of tension usually increase rapidly until the movement has to be repeated. They are more marked under conditions of stress than when the child is relaxed or can be distracted. If the child is asked to perform a task the tic often stops, which will not happen in the case of chorea or benign familial tremor. Evidence of some underlying emotional disturbance can usually be elicited, quite often related to domestic difficulties or unhappiness at school. However, this is not always obvious as the fault may lie more in the seed than in the soil. The child may be of a nervous disposition, tense, anxious and excitable.

Occasionally the tic is of a more complex nature, as in the Gilles de la Tourette syndrome. These tics more frequently persist among boys, and as the child grows older the motor movements are often associated with compulsive utterance of sounds or words which are often obscene (Corbett et al., 1969). Differentiation from involuntary movements, such as chorea or myoclonus, can be difficult, but these movements tend to affect larger areas of the body and not to be so stereotyped. Also, there are likely to be other abnormalities, such as hypotonia and inco-ordination. There is evidence that in the case of complex tics, anyhow, there may be a disturbance of dopaminergic and noradrenergic pathways. There is sometimes a positive family history which does suggest a disturbance of transmitter substances (Nomura and Segawa, 1979).

The tic is often more disturbing to the parents than the child, and if tensions within the family or at school can be reduced this may be of considerable benefit. The social worker can have an essential part to play in trying to resolve the problems that may exist in the home, and it will be important to enquire from the school about possible learning difficulties. If such measures and the reassurance that must accompany them fail to cure the tic, the use of tranquillizers, such as chlordiazepoxide, can be used for a while, and haloperidol has also been tried, especially in the more complex varieties such as the Gilles de la Tourette syndrome (Corbett et al., 1969), although there is a risk of tardive dyskinesia with this drug. Clonidine and pimozide also seem to help some children with Tourette's syndrome (Cohen et al., 1979). If the symptom persists it may well be necessary to obtain psychiatric advice on the management of the anxieties of the child and the family.

Nocturnal enuresis

Incontinence of urine during childhood, whether it occurs by day or by night, may be due to disorders of function, or structure, or both. If there are no obvious indications for further tests (e.g. the presence of a urinary infection or of neurological signs suggesting a spinal cord lesion) it is justifiable to pursue conservative treatment for several months before reassessing the situation and deciding on the need for intensive investigations (Apley and MacKeith, 1968). Nocturnal enuresis presents a diverse problem. The majority of children are dry at night by the age of 4 or 5 years, and if this happy state has not been reached by then the explanation may lie in delayed development. Many other skills are gained by children at different ages and, when they are selectively delayed, can earn the status of a specific disorder. MacKeith (1968) has suggested that anxiety occurring around the age of 3 years, for instance the anxiety caused by the arrival of a new baby, may interfere with a 'sensitive' period of learning as far as the gaining of bladder control is concerned. Certainly, when the child starts to wet the bed after being dry for a while, anxiety is a very likely cause; and diurnal incontinence, when not due to an organic lesion, is frequently related to psychogenic disorders. Admission of a young child to hospital will often cause a relapse of bladder control.

If the child fails to gain bladder control at the expected age, emotional complications are likely to occur. The mother will become increasingly upset, either from her sense of failure to train the child or from the extra work entailed. The child will begin to feel ashamed and possibly guilty, and these feelings will be made worse if punishments are used as a means of treatment. The family situation will have to be assessed, and, if tensions and pressures are present, discussion with the parents and child will have to take place on a number of occasions.

Apart from explanations of the likely nature of the condition, it is important to stress that it is no one's fault and that the vast majority of children gain bladder control in a very short space of time. Various suggestions can be made if they have not been tried already; for example, restriction of fluids in the evening and rousing the child after a few hours of sleep. Drug treatment is of limited value, although there may be some evidence in favour of the beneficial action of imipramine given in a dose of 25 mg in the evening to children under the age of 12 years, and in double the dose to older children (Poussaint and Ditman, 1965). Amitryptyline is recommended in a dose of 10 mg at night for children under the age of 6 years, increasing to 20 mg in older children (Poussaint, Ditman and Greenfield, 1966). It is difficult to know if these antidepressant agents do have a specific action in a condition which may cease at any time and is so susceptible to suggestion (Forsythe and Redmond, 1974).

If enuresis continues in spite of such advice and treatment, and the child is over the age of 7 years, the use of an electric alarm buzzer may well be successful (Werry, 1966). Sometimes it fails, or it wakes the rest of the family but not the affected child, but the failure is most often due to lack of attention to detail. Among children of average intelligence the method can sometimes be used down to the age of 5 years; and the child must take as much responsibility as possible for organizing and carrying out the treatment (Meadow, 1977). The buzzer may work by some kind of conditioning, possibly the avoidance of being woken by the establishment of bladder control. If nocturnal enuresis persists in the older child unresponsive to treatment, and no abnormalities are found, particularly of bladder function, a trial of a vasopressin analogue given by nasal spray may be justifiable.

Encopresis

Faecal soiling in a child of school age, although less common than urinary incontinence, is a greater source of embarrassment, and is likely to be associated with severer emotional disturbances. Affected children often seem blandly indifferent to the problem, which adds to parental exasperation. Social factors such as overcrowding, lack of parental supervision of toilet habits and absence of an inside lavatory are commonly associated with this complaint, as well as psychiatric illness. Personality disorders among the mothers and social incompetence of the families are common findings (Olatawura, 1973). Constipation with overflow must always be considered and checked by abdominal and rectal examination. These children often show evidence of slow development in other spheres, although a low IQ in itself need be no barrier to successful toilet training of the preschool child. Treatment of constipation may be needed, and regular toilet habits must be established.

References

Apley, J. and MacKeith. R. 1968) *The Child and His Symptoms*, Blackwell Scientific, Oxford

Barker, P.A. (1971) *Basic Child Psychiatry*, Staples Press, London

Betts, T.A. (1982) Psychiatry and epilepsy. In *A Textbook of Epilepsy* (eds. J. Laidlaw and A. Richens), Churchill Livingstone, Edinburgh

Cohen, D.J., Young, J.G., Nathanson, J.A. and Shaywitz, B.A. (1979) Clonidine in Tourette's syndrome. *Lancet*, **ii**, 551

Corbett, J.A., Matthews, A.M., Connell, P.H. and Shapiro, D.A. (1969) Tics and Gilles de la Tourette's syndrome: a follow-up study and critical review. *British Journal of Psychiatry*, **115**, 1229

Corfariu, O. and Popoviciu, L. (1974) Clinical and polygraphic study of the cataplectic attack. *Revue Roumaine de Neurologie*, **11**, 1

Evans-Jones, L.G. and Rosenbloom, L. (1978) Disintegrative psychosis in childhood. *Developmental Medicine and Child Neurology*, **20**, 462

Forsythe, W.I. and Redmond, A. (1974) Enuresis and spontaneous cure rate. *Archives of Disease in Childhood*, **49**, 259

Gordon, N. (1970) Faints in early adolescence. *British Journal of Clinical Practice*, **24**, 34

Green, J. (1990) Is Asperger's a syndrome. *Developmental Medicine and Child Neurology*, **32**, 743

Guilleminault, C., Carskadon, M. and Dement, W.C. (1974) On the treatment of rapid eye movement narcolepsy. *Archives of Neurology*, **30**, 90

MacKeith, R. (1968) A frequent factor in the origins of primary nocturnal enuresis: anxiety in the third year of life. *Developmental Medicine and Child Neurology*, **10**, 465

Meadow, R. (1977) How to use buzzer alarms to cure bed wetting. *British Medical Journal*, **ii**, 1073

Nomura, Y. and Segawa, M. (1979) Gilles de la Tourette syndrome in oriental children. *Brain and Development*, **1**, 103

Olatawura, M.O. (1973) Encopresis: a review of thirty-two cases. *Acta Paediatrica Scandinavica*, **62**, 358

Parks, J.D. (1977) The sleepy patient. *Lancet*, **i**, 990

Poussaint, A.F. and Ditman, K.S. (1965) A controlled study of imipramine (Tofranil) in the treatment of childhood enuresis. *Journal of Pediatrics*, **67**, 283

Poussaint, A.F., Ditman, K.S. and Greenfield, R. (1966) Amitryptiline in childhood enuresis. *Clinical Pharmacology and Therapeutics*, **7**, 21

Szatmari, P., Bremner, R. and Nagy, J. (1989) Asperger's syndrome: a review of clinical features. *Canadian Journal of Psychiatry*, **34**, 554

Rutter, M., Graham, P. and Yule, W. (1970) *A Neuropsychiatric Study in Childhood*, Clinics in Developmental Medicine, Nos. 35/36, SIMP, William Heinemann, London

Taylor, D.C. (1982) The components of sickness: diseases, illnesses and predicaments. In *One Child* (eds. J. Apley and C. Ounsted), Heinemann, Tadworth

Taylor, D. (1986) The sick child's predicament. In *Neurologically Handicapped Children: Treatment and Management* (eds. N. Gordon and I. McKinlay), Blackwood Scientific, Oxford

Werry. J.S. (1966) The conditioning treatment of enuresis. *American Journal of Psychiatry*, **123**, 226

14 Envoi

If it is accepted that paediatric neurology is a broad specialty, it is to be hoped that in future it will command increasing resources in terms of service commitments, training facilities and opportunities for research. It can reasonably be claimed that neurological disorders, acute and chronic diseases and disabilities of one kind and another, constitute a major part of paediatrics. This is not to claim that more than a small fraction of the work should be done by paediatric neurologists, but it does suggest that, with few exceptions, academic departments of paediatrics have not given it the attention it deserves. If any such department in the future does not have at least one member of its staff with a major interest and training in paediatric neurology, there is a case for maintaining that it is not doing its duty.

Training in paediatric neurology will differ in various centres and in different countries, and this is to be encouraged. However, for the average person, adequate experience in both paediatrics and neurology is surely essential for those working in this field. Training should not be merely the acquisition of facts; these can always be looked up in books, but it is a way of thought. To develop this, there must be a commitment of sufficient depth, and a willingness to regard the learning process as a discipline in the old-fashioned sense of the word. For example, it is only when the average person has accepted the rigours of taking a detailed history and meticulously carrying out the neurological examination time and time again until it becomes 'second-nature' that the experience is gained which makes it safe to take short-cuts.

There will be at least two exceptions to this statement: the few individuals of such talent that they will succeed without apparent effort in whatever tasks they are involved, and those who, by their research into a particular aspect of a subject, make a major contribution to the whole.

If paediatric neurology is the child of both paediatrics and neurology it must be educated by both its parents, and to exclude one or other is to be guilty of narrow-mindedness. As far as individuals are concerned, one or other may have had a major influence in training, but for the future it is to be hoped that there will be increasing opportunities for experience in both disciplines, and that a more equal contribution to knowledge will be made by them.

Specialization within the field of neurology among adults is well recognized, for example in epilepsy, neuro-ophthalmology, or in disorders of the peripheral nerves and muscles. The increase in knowledge is such that the same must happen in paediatric neurology, and there is no reason why one paediatric neurologist should not have a special knowledge of metabolic disorders, another of neonatal neurology, and another of learning disorders, and so on. Also, within this field, there is a need for two types of specialist; the paediatric neurologist dealing with a wide variety of problems, both acute and chronic, as considered in this book; and the habilitationist who is concerned mainly with the assessment and day-to-day care and treatment of physically and mentally handicapped children. Such a specialist will need a knowledge of physical medicine, paediatrics, particularly developmental paediatrics, and of community services. Habilitation, whether medical, psychological, educational or social, often seems to work best if based on an assessment centre or special school, and this is one way to ensure a close liaison between the doctor, the various therapists, the teacher and the parents.

The work of the paediatric neurologist and habilitationist must obviously overlap, and ideally they should hold joint clinics. In turn their work will overlap that of many paediatricians, especially those working in the community. It is probably better to emphasize this overlapping of commitments than to try to define the exact role of the individual expert. Also, it would be presumptuous to say exactly when a child should be referred to the paediatric neurologist. If a problem exists, and if someone is known to have a special knowledge of it, then there is every chance that his or her opinion will be sought. The exceptions to this are more likely to occur among chronic than among acute disorders. For example, among children with learning disorders, those whose parents are vocal and place education high on their list of priorities are most likely to be seen in the neurology clinic. The remedy seems to lie in 'education' of those concerned with the care of children, i.e. doctors, teachers and parents; and in taking the services to the children in the community rather than bringing the children to the hospital.

Should there be special clinics for particular disabilities such as epilepsy, speech and language defects, cerebral palsy, spina bifida and other disorders? It depends to a certain extent on the resources available, but the role of such clinics must be defined carefully. To take the example of epilepsy, confusion has arisen between diagnostic and therapeutic clinics. If anyone develops epilepsy it will be best if they are investigated by a good general physician; he or she may be a neurologist, and may need all the diagnostic resources of the hospital service at his or her disposal. However, when it has been found that the epilepsy is not a symptom of a metabolic disorder, a tumour, nephritis, infections or any other condition likely to respond to specific treatment, the position is different. When the cause is unknown or irremediable, and the possibility of a life-long disability has to be faced, special expertise is needed, and often not provided. The control of long-term anti-epileptic treatment with drugs must be improved if unacceptable side-effects are to be avoided. Quite apart from the medical problems, help is often required from an experienced social worker, as well as advice from educational and vocational experts. It may only be by organizing a special clinic around such personnel that the patient can be given an efficient long-term service.

Similar arguments can be made in favour of clinics for other disabilities, when this is practical. One has only to assess the work of someone with many years of experience of the problems of children with cerebral palsy, or blind children for instance, to realize that very often the help offered by such people and their colleagues is unique.

What of the future? As far as diagnosis is concerned there is no doubt that the scene has been changed by the advent of CT and MRI scanning and other techniques such as single proton emission computed tomography (SPECT) and positron emission tomography (PET). It will make the identification of lesions of the CNS much easier, and with little discomfort to the patient. Also, it will mean that the monitoring of possibly progressive lesions such as hydrocephalus and demyelinating diseases will be simplified, and that metabolic disorders which cause changes in the density of tissues can be studied. No doubt the identification of metabolic disorders and the elucidation of their cause, particularly enzyme deficiencies, will continue; and the advances in the field of genetics are also going to make enormous contributions to the management of neurological disease, especially DNA studies.

Much has been done to prevent brain damage from perinatal and postnatal causes, and now the maximum effort in research is required to identify more of the prenatal causes. Effective antiviral treatment will make a great contribution to preventing brain damage before birth.

Without decrying in any way the importance of medical treatment for infections, metabolic disorders, and the increasing number of conditions which can now be prevented and cured, there is an equally important role for the paediatric neurologist in helping the child with long-term disabilities. Even the more subtle difficulties of learning can cause a major degree of suffering to the child, and often to the family as well. The very diversity of the subject, as well as the challenge of so many problems yet unsolved, and the need for research into these, should attract more people into this field if medicine still maintains its ideals. If this does not happen, the teachers of medicine will be largely to blame.

The changes that have occurred in medicine, and particularly in paediatrics, in the past 50 years since the author qualified, have been truly amazing; and surely the advances in the next 50 years will be beyond our imagination. These are exciting times; in spite of the disappointments that undoubtedly occur, particularly from financial restraints and misguided management. The abolition of special services such as regional units may not immediately cause problems, and in the short-term will no doubt help to balance a budget. However, in the long-term, it is likely to cost the community dearly; quite apart from the distress to the child and the family. It may be difficult to persuade those responsible of the truth of this dictum, but this is no excuse for not trying. The hope is that there are sufficient people with the imagination to realize the possibilities that are there for the taking, if the opportunities are made available.

Index